Communication and Swallowing in Parkinson Disease

Communication and Swallowing in Parkinson Disease

DEBORAH THEODOROS, PhD
LORRAINE RAMIG, PhD

PLURAL PUBLISHING
INC.
SAN DIEGO
OXFORD
BRISBANE

PLURAL PUBLISHING
INC.

5521 Ruffin Road
San Diego, CA 92123

e-mail: info@pluralpublishing.com
Web site: http://www.pluralpublishing.com

49 Bath Street
Abingdon, Oxfordshire OX14 1EA
United Kingdom

Typeset in 11/14 Garamond by Flanagan's Publishing Services, Inc.
Printed in the United States of America by McNaughton and Gunn.

Library of Congress Cataloging-in-Publication Data:

Theodoros, Deborah G.
Communication and swallowing in Parkinson disease / Deborah Theodoros and Lorraine Ramig.
p. ; cm.
Includes bibliographical references.
ISBN-13: 978-1-59756-205-8 (alk. paper)
ISBN-10: 1-59756-205-X (alk. paper)
1. Parkinson's disease—Complications. 2. Communicative disorders—Treatment. 3. Deglutition disorders—Treatment. I. Ramig, Lorraine O. II. Title.
[DNLM: 1. Communication Disorders—therapy. 2. Deglutition Disorders—therapy. 3. Parkinson Disease—complications. WL 340.2]
RC382.T42 2011
616.8'33—dc22

2011001752

Contents

Foreword

There are but a few critical functions that distinguish existence: cognition, communication, and the capacity to be well nourished are among the most important. Unfortunately, areas of the brain responsible for control, coordination, and integration of these key areas become dysfunctional in neurodegenerative disorders such as Parkinson disease (PD).

In his original description of the disease named after him, James Parkinson reflected:

> *"His words are now scarcely intelligible; and he is . . . no longer able to feed himself . . ."*
>
> (Parkinson, 2002, p.225).

Loss of these functions therefore threatens the experience of life.

The pillars of medical care include understanding disease, relieving suffering, and improving quality of life; the latter is the real paramount tangible goal. Notwithstanding that there is currently no cure for Parkinson disease, research during the 20th century produced a wealth of new tools that resulted in practical knowledge on the pathophysiology of PD and, consequently, highly effective symptomatic therapies. These tools have prepared the scientific community to readdress the important goal of neuroprotective treatments. We acknowledge that currently available therapies are not sufficient, and there is a long road ahead.

The authors of this book have dedicated much of their personal time and professional careers to understanding, assessing, and treating the communication and swallowing disorders affecting people with PD, and have chosen to share their extensive knowledge. This book is designed to provide the reader with a comprehensive insight into the underlying neuropathophysiology of the communication and swallowing difficulties experienced by people with PD; the challenging and perplexing characteristics of the speech, language, and swallowing disorders; and the current treatments required to address these taxing symptoms.

Such information is important for all health professionals in order to facilitate the maintenance of a high quality of life for people with PD and their families. This book, the first of its kind to provide a complete account of communication and swallowing in PD, will go a long way toward supporting people with PD, and the professionals who work with them on this journey.

Mitchell F. Brin, MD

Contributors

Andrew Blitzer, MD, DDS
Professor of Clinical Otolaryngology
Columbia University College of Physicians and Surgeons
Director, New York Center for Voice and Swallowing Disorders
President, American Laryngological Association
New York, NY
Chapter 1

Mitchell F. Brin, MD
Clinical Professor of Neurology
University of California, Irvine
Senior Vice President. Global Drug Development
Allergan, LLC
Irvine, CA
Chapter 1

Michelle Ciucci, PhD, CCC-SLP
Assistant Professor
Department of Surgery
Division of Otolaryngology-Head and Neck Surgery
Department of Communicative Disorders
University of Wisconsin
Madison, WI
Chapter 7

Cynthia Marie Fox, PhD, CCC-SLP
Research Associate
National Center for Voice and Speech
University of Colorado
Boulder, CO
Chapter 4

Adrienne B. Hancock, PhD
Assistant Professor
Department of Speech and Hearing
George Washington University
Washington, DC
Chapter 5

Leonard LaPointe, PhD
Francis Eppes Distinguished Professor
School of Communication Science and Disorders
Florida State University
Tallahassee, FL
Chapter 5

David H. McFarland, PhD
Professor, Faculties of Medicine
Université de Montréal and McGill University
Montréal, Québec
Canada
Chapter 7

Leslie A. Mahler, PhD
Assistant Professor
Department of Communicative Disorders
University of Rhode Island
Kingston, RI
Chapter 7

Lorraine Ramig, PhD
Department of Speech-Language and Hearing Science
University of Colorado
Boulder, CO
National Center for Voice and Speech
Denver, CO
Chapter 4

Shimon Sapir, PhD, CCC-SLP
Associate Professor
Department of Communication Sciences and Disorders
University of Haifa
Mount Carmel
Haifa, Israel
Chapter 4

Geralyn Schulz, PhD, CCC-SLP
Associate Dean for Research
Professor of Speech and Hearing Science
Columbian College of Arts and Sciences
George Washington University
Washington, DC
Chapter 2

Deborah Theodoros, PhD
Professor and Head
Division of Speech Pathology
School of Health and Rehabilitation Sciences
University of Queensland
Brisbane
Australia
Chapter 3

Miodrag Velickovic, MD
Assistant Professor of Neurology
Movement Disorders Center
Mt Sinai School of Medicine
New York, NY
Chapter 1

Brooke-Mai Whelan, PhD
Senior Research Fellow
Division of Speech Pathology
School of Health and Rehabilitation Sciences
University of Queensland
Brisbane
Australia
Chapters 5 and 6

We dedicate this book to our clients with Parkinson disease
whose courage inspires us daily.
Our lives have been enriched by your efforts to improve your speech.
We admire your persistence and patience as we
continually learn from you.

1

Parkinson Disease: Symptoms and Medical Management

ANDREW BLITZER
MITCHELL F. BRIN
MIODRAG VELICKOVIC

Parkinsonism is a neurologic syndrome with the following cardinal features: (a) bradykinesia, (b) postural instability, (c) rigidity, (d) rest tremor, and (e) freezing (motor blocks) (Fahn, 1986, 1989). At least two of these five cardinal features should be present, with one of them being either tremor or rigidity. As a syndrome, parkinsonism can be caused by: (a) idiopathic Parkinson disease (PD) including sporadic disease and cases with known gene mutation causing symptoms of PD only; (b) secondary (symptomatic) PD caused by a known and identifiable cause; (c) Parkinson-plus syndromes where symptoms of parkinsonism may

Cardinal Features of Parkinsonism

- Bradykinesia
- Postural instability
- Rigidity
- Rest tremor
- Freezing (motor blocks)

be caused by a known gene defect and have a distinctive pathology (Table 1–1). The specific diagnosis depends on details of the clinical history, neurologic examination, and laboratory tests.

Parkinson disease is the most common type of parkinsonism. It is a progressive disorder of unknown etiology, and the diagnosis is usually made by excluding known causes of parkinsonism (Table 1–2). Some patients, however, who present with a classical phenotype, have a genetic history. So far, there are nearly a dozen gene mutations that can cause symptoms of PD indistinguishable from sporadic disease (Schiesling, Kieper, Seidel, & Krüger, 2008). In certain populations these mutations can account for 40% of cases of PD.

Table 1–1. Classification of Parkinsonism

I. Idiopathic (primary)
   Parkinson Disease

II. Symptomatic (secondary)
   A. Drugs—neuroleptics
   B. Postencephalitic
   C. Toxins—Mn, CO, MPTP, cyanide
   D. Vascular
   E. Brain tumor
   F. Head trauma

III. Parkinson-plus Syndromes
   A. Progressive supranuclear palsy
   B. Multiple system atrophy
      1. Pyramid type (formerly known as striatonigral degeneration)
      2. Cerebellar type (formerly known as olivopontocerebellar [OPCA] degeneration)
   C. Dementia syndromes
      1. Alzheimer disease
      2. Normal pressure hydrocephalus
      3. Frontotemporal dementia
   D. Hereditary disorders
      1. Wilson disease
      2. Huntington disease
      3. Pantothenate kinase-associated neurodegeneration (formerly known as Hallervorden-Spatz disease)

Mn: manganese; CO: carbon monoxide; MPTP: 1-Methyl-4-phenyl-1,2,3,6-tetrahydropyridine.

Table 1–2. Exclusion Criteria for Diagnosis of Parkinson Disease

1. History of:
   encephalitis
   exposure to carbon monoxide, manganese, MPTP, or other toxins
   recent exposure to neuroleptic medication
2. Onset of parkinsonian symptoms following:
   head trauma
   stroke
3. Presence on examination of:
   cerebellar ataxia
   loss of downward ocular movements
   pronounced postural hypotension not due to concurrent medication
   vocal fold paralysis
4. Magnetic resonance imaging or computed tomography of the head revealing:
   lacunar infarcts
   capacious cerebral ventricles
   cerebellar atrophy
   atrophy of the midbrain or other parts of the brainstem
5. Failure to respond to levodopa therapy

Source: Modified with permission from Fahn, S. (1988). Disorders with parkinsonian features. In J. W. Hurst (Ed.), *Medicine for the practicing physician* (2nd ed., pp. 1522–1525). Boston, MA: Butterworth.

Symptoms of Parkinson Disease

The disease usually begins insidiously. Nonmotor symptoms such as loss of sensation of smell, Rapid Eye Movement sleep behavioral disorder, and constipation might precede motor symptoms of PD by many years, possibly decades (Langston, 2006). Resting tremor is usually the first symptom recognized by the patient. The majority of patients have asymmetric symptoms, and good response to levodopa for many years. Although speech and voice changes, swallowing difficulty, shuffling gait, and falls eventually will occur in the majority of patients they usually are not present during the first year of the disease (Müller et al., 2000, 2001). Resting tremor and responsiveness of PD symptoms to levodopa (LD) actually are not uncommon in the other types of parkinsonism.

For instance, resting tremor was present in 39% of pathologically proven cases of multiple system atrophy (MSA) (Wenning, Tison, Ben Shlomo, Daniel, & Quinn, 1997) and 20% of progressive supranuclear palsy (PSP) cases (Williams et al., 2005). Response to LD was present in 28 to 49% of the patients with pathologically proven Parkinson-plus syndrome (Müller et al., 2001; Wenning et al., 1997; Williams et al., 2005). On the other hand, a lack of LD responsiveness has been documented in pathologically proven cases of idiopathic PD (Mark, Sage, Dickson, Schwarz, & Duvoisin, 1992).

Tremor of approximately 3 Hz is present in the distal parts of the extremities and the lips, while the involved body part is at rest. "Pill-rolling" tremor of the hands is the most common. The tremor is suppressed with active movement of the limb in most cases. Resting tremor must be differentiated from postural and kinetic tremors that appear only when the arm is used. These tremors typically are caused by other disorders such as essential tremor or cerebellar disorders. However, after maintaining outstretched hands for a few seconds, some patients have a re-emergence of the resting tremor at 3 Hz.

Bradykinesia is manifest by a masked face; decreased blinking; drooling of saliva due to decreased spontaneous swallowing; loss of spontaneous movements such as gesturing; small and slow handwriting (micrographia); difficulty with hand dexterity (for shaving, brushing of teeth, putting on makeup); shuffling gait with decreased arm swing; and difficulty getting up and out of a chair, car, or bed. Bradykinesia encompasses a loss of automatic movements as well as slowness in initiating movement on command, and a reduction in amplitude of the voluntary movement (hypokinesia) as demonstrated by decrementing amplitude with repetitive finger tapping or foot tapping.

Rigidity is an increased resistance to passive movement, equal in all directions, and usually manifested by a ratchety "give" in the range of motion (cogwheel rigidity). Eventually, the patient assumes a stooped posture and begins to lose balance, with a tendency to fall due to loss of postural reflexes. The loss of postural reflexes combined with the stooped posture leads to a festinating gait with faster and faster small steps.

In addition to these motor signs, most patients with PD have behavioral signs as well. The patient slowly becomes more dependent, fearful, indecisive, and passive. The significant other gradually makes more of the decisions and becomes the dominant decision maker. Eventually, the patient will sit much of the day unless encouraged to exercise. Passivity also expresses itself by the patient not wishing to attend social events. Depression is frequent in patients with PD. Dementia occurs in about 30% of patients with PD and is nearly universal in the bed-bound

Characteristics of Parkinson Disease

- Resting tremor
- "Pill-rolling" tremor of hands
- Festinating and/or shuffling gait
- Stooped posture
- Cogwheel rigidity of limbs
- Decreased arm swing when walking
- Unstable balance
- Masked facial appearance
- Decreased eye blinking
- Loss of spontaneous movement (e.g., gesturing)
- Micrographia
- Reduced hand dexterity
- Speech and voice impairment
- Swallowing difficulty
- Slowness in initiating movement, thought, and speech
- Depression
- Dementia—30%

patient. More common is bradyphrenia, in which the patient is slow to respond to questions, but has intact cognitive function.

Clinical presentation offers insight into the rate of progression and survival in PD. Patients with tremor predominant PD, and absence of dementia have a milder course of the disease and longer survival (Jellinger, Seppi, Wenning, & Poewe, 2002). Patients who develop disease at the younger age also have longer survival (Jellinger et al., 2002).

Pathology and Biochemistry of PD

The pigmented nuclei of the brainstem, namely, the pars compacta of the substantia nigra (SNc), the locus coeruleus, and the dorsal motor nucleus of the vagus are affected in PD. There is loss of nerve cells and increased gliosis in these nuclei. The cytoplasm of intact neurons often shows eosinophilic inclusions called "Lewy bodies" (Forno, 1982) (Figure 1–1). These inclusions are most likely not a cause of cell death, but a sign that the cell's mechanism for clearance of unwanted (damaged or mutated) proteins is failing (Olanow, Perl, DeMartino, & McNaught, 2004).

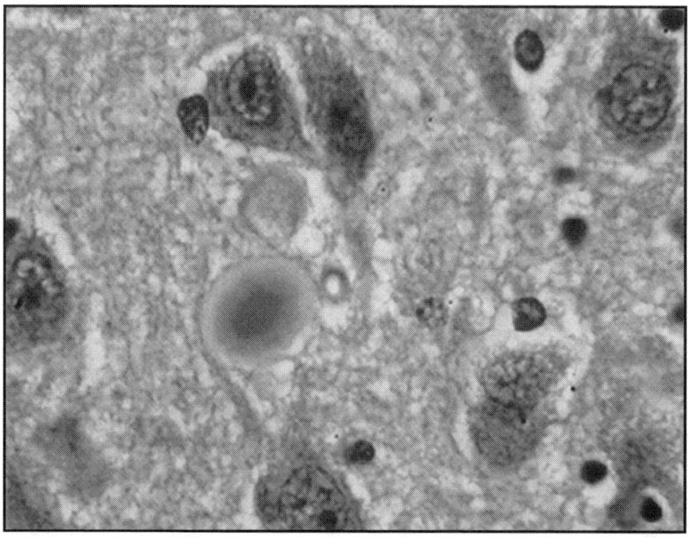

FIGURE 1–1. Lewy bodies. Photo courtesy of Kondi Wong, Armed Forces Institute of Pathology. (http://www.genome.gov)

The substantia nigra neurons contain dopamine; the locus coeruleus contain norepinephrine; and other pigmented neurons contain serotonin. Thus, the loss of these neurons results in a loss of these monoamine neurotransmitters in their nerve terminals. The most consistent biochemical alteration in PD is a marked depletion of dopamine in the neostriatum (Agid et al., 1989). Most symptoms of PD can be directly related to the loss of striatal dopamine. However, some of the motor (e.g., postural instability) and nonmotor (e.g., dementia, depression) features are either incompletely or totally unresponsive to dopamine replacement therapy, suggesting that other neurotransmitter systems are involved (Chaudhuri, Healy, & Schapira, 2006; Muller, 2002).

Historically, environmental factors were deemed to be the primary cause of the condition. Twenty years ago, literature began to appear suggesting that PD could have a genetic basis (Barbeau & Roy, 1984). The role of genetics in this condition was hotly debated with the primary example appearing in twin studies. Subsequently, with advances in molecular biology nearly a dozen loci have been identified (Farrer, 2006; Muller, 2002). Experience with the neuropathology of patients subsequent to grafting presumably normal nigral neurons into select areas of the brain is refocusing attention on local cellular environmental factors. Abnormal protein aggregations closely resembling Lewy bodies were found in grafted nigral cells implanted into PD patients' striatum 11 to 16 years earlier (Kordower, Chu, Hauser, Freeman, & Olanow, 2008; Li et al., 2008). Although another report published at the same time had contradicted these findings (Mendez et al., 2008), re-examination of the tissue revealed the presence of Lewy bodies (Olanow, personal communication). Clinically, all patients demonstrated initial improvement followed by deterioration of their condition, suggesting an ongoing pathologic process affecting the grafted neurons. These reports also implied that the pathologic process was widespread, and did not affect only the pigmented neurons of SNc (Kordower et al., 2008; Li et al., 2008). Consistent with Barbeau's hypothesis (Barbeau & Roy, 1984), both external environmental factors and internal local cellular factors likely impact on primary cellular underlying metabolic function and consequent neurodegeneration. Consequently one cannot discount the contributions of nongenetic factors on the underlying metabolic (genetic) fabric of the individual. In individual cases, however, it may be impossible to tease out the relative contributions of nature and nurture. Nevertheless, these insights may lead to new strategies for both symptom relief and neuroprotection with the hope for more effective therapies in the future.

Multiple system atrophy is one of the Parkinson-plus syndromes and may affect the larynx during speech and breathing. Autonomic dysfunction is one of the hallmarks of the disorder. In the parkinsonism type of MSA (MSA-p), formerly known as striatonigral degeneration, the vocal folds may be paralyzed or weakened (Fahn & Greeberg, 1972). Ataxic dysarthria is present in the cerebellar type of MSA (MSA-c), formerly known as olivopontocerebellar atrophy. There also may be a sensory aberration causing diminished or absent cough reflexes with intermittent aspiration. The laryngeal and respiratory function may deteriorate during sleep with stridor and obstructive events that may become life threatening and result in sudden death (Nagashima et al., 1993; Silber & Levine et al., 2000). Consequently, a sleep study and appropriate consultations should be given to all patients who have signs or symptoms of stridor, sleep disturbance, or respiratory dysfunction. In some patients, a tracheostomy may be required. Surgery may be complicated by severe blood pressure fluctuations that are common in MSA patients.

Management

Drug Therapy

The patients with idiopathic PD (IPD) usually have an improvement of symptoms using dopamine precursors (levodopa with carbodopa) either alone or in combination with a catechol-o-methyl transferase inhibitor (entacapone, tolcapone), or dopamine agonists (bromocriptine, pergolide mesylate, ropinirol, pramipexole). Patients with secondary parkinsonism typically are resistant to medication. Propargylamines including selegiline (Shoulsen, Fahn, & Parkinson Study Group, 1989) and rasagiline (Parkinson Study Group) have been reported, although not confirmed, to slow progression of IPD if added early in the course of the disease. The patients' symptomatic relief seems to be from the inhibition of monoamine oxidase type B enzyme (MAO-B). Some dopamine agonists may slow the progression of IPD but because of the challenges of distinguishing symptomatic benefit from delayed neurodegeneration, conclusive data are not available (Schapira, 2004; Schapira & Olanow, 2004).

Long-term levodopa therapy often leads to complications, which include oscillations, dyskinesias, and drug-induced psychiatric effects. Most patients have continuous benefit from levodopa (3 to 4 doses) early in their disease. The response oscillations typically develop within 5 years of beginning treatment (Hurtig, 1997). Some patients develop unpredictable oscillations with no apparent relationship to their dosing pattern. The response oscillations may be accompanied by dyskinesias, or choreas with or without dystonia, especially at the time of peak drug levels. Although dose reduction may be effective for peak-dose dyskinesias, many patients have a very narrow window, and titration may be difficult. The strategies to deal with this problem include sustained-release preparations, co-administration of dopamine agonists, liquid preparations, metabolic inhibitors such as catechol-o-methyl-transferase inhibitors and MAO-B inhibitors, or subcutaneous apomorphine (Pahwa et al., 1997). Delayed gastric emptying may be the cause of the problem in dosing in some cases. Cisapride had been used in these patients in the past, but was removed from the U.S. market by the FDA due to its cardiac side effects. Mosapride, a similar type agent, may be used in some cases (Djaldetti, Koren, Ziv, Achiron, & Melamed, 1995). Continuous enteric delivery of aqueous preparation of levodopa (Nyholm et al., 2005), or continuous subcutaneous delivery of apomorphine (Garc›a Ruiz et al., 2008), or lisuride (Stocchi, Ruggieri, Vacca, & Olanow, 2002) can be beneficial in PD who have developed oscillations. Patients in these studies have spent less time in "off" state, had less severe dyskinesia, and had more "on" time.

There are a number of psychiatric side effects to using levodopa and any dopamine agonist, including vivid dreams, hallucinations, and an exacerbation of memory loss, confusion, and anxiety. Some of these side effects can be treated symptomatically, whereas others may require a reduction of levodopa (or the dopamine agonist) (Chaudhuri et al., 2006; Djaldetti et al., 1995; Fernandez, Donnelly, & Friedman, 2004).

Many oral agents that result in stimulation of dopamine receptors (e.g., levodopa, dopamine agonists, dopamine releasers) have demonstrated an overall improvement in general motor function, as well as speech (Goberman & Coelho, 2002). Many of the characteristics of speech including respiration, phonation, and articulation may be paradoxically changed by levodopa-related fluctuations. Some of the medications also worsen speech by increasing rate, decreasing distinction, and causing "palilalia" (repetition of syllables and phrases) (Ackerman, Ziegler, & Oertel, 1989). (See Chapter 3 for greater detail on the effects of medications on speech).

Neurosurgical Intervention

Early in the 20th century, neurosurgeons lesioned the motor cortex in an attempt to decrease hyperkinetic movements, including the tremor associated with PD (Bucy & Case, 1939; Klemme, 1940). These operations, however, often led to a spastic hemiparesis as a substitute for the dyskinesia. In the 1940s, Meyers (1940, 1951) described pallidotomy for PD, later showing that dyskinesias can be improved with this procedure without pyramidal tract damage. During a surgical procedure in a patient with postencephalitic PD, Cooper (1954, 1956) accidentally severed the anterior choroidal artery, which feeds the medial globus pallidus and lateral ventral thalamus, and discovered marked improvement in the patient's tremor and rigidity. Cooper also reported that dystonic posturing in PD patients improved with anterior choroidal artery ligation, and he began to operate on primary dystonia patients. Cooper performed lesions in the pallidum and thalamus with improved tremor control. With bilateral procedures, however, there was a significant morbidity due to dysarthria and dysphagia. Once levodopa became available in the late 1960s, surgical interventions were rarely performed.

During the past two decades, there has been a resurgence of interest in surgery for PD. This was prompted by the fact that chronic levodopa therapy resulted in motor fluctuations, beginning in the first 3 to 5 years (Fahn, 1992). Strategies have developed to delay the onset of the motor fluctuations, but they emerge ultimately in most patients. Advances in neuroimaging, stereotactic neurosurgery and microelectrode intraoperative recording have permitted improved localization of the surgical targets and placement of lesions or electrodes. The understanding of the organization of the basal ganglia and the pathways important to the physiology of PD has led to a more rational approach to surgical target selection (Delong, 1990; Delong, Crutcher, & Georgopoulopos, 1985;

Gironell, Amirian, Kulisevsky, & Molet, 2005). The current neurosurgical procedures are broadly classified as: (1) ablative, (2) stimulation procedures, and (3) potentially restorative procedures.

Ablative

These procedures are performed in the thalamus and internal segment of the pallidum. Thalamotomy can be performed with modest morbidity, and may improve contralateral tremor and possibly rigidity in up to 90% of the patients (Fox, Ahlskog, & Kelly, 1991; Tasker, 1990). In most cases, however, there is no improvement in bradykinesia, postural instability, or ipsilateral tremor. The current mortality rate is less than 1% and the complications include contralateral hemiparesis, seizures, paresthesias, ataxia, apraxia, hypotonia, abulia, and gait disturbances (Tasker, Siqueira, Hawrylyshyn, & Organ, 1983).

Pallidotomy involves lesioning the posteroventral portion of the internal segment of the globus pallidus (GPi). This procedure can result in long-lasting improvement in tremor, rigidity, hypokinesia, gait, dystonia, and levodopa-induced dyskinesias. Using microelectrode recordings for targeted localization in pallidotomy, many reports show impressive improvements in dyskinesias, with modest improvements in the cardinal signs of PD (Lang et al., 1997; Lozano et al., 1996).

Deep Brain Stimulation (DBS)

Deep brain stimulation (DBS) was explored, initially by Benabid et al. (1991) for the management of PD. They showed that high-frequency (>100 Hz) low-voltage (<5 V) electrical stimulation of the ventro intermediate nucleaus (Vim) of the thalamus improved tremor in PD and essential tremor patients (Benabid et al., 1991). Based on a growing understanding of the neural networks controlling basal ganglia function in PD and other disorders, attention shifted to stimulating the globus pallidus interna (GPi) and subthalamic nucleus (STN) in patients with intractable PD. The early trials showed a benefit not only for tremor, but improvement in bradykinesia, gait disturbance, rigidity, and balance (Limousin et al., 1995; Pahwa et al., 1997). A 4-year follow-up study of DBS of GPi and STN revealed persistent improvement in cardinal features of PD and activities of daily living in PD patients compared to their preoperative state when they were off medications (Rodriguez-Oroz et al., 2005). The exact mechanism of DBS is unknown. High-frequency stimulation most likely electrically interferes with pathologic oscillatory activity present in basal ganglia of PD patients, making it more regular (Hammond, Ammari, Bioulac, & Garcia, 2008). Bilateral DBS of the STN increases the regional cerebral blood flow (rCBF) to both thalami correlating to an improvement in bradykinesia, and decreases the rCBF to the supplemental motor area correlating with an improvement of rigidity (Karimi et al., 2008). Decreased rCBF was seen in pedunculopontine nuclei correlating with improvement in postural reflexes (Karimi et al., 2008). Increased rCBF was also observed in the globus pallidus (GP) area (Hilker et al., 2008).

Transplantation

Transplantation is an experimental procedure whereby dopamine-containing cells are transplanted into the nigral targets of patients with intractable PD. This is based on the observation that PD is associated with specific degeneration of the dopaminergic nigrostriatal neurons, and that dopamine replacement seemed to improve motor signs and symptoms of PD. The tissues that can be used as transplants include adrenal, fetal nigral, retinal pigment epithelial, stem cells, and so forth. The results also are related to the density and quantity of transplanted tissue, the locations of the transplant and the immunosuppressive therapy. The initial transplants conducted by Madrazo et al. (1987) were adrenal medullary cells inserted into the caudate nucleus. Although the initial results were good they were not reproduced by other investigators. Fetal nigral cells were then transplanted into the posterior putamen (Freed et al., 2001; Hauser et al., 1999; Wenning et al., 1997), and patients seemed to demonstrate an improvement in symptoms. Postmortem studies showed that with some of the protocols, implanted cells survived in large numbers and reinnervated the striatum in an organotypic fashion (Kordower et al., 1996).

One double-blind study demonstrated benefit in younger patients (under age 60). There was a marked placebo effect and some patients developed a severe dyskinesia when not on medication, which could not be ameliorated by decreasing dopamine therapy (Freed et al., 1992). The second study (Kordower et al., 1995) showed no overall treatment effect, but milder patients did show significant improvement. Neuroimaging demonstrated transplant survival as did postmortem exams up to 4 years after the transplant (Kordower et al., 1995; Mendez et al., 2005). However, as mentioned above, the most recent studies have revealed the presence of Lewy bodies even in grafted cells (Kordower et al., 2008; Li et al., 2008) implying an ongoing neuropathologic process.

Restorative Approaches

A number of novel treatment approaches have been tried. These include: implantation of human retinal pigment epithelial cells, attached to an excipient part of cross-linked porcine gelatin microcarrriers (spheramine) (Stover & Watts, 2008); infusion of an adenoassociated viral (AAV) vector containing the human aromatic l-amino acid decarboxylase (hAADC) gene (Eberling et al., 2008) or serotype 2-neurturin (CERE-120) (Marks et al., 2008) into the putamen of PD patients; or injection of glutamic acid decarboxylase (GAD) gene with AAV into the STN of patients with advanced PD (Kaplitt et al., 2007). Further studies are necessary to confirm clinical benefits observed in initial trials.

It should be noted that all forms of neurosurgical intervention for PD can contribute to speech disorders by impacting the motor and language circuits. This issue must be taken into consideration when evaluating a patient who has had CNS surgery.

Vocal Fold Augmentation

Vocal fold augmentation has been used successfully in some patients who have vocal fold bowing and hypophonia secondary to an open glottis. The phonatory results, however, may still be poor as many PD patients have discoordination of respiratory effort and speaking, thereby decreasing the amount of air presented to the closed glottis. Therefore, good pulmonary function tests should be included in the evaluation before any augmentation is performed (Berke, Gerratt, Kreiman, & Jackson, 1999).

Summary

Parkinsonism is a neurologic syndrome consisting of bradykinesia, postural instability, rigidity, resting tremor, and/or freezing (motor blocks). Patients also may have additional symptoms in Parkinson-plus syndromes. Some patients may have additional autonomic dysfunction as seen in multiple system atrophy that may affect the larynx during speech and breathing. The management of parkinsonism is both complex and challenging. Interventions may include drug therapy, and surgical interventions such as pallidotomy, thalmotomy, deep brain stimulation, transplantation, novel restorative procedures, and vocal fold augmentation.

Management of Parkinson Disease

I. Drug Therapy

- Dopamine precursors (Levodopa with carbodopa) alone or combined with:
  - Catechol-o-methyl transferase inhibitors (entacapone, tolcapone) or dopamine agonists (bromocriptine, pergolide mesylate, ropinirol, pramipexole)

II. Surgical Intervention

- Thalamotomy
- Pallidotomy
- Deep Brain Stimulation (DBS)
  - Subthalamic Nucleus (STN)
  - Globus Pallidus Interna (GPi)
- Transplantation
  - Dopamine-containing cells (adrenal, fetal nigral, retinal pigment epithelial, stem cells)
- Novel/Restorative approaches
- Vocal fold augmentation

References

Ackermann, H., Ziegler, W., & Oertel, W. H. (1989). Palilalia as a symptom of levodopa induced hyperkinesia in Parkinson's disease. *Journal of Neurology, Neurosurgery and Psychiatry, 52*, 805–807.

Agid, Y., Cervera, P., Hirsch, E., Javoy-Agi,d F., Lehericy, S., Raisman, R., & Ruberg, M. (1989). Biochemistry of Parkinson's disease 28 years later: A critical review. *Movement Disorders, 44*, S126–S144.

Barbeau, A., & Roy, M. (1984). Familial subsets in idiopathic Parkinson's disease. *Canadian Journal of Neurological Sciences, 11*, 144–150.

Benabid, A. L., Pollak, P., Gervason, C., Hoffman, D., Gao, D. M., Hommel, M., . . . De Rougemont, J. (1991). Long-term suppression of tremor by chronic stimulation of the ventral intermediate thalamic nucleus. *Lancet, 337*, 403–406.

Berke, G. S., Gerratt, B., Kreiman, J., & Jackson, K. (1999). Treatment of Parkinson hypophonia with percutaneous collagen augmentation. *Laryngoscope, 109*, 1295–1299.

Bucy, P. C., & Case, J. T. (1939). Tremor: Physiologic mechanism and abolition by surgical means. *Archives of Neurology and Psychiatry, 41*, 721–746.

Chaudhuri, K. R., Healy, D. G., & Schapira, A. H. (2006). Non-motor symptoms of Parkinson's disease: Diagnosis and management. *Lancet Neurology, 5*, 235–245.

Cooper, I. S. (1954). Surgical alleviation of parkinsonism: Effects of occlusion of the anterior choroidal artery. *Journal of the American Geriatric Society, 11*, 691–717.

Cooper, I. S. (1956). An investigation of neurosurgical alleviation of parkinsonism, chorea, athetosis and dystonia. *Annals of Internal Medicine, 45*, 381–392.

DeLong, M. R. (1990). Primate models of movement disorders of basal ganglia origin. *Trends in Neuroscience, 13*, 281–285.

DeLong, M. R., Crutcher, M. D., & Georgopoulopos, A. P. (1985). Primate globus pallidus and subthalamic nucleus: Functional organisation. *Journal of Neurophysiology, 53*, 530–543.

Djaldetti, R., Koren, M., Ziv, I., Achiron, A., & Melamed, E. (1995). Effect of cisapride on response fluctuations in Parkinson's disease. *Movement Disorders, 10*, 81–84.

Eberling, J. L, Jagust, W. J., Christine, C. W., Starr, P., Larson, P., Bankiewicz, K. S., & Aminoff, M. J. (2008). Results from a Phase I safety trial of hAADC gene therapy for Parkinson disease. *Neurology, 70*, 1980–1983.

Fahn, S. (1986). Parkinson's disease and other basal ganglion disorders. In A. K. Asbury, G. M. McKhann, & W. I. McDonald (Eds.), *Diseases of the nervous system: Clinical neurobiology* (pp. 1217–1228). Philadelphia, PA: Ardmore Medical Books.

Fahn, S. (1988). Disorders with parkinsonian features. In J. W. Hurst (Ed.), *Medicine for the practicing physician* (2nd ed., pp. 1522–1525). Boston, MA: Butterworth.

Fahn, S. (1989). The history of parkinsonism. *Movement Disorders, 4*(Suppl. 1), S2–S10.

Fahn, S. (1992). Adverse effects of levodopa. In C. W. Olanow & A. N. Lieberman (Eds.), *The scientific basis for the treatment of Parkinson's disease* (pp. 89–112). Lancashire, UK: Parthenon.

Fahn, S., & Greenberg, J. (1972). Striatonigral degeneration. *Transactions of the American Neurological Association, 97*, 275–277.

Farrer, M. J. (2006). Genetics of Parkinson disease: Paradigm shifts and future prospects. *Nature Reviews Genetics, 7*, 306–318.

Fernandez, H. H., Donnelly, E. M., & Friedman, J. H. (2004). Long-term outcome of clozapine use for psychosis in parkinsonian patients. *Movement Disorders, 19*, 831–833.

Forno, L. S. (1982). Pathology of Parkinson's disease. In C. D. Marsden & S. Fahn (Eds.), *Movement disorders* (pp. 25–40). London, UK: Butterworth Scientific.

Fox, M., Ahlskog, J. E., & Kelly, P. J. (1991). Stereotactic ventrolateralis thalamotomy for medically refractory tremor in post-levodopa era Parkinson's disease patients. *Journal of Neurosurgery, 75*, 723–730.

Freed, C. R., Breeze, R. E., Rosenberg, N. L., Schneck, S. A., Kriek, E., Qi, J. X., . . . Wells, T. H. (1992). Survival of implanted fetal dopamine cells and neurologic improvement 12 to 46 months after transplantation for Parkinson's disease [See comments]. *New England Journal of Medicine, 327*, 1549–1555.

Freed, C. R., Greene, P. E., Breeze, R. E., Tsai, W. Y., DuMouchel, W., Kao, R., . . . Fahn, S. (2001). Transplantation of embryonic dopamine neurons for severe Parkinson's disease. *New England Journal of Medicine, 344*, 710–719.

García Ruiz, P. J., Sesar Ignacio, A., Ares Pensado, B., Castro García, A., Alonso Frech, F., Alvarez López, M., . . . Zamarbide Capdepon, I. (2008). Efficacy of long-term continuous subcutaneous apomorphine infusion in advanced Parkinson's disease with motor fluctuations: A multicenter study. *Movement Disorders, 23*, 1130–1136.

Gironell, A., Amirian, G., Kulisevsky, J., & Molet, J. (2005). Usefulness of an intraoperative electrophysiological navigator system for subthalamic nucleus surgery in Parkinson's disease. *Stereotactic and Functional Neurosurgery, 83*, 101–107.

Goberman, A. M., & Coelho, C. (2002). Acoustic analysis of parkinsonian speech II: L-Dopa related fluctuations and methodological issues. *NeuroRehabilitation, 17*, 247–254.

Hammond, C., Ammari, R., Bioulac, B., & Garcia, L. (2008). Latest view on the mechanism of action of deep brain stimulation. *Movement Disorders, 23*, 2111–2121.

Hauser, R. A., Freemanm T. B., Snow, B. J., Nauert, M., Gauger, L., Kordower, J. H., & Olanow, C. W. (1999). Long-term evaluation of bilateral fetal nigral transplantation in Parkinson disease. *Archives of Neurology, 56*, 179–187.

Hilker, R., Voges, J., Weber, T., Kracht, L. W., Roggendorf, J., Baudrexel, S., . . . Heiss, W. D. (2008). STN-DBS activates the target area in Parkinson disease: An FDG-PET study. *Neurology, 71*, 708–713.

Hurtig, H. I. (1997). Problems with current pharmacologic treatment of Parkinson's disease. *Experimental Neurology, 144*, 10–16.

Jellinger, K. A., Seppi, K., Wenning, G. K., & Poewe, W. (2002), Impact of coexistent Alzheimer pathology on the natural history of Parkinson's disease. *Journal of Neural Transmission, 109*, 329–339.

Kaplitt, M. G., Feigin, A., Tang, C., Fitzsimons, H. L., Mattis, P., Lawlor, P. A., . . . During, M. J. (2007). Safety and tolerability of gene therapy with an adeno-associated virus (AAV) borne GAD gene for Parkinson's disease: An open label, Phase I trial. *Lancet, 369*, 2056–2058.

Karimi, M., Golchin, N., Tabbal, S. D., Hershey, T., Videen, T. O., Wu, J., . . . Perlmutter, J. S. (2008). Subthalamic nucleus stimulation-induced regional blood flow responses correlate with improvement of motor signs in Parkinson disease. *Brain, 131*, 2710–2719.

Klemme, R. M. (1940). Surgical treatment of dystonia, paralysis agitans and athetosis. *Archives of Neurology, and Psychiatry, 44*, 26.

Kordower, J. H., Chu, Y., Hauser, R. A., Freeman, T. B., & Olanow, C. W. (2008). Lewy body-like pathology in long-term embryonic nigral transplants in Parkinson's disease. *Nature Medicine, 14*, 504–506.

Kordower, J. H., Freeman, T. B., Snow, B. J., Vingerhoets, F. J., Mufson, E. J., Sanberg, P. R., . . . Olanow, C. W. (1995). Neuropathological evidence of graft survival and striatal reinnervation after the transplantation of fetal mesencephalic tissue in a patient with Parkinson's disease. *New England Journal of Medicine, 332*, 1118–1124.

Kordower, J. H., Rosenstein, J. M., Collier, T. J., Burke, M. A., Chen, E. Y., Li, J. M., . . . Olanow, C. W. (1996). Functional fetal nigral grafts in a patient with Parkinson's disease: Chemoanatomic, ultrastructural, and metabolic studies. *Journal of Comparative Neurology, 370*, 203–230.

Lang, A. E., Lozano, A. M., Montgomery, E., Duff, J., Tasker, R., & Hutchinson, W. (1997). Posteroventral medial pallidotomy in advanced Parkinson's disease. *New England Journal of Medicine, 337*, 1036–1042.

Langston, J. W. (2006). The Parkinson's complex: Parkinsonism is just the tip of the iceberg. *Annals of Neurology, 59*, 591–596.

Li, J. Y., Englund, E., Holton, J. L., Soulet, D., Hagell, P., Lees, A. J., . . . Brundin, P. (2008). Lewy bodies in grafted neurons in subjects with Parkinson's disease suggest host-to-graft disease propagation. *Nature Medicine, 14*, 501–503.

Limousin, P., Pollak, P., Benazzouz, A., Hoffmann, D., Broussolle, E., Perret, J. E., & Benabid, A. L. (1995). Bilateral subthalamic nucleus stimulation for severe Parkinson's disease. *Movement Disorders, 10*, 672–674.

Lozano, A., Hutchison, W., Kiss, Z., Tasker, R., Davis, K., & Dostrovsky, J. (1996). Methods for microelectrode-guided posteroventral pallidotomy. *Journal of Neurosurgery, 84*, 194–202.

Madrazo, I., Drucker-Colin, R., Diaz, V., Martinez-Mata, J., Torres, C., & Becerril, J. J. (1987). Open microsurgical autograft of adrenal medulla to the right caudate nucleus in two patients with intractable Parkinson's disease. *New England Journal of Medicine, 316*, 831–834.

Mark, M. H., Sage, J. I., Dickson, D. W., Schwarz, K. O., & Duvoisin, R. C. (1992). Levodopa-nonresponsive Lewy body parkinsonism: Clinicopathologic study of two cases. *Neurology, 42*, 1323–1327.

Marks, W. J., Jr., Ostrem, J. L., Verhagen, L., Starr, P. A., Larson, P. S., Bakay, R. A., . . . Bartus, R. T. (2008). Safety and tolerability of intraputaminal delivery of CERE-120 (adeno-associated virus serotype 2-neurturin) to patients with idiopathic Parkinson's disease: An open-label, Phase I trial. *Lancet Neurology, 7*, 375–376.

Mendez, I., Sanchez-Pernaute, R., Cooper, O., Viñuela, A., Ferrari, D., Björklund, L., . . . Isacson, O. (2005). Cell type analysis of functional fetal dopamine cell suspension transplants in the striatum and substantia nigra of patients with Parkinson's disease. *Brain, 128*, 1498–1510.

Mendez, I., Viñuela, A., Astradsson, A., Mukhida, K., Hallett, P., Robertson, H., . . . Isacson, O. (2008). Dopamine neurons implanted into people with Parkinson's disease survive without pathology for 14 years. *Nature Medicine, 14*, 507–509.

Meyers, R. (1940). Surgical procedure for postencephalitic tremor, with notes on the physiology of premotor fibres. *Archives of Neurology and Psychiatry, 44*, 455–457.

Meyers, R. (1951). Surgical experiments in therapy of certain "extrapyramidal" diseases: Current evaluation. *Acta Psychiatrica et Neurologica Scandinavica Supplementum, 67*, 1–42.
Muller, T. (2002). Drug treatment of non-motor symptoms in Parkinson's disease. *Expert Opinion on Pharmacotherapy, 3*, 381–388.
Müller, J., Wenning, G. K., Jellinger, K., McKee, A., Poewe, W., & Litvan, I. (2000). Progression of Hoehn and Yahr stages in parkinsonian disorders: A clinicopathologic study. *Neurology, 26*, 888–891.
Müller, J., Wenning, G. K., Verny, M., McKee, A., Chaudhuri, K. R., Jellinger, K., . . . Litvan, I. (2001). Progression of dysarthria and dysphagia in postmortem-confirmed parkinsonian disorders. *Archives of Neurology, 58*, 259–264.
Nagashima, T., Oda, M., Tanabe, H., Morimatsu, Y., Inoue, Y., Sasaki, H., . . . Ohkawa, M. (1993). Sleep apnea and sudden death in multiple system atrophy: Polysomnographic studies and brain stem neuropathology. In K. Togawa, S. Katayama, Y. Hishikawa, Y. Ohta, & T. Horie (Eds.), *Sleep apnea and rhonchopathy* (pp. 128–131). Basel, Switzerland: S. Karger.
Nyholm, D., Nilsson Remahl, A. I., Dizdar, N., Constantinescu, R., Holmberg, B., Jansson, R., . . . Askmark, H. (2005). Duodenal levodopa infusion monotherapy vs. oral polypharmacy in advanced Parkinson disease. *Neurology, 64*, 216–223.
Olanow, C. W., Perl, D. P., DeMartino, G. N., & McNaught, K. S. (2004). Lewy-body formation is an aggresome-related process: A hypothesis. *Lancet Neurology, 3*, 496–503.
Pahwa, R., Wilkinson, S., Smith, D., Lyons, K., Miyawaki, E., & Koller, W. C. (1997). High-frequency stimulation of the globus pallidus for the treatment of Parkinson's disease. *Neurology, 49*, 249–253.
Parkinson Study Group. (2004). A controlled, randomized, delayed-start study of rasagiline in early Parkinson disease. *Archives of Neurology, 61*, 561–566.
Rodriguez-Oroz, M. C., Obeso, J. A., Lang, A. E., Houeto, J. L., Pollak, P., Rehncrona, S., . . . Van Blercom, N. (2005). Bilateral deep brain stimulation in Parkinson's disease: A multicentre study with 4 years follow-up. *Brain, 128*, 2240–2249.
Schapira, A. H. (2004). Disease modification in Parkinson's disease. *Lancet Neurology, 3*, 362–368.
Schapira, A. H., & Olanow, C. W. (2004). Neuroprotection in Parkinson disease: mysteries, myths, and misconceptions. *Journal of the American Medical Association, 291*, 358–364.
Schiesling, C., Kieper, N., Seidel, K., & Krüger, R. (2008). Review: Familial Parkinson's disease—genetics, clinical phenotype and neuropathology in relation to the common sporadic form of the disease. *Neuropathology and Applied Neurobiology, 34*, 255–271.
Schoenberg, B. S. (1987). Epidemiology of movement disorders. In C. D. Marsden & S. Fahn (Eds.), *Movement disorders* (pp. 17–32). London, UK: Butterworth.
Shoulson, I., Fah, S., & Parkinson Study Group. (1989). Effect of deprenyl on the progression of disability in early Parkinson's disease. *New England Journal of Medicine, 321*, 1364–1371.

Silber, M. H., & Levine, S. (2000). Stridor and death in multiple system atrophy. *Movement Disorders, 15,* 699–704.

Stocchi, F., Ruggieri, S., Vacca, L., & Olanow, C. W. (2002). Prospective randomized trial of lisuride infusion versus oral levodopa in patients with Parkinson's disease. *Brain, 125,* 2058–2066.

Stover, N. P., & Watts, R. L. (2008). Spheramine for treatment of Parkinson's disease. *Neurotherapeutics, 5,* 252–259.

Tasker, R. R. (1990). Thalamotomy. *Neurosurgery Clinics of North America, 1,* 841–864.

Tasker, R. R., Siqueira, J., Hawrylyshyn, P., & Organ, L. W. (1983). What happened to VIM thalamotomy for Parkinson's disease? *Applied Neurophysiology, 46,* 68–83.

Wenning, G. K., Odin, P., Morrish, P., Rehncrona, S., Widner, H., Brundin, P., . . . Lindvall, O. (1997). Short- and long-term survival and function of unilateral intrastriatal dopaminergic grafts in Parkinson's disease. *Annals of Neurology, 42,* 95–107.

Wenning, G. K., Tison, F., Ben Shlomo, Y., Daniel, S. E., Quinn, N. P. (1997). Multiple system atrophy: A review of 203 pathologically proven cases. *Movement Disorders, 12,* 133–147.

Williams, D. R., de Silva, R., Paviour, D. C., Pittman, A., Watt, H. C., Kilford, L., . . . Lees, A. J. (2005). Characteristics of two distinct clinical phenotypes in pathologically proven progressive supranuclear palsy: Richardson's syndrome and PSP-parkinsonism. *Brain, 128,* 1247–1258.

2

Neuropathologic Bases for Communication and Swallowing Disorders in Parkinson Disease

GERALYN SCHULZ

From the time that James Parkinson published his seminal "Essay on the Shaking Palsy" in 1817 (Parkinson, 2002) the cardinal signs of Parkinson disease (PD) have been described as resting tremor, muscle stiffness (rigidity) and weakness, with reduced and slow movements (hypokinesia and bradykinesia). In his original essay Parkinson described speech and swallowing impairments as appearing when the disease progressed to the point that the patient could no longer ambulate unassisted,

> His words are now scarcely intelligible; and he is not only no longer able to feed himself, but when the food is conveyed to the mouth, so much are the actions of the muscles of the tongue, pharynx, etc. impeded by impaired action and perpetual agitation, that the food is with difficulty retained in the month until masticated; and then as difficultly swallowed. Now also, from the same cause, another very unpleasant circumstance occurs: the saliva fails of being directed to the back part of the fauces, and hence is continually draining from the mouth, mixed with the particles of food, which he is no longer able to clear from the inside of the mouth. (Parkinson, 2002, p. 225)

Parkinson attributed the cause of the disorder to the result of impairments to the cervical spine and the medulla. However, it is now known that there is a degeneration of dopaminergic neurons in a midbrain region, the substantia nigra pars compacta (SNc), that is the major cause of PD. Based on years of anatomic and neurophysiologic studies, the dopaminergic pathways emanating from the SNc travel to a group of subcortical nuclei, the basal ganglia (BG), and have been mapped out, as have been the connections to and from BG nuclei to other cortical and subcortical areas (for an excellent review of the history of the involvement of dopamine see Marsden, 2006). The basic model for the motor disturbances in PD is that the lack of dopamine to subcortical nuclei in the BG results in disruptions to other areas involved in motor control including the thalamus, cortex, cerebellum, and areas of the brainstem. In particular, the net effect of the diminution in the flow of dopamine through the BG results in the underactivation of the thalamus which then results in an underactivation of cortical motor areas resulting in reduced and slowed movements that are hallmarks of PD (Marsden, 1994). Thus, PD was viewed as a disruption of the basal ganglia-thalamocortical circuits/loops. Since the 1970s our understanding of the neuropathophysiology of PD has expanded on this basic model based in large part on three advances, the discovery of toxins that selectively cause dopamine loss in animals (Burns et al., 1983), the advent and development of neurosurgical techniques and treatments for PD particularly deep brain stimulation (Li, Zhuang, & Li, 2008), and by advances in neuroimaging (Grafton, 2004).

The purpose of this chapter is to review the traditional circuit anatomy model and newer models of PD that emphasize altered neuronal firing, oscillatory neural activity, and synchronous (or dyssynchronous) firing of various cortical and subcortical areas (Montgomery, 2007; Stoffers et al., 2007). With the incorporation of in vivo electrophysiologic data PD is now viewed as a complex network disorder in which abnormal activity of neurons in the BG affects electrophysiologic activity in various thalamic, cortical, and subcortical areas that are involved in motor, executive, limbic, and sensory processing (Galvan & Wichmann, 2008). The neuropathophysiology of speech, language, and swallowing disorders in PD is reviewed within the traditional circuit model framework and within the oscillatory network model.

Circuit Anatomy Model of PD

Abnormalities in the functioning of the BG underlie the primary motor disorders of PD. The BG consist of several subcortical nuclei including the neostriatum (caudate nucleus and putamen), the external and internal globus palladus (GPe and GPi), the subthalamic nucleus (STN), and the substantia nigra pars reticular (SNr) and pars compacta (SNc). Input to the BG (neostriatum) comes from various motor and frontal areas in the cortex and BG output nuclei (GPi/SNr) are functionally and physiologically connected to other subcortical structures (predominantly the thalamus and pedunculopontine nucleus (PPN) which then send projections back to the various motor and frontal areas of the cortex from which they originated to form functional loops (Akkal, Dum, & Strick, 2007; Alexander, Crutcher, & DeLong, 1990; Alexander, DeLong, & Strick, 1986). These loops form functionally segregated, parallel circuits and are divided according to the area of cortex that is involved; "motor," "oculomotor," "prefrontal," and "limbic" (Alexander et al., 1990; Middleton & Strick, 2000). By far, the most well studied of these is the motor circuit loop, and disruptions to this loop traditionally have been invoked as causing the speech and voice disorders, collectively known as hypokinetic dysarthria (Darley, Aronson, & Brown, 1969a). The features of hypokinetic dysarthria are described in detail in Chapter 3.

Motor Circuit Loop

This circuit involves BG nuclei receiving input from motor areas of the cortex and from the dopamine-producing SNc, and then sending output to motor areas of the thalamus and brainstem which in turn send output back to the motor areas of the cortex from which they originated to complete the loop. Specifically, motor areas of the cortex (primary motor and somatosensory cortex, premotor, PMA, and supplementary motor areas, SMA) send excitatory glutamatergic afferents to the BG input nuclei, the striatum and STN. The striatum and STN also receive inhibitory dopaminergic projections directly (striatum) or indirectly (STN) from SNc. Information is then transferred to the output nuclei of the BG, GPi, and SNr, which send inhibitory GABAergic output predominantly to the ventroanterior (VA) and ventrolateral (VL) nuclei of the thalamus, and to a lesser extent to brainstem nuclei such as the pedunculopontine nucleus (PPN). Figure 2–1, adapted from Galvan and Wichmann (2008), depicts this corticobasal ganglia-thalamocortical circuitry. It should be noted that the pathways in this circuit retain the somatotopic organization that has been well documented in primary motor and somatosensory cortex (Alexander et al., 1986); that is, there are functionally segregated "leg," "face," and "arm" projections from cortex to striatum (mainly to the putamen), and from the striatum to the thalamus via BG output nuclei, and from thalamus back to cortical motor areas (SMA). Although there appears to be a more strict point to

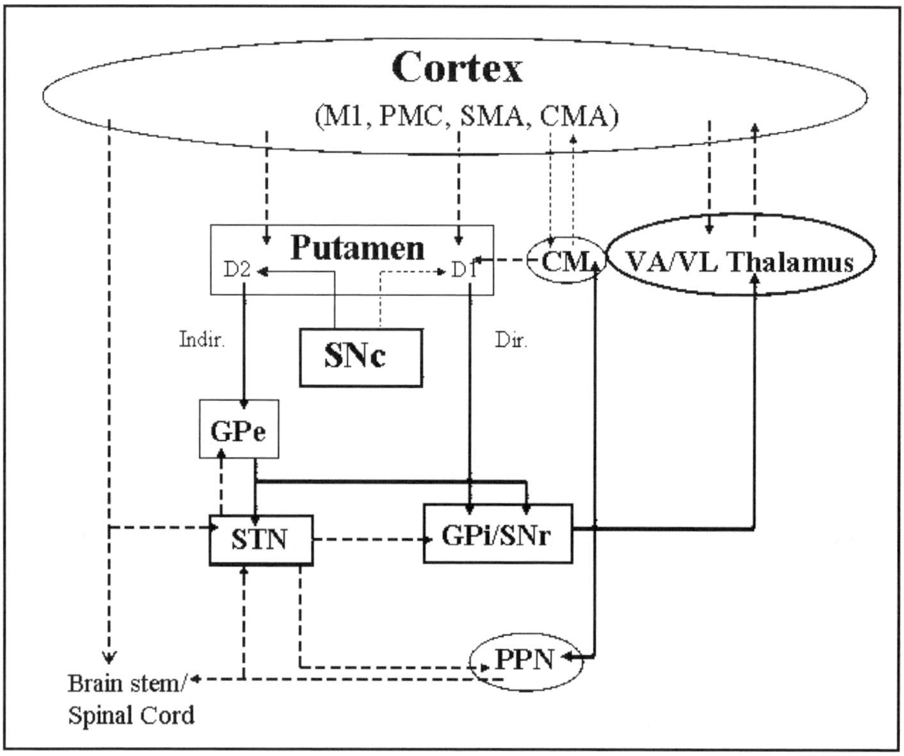

FIGURE 2–1. Normal motor circuit function of the basal ganglia. Excitatory pathways depicted in dotted lines and inhibitory pathways depicted in solid lines. Abbreviations: SM1, primary sensorimotor cortex; PMA, premotor cortex; SMA, supplementary motor area; VA/VL thalamus, ventroanterior and ventrolateral; CM, centromedian nucleus of the thalamus; SNc, substantia nigra pars compacta; SNr, substantia nigra pars recticular; STN, subthalamic nucleus; GPe, external segment of the globus pallidus; GPi, internal segment of the globus pallidus; PPN, pedunculopontine nucleus. Adapted from: *Clinical Neurophysiology, 119,* Galvan, A., & Wichmann, T., Pathophysiology of Parkinsonism, pp. 1459–1474, Copyright (2008), with permission from Elsevier.

point topography from the primary motor cortex to the putamen, projections within basal ganglia nuclei and the thalamus have been found to be more interdigitated. However, functional specificity nevertheless is maintained (Alexander et al., 1990).

As noted, connections within the BG are direct (striatum → GPi/SNr) or indirect (striatum → GPe → STN → GPi/SNr). These two pathways have opposing actions on the striatum such that the output of the basal ganglia (GPi/SNr) in the nonimpaired brain is reduced so that the activity in the thalamocortical pathway is enhanced, thus facilitating movement (DeLong, 1990; DeLong & Wichmann, 2007). More specifically, nigrostriatal dopamine facilitates transmission of corticostriatal synapses on striatal output neurons (which carry D1 dopamine receptors) in the direct pathway. Nigrostrial dopamine, however, inhibits transmission of corticostriatal synapses on striatal output neurons of the indirect pathway (which carry D2 dopamine receptors). Thus, the inhibitory GABAergic output of the BG (GPi/SNr) is regulated by the inhibitory activity in the direct pathway and by facilitating activity in the indirect pathway. In the normal functioning BG, the output of the GPi/SNr which tonically inhibits thalamocortical neurons in VA/VL thalamus is regulated so that the motor areas of the cortex receive the "right amount" of facilitation from VA/VL thalamus to allow correctly scaled movements (DeLong & Wichmann, 2007).

Parkinson Disease as a Dysregulation in the Motor Circuit

Parkinson disease is now known to be caused by a degeneration of DA-producing cells in the SNc which project to the sensorimotor areas of the striatum (Bernheimer, Birkmayer, Hornykiewicz, Jellinger, & Seitelberger, 1973; Kish, Shannak, & Hornykiewicz, 1988). As a consequence of reduced dopamine in the striatum, the major effect on the motor circuit is an increase in inhibitory outflow from the GPi/SNr to the thalamus which results in a reduction of excitatory output to the cortical motor areas (Figure 2–2). These areas are seen to be underexcited resulting in a reduced excitatory output back to the BG and also to the brainstem and spinal cord. Thus, the resulting movements are "underscaled" (DeLong & Wichmann, 2007). More specifically, reductions in nigrostriatal dopamine result in increased activity in the indirect striatal pathway which results in increased inhibition of GPe, and disinhibition of STN. Consequently, there is increased excitation of GPi/SNr and decreased activity of the direct striatal pathway which results in reduced inhibitory outflow to the GPi/SNr. The combined effect of these is to increase the normally inhibitory output of the GPi/SNr which thus decreases the activity in VA/VL thalamic neurons (see Figure 2–2) (DeLong & Wichmann, 2007). These, in turn, send reduced activation to cortical motor areas such as the primary motor, SMA, and premotor areas (Hoover & Strick, 1993, 1999; Middleton & Strick, 2000).

Implicit in this model is the notion of rate of neuronal firing. That is, the increased outflow from the BG is actually an increase in the rate of firing of inhibitory GPi/SNr neurons that are projecting to the thalamus, resulting in a reduced rate of firing of thalamic excitatory neurons that project to cortical motor areas, followed by a reduced rate of firing of

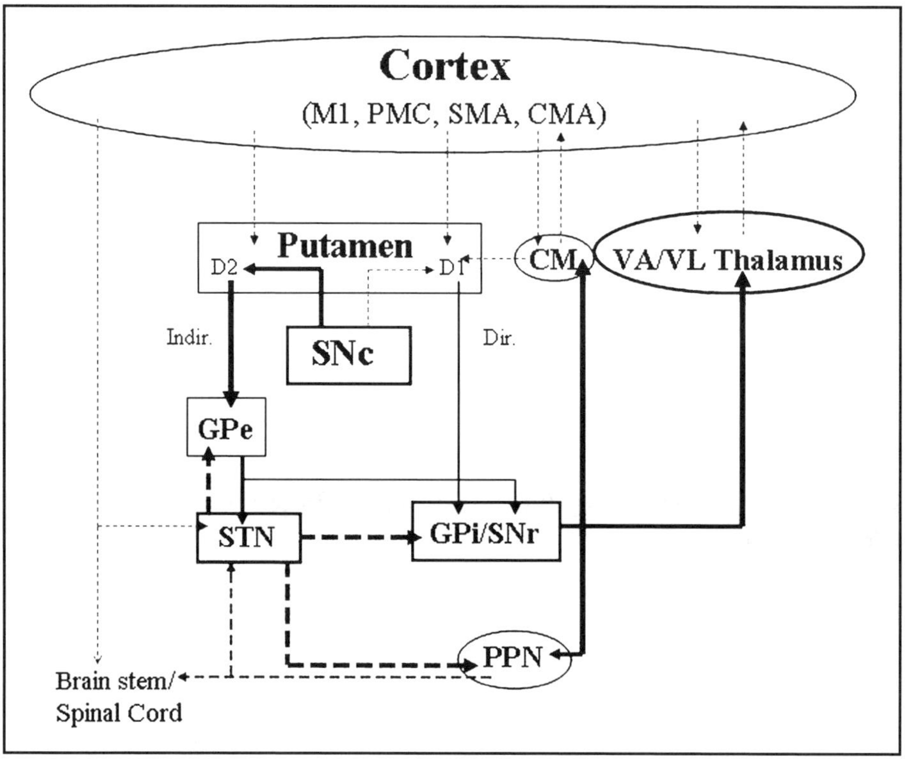

FIGURE 2–2. Motor circuit function of the basal ganglia in Parkinson disease. Excitatory pathways depicted in dotted lines and inhibitory pathways depicted in solid lines; thickness of the lines and arrows indicates altered (diminished or enhanced) activity (rate of firing) in the pathway. Abbreviations: SM1, primary sensorimotor cortex; PMA, premotor cortex; SMA, supplementary motor area; VA/VL thalamus, ventroanterior and ventrolateral; CM, centromedian nucleus of the thalamus; SNc, substantia nigra pars compacta; SNr, substantia nigra pars recticular; STN, subthalamic nucleus; GPe, external segment of the globus pallidus; GPi, internal segment of the globus pallidus; PPN, pedunculopontine nucleus. Adapted from: *Clinical Neurophysiology, 119,* Galvan, A., & Wichmann, T., Pathophysiology of Parkinsonism, pp.1459–1474, Copyright (2008), with permission from Elsevier.

excitatory cortical motor neurons that project to brainstem and spinal cord motor neurons (Berardelli, Rothwell, Thompson, & Hallett, 2001; DeLong & Wichmann, 2007). The reduced and slow movement, akinesia, and bradykinesia, observed in PD is thus explained as result of the cortical motor areas being excessively inhibited and thus not sending sufficient excitation to the muscles (Berardelli et al., 2001). Support for this model is found from lesioning and/or stimulation studies of the STN and GPi that result in significant improvements in motor functioning (Esselink et al., 2004).

Neuropathophysiologic Bases of Speech and Swallowing Disorders in PD as a Function of Disruption to the Motor Circuit

In their seminal work investigating the perceptual attributes of the dysarthrias, Darley et al. (1969a, 1969b) described five types of dysarthria caused by central or peripheral nervous system disorders that impair the movement of the muscles involved in producing speech. They explicitly stated that there was a direct association between the damage to the nervous system and the resulting impairments of movement, and that the impairments observed in speech would be of the same nature as that observed in the limbs, "Speech indeed follows neuroanatomy and neurophysiology. There are multiple types or patterns of dysarthria, each of which mirrors a different kind of abnormality of motor functioning" (Darley et al.,1969b). Indeed, they claimed as did Grewel (1957) that one could localize the neurologic disorder on the basis of the particular clustering of deviant perceptual dimensions of speech and that if you understood the neurologic bases of motor control you would be able to predict the cluster of deviant perceptual dimensions of speech (Darley et al., 1969a).

Using this logic, they described the cluster of deviant perceptual dimensions of speech in PD as resulting from the same movement abnormality as occurs in the limbs, hypokinesia; that is, a slowness and limited range of movement and so named the type of dysarthria in PD as "hypokinetic" (Darley et al., 1969b). The perceptual dimensions of speech that were rated as most deviant in hypokinetic dysarthria were monopitch, reduced stress, monoloudness, imprecise consonants, inappropriate silences, short rushes of speech, and harsh and breathy voice quality. Support for the similarity of speech motor abnormalities and limb motor abnormalities has come from a variety of studies (e.g., (Ackermann & Ziegler, 1991; Forrest, Weismer, & Turner, 1989; Hirose, Kiritani, Ushijima, Yoshioka, & Sawashima, 1981; Solomon & Hixon, 1993). Refer to Chapter 3 for further details concerning speech disorder in PD.

Some of the same laryngeal movement disorders that negatively affect phonation may also negatively affect swallowing (e.g., (Blumin, Pcolinsky, & Atkins, 2004; Bushmann, Dobmeyer, Leeker, & Perlmutter, 1989; Leopold & Kagel, 1997; Miller et al., 2009). (See Chapter 7 for further details.) Additionally, PD patients with more advanced disease and/or longer disease duration have greater laryngeal movement deficits and therefore more frequent and severe dyphagia (Coates & Bakheit, 1997;

Leopold & Kagel, 1997; Logemann, Blonsky, & Boshes, 1975; Manor, Balas, Giladi, Mootanah, & Cohen, 2009; Miller et al., 2009).

The general conclusion reached by many of these authors was consistent with the conclusion reached by Darley and colleagues that as the movement abnormalities underlying limb, speech, voice, and swallowing disorders observed in PD were similar they must be caused by the same underlying BG dysfunction. That is, dysfunction in the motor circuit with the slight variation being that the speech, voice and swallowing movement disorders were due to damage to the "face" projections from sensorimotor cortex/SMA, whereas the limb movement disorders were due to damage in the "arm" and "leg" projection pathways.

On the bases that the speech, voice, and swallowing symptoms and the limb motor symptoms of PD have the same neuropathologic basis, the next logical assumption would be that the speech, voice, and swallowing symptoms would demonstrate similar improvements to the limb symptoms of bradykinesia and rigidity, in response to dopaminergic medication. However, the impact of dopamine replacement on voice, speech, and swallowing symptoms in PD is not as clearly beneficial as such medication on limb movements (Schulz & Grant, 2000; Spencer, Morgan, & Blond, 2009). Positive dopaminergic effects have been reported for lip and tongue functions (Cahill et al., 1998), word intelligibility (De Letter et al., 2007), and gross assessment of swallowing (from the Activities of Daily Living section of the UPDRS rating scale) (Bejjani et al., 2000). Conflicting dopaminergic effects have been reported for prosody (Ho, Bradshaw, & Iansek, 2008) and for individual patient's swallowing functions (Bushmann et al., 1989). Finally, most acoustic studies report no changes with dopaminergic medication (Goberman, Coelho, & Robb,

Basic Model of PD as a Disruption of the Basal Ganglia-Thalamocortical Motor Circuits/Loops

Loss of Dopaminergic Cells in Substantia Nigra Pars Compacta →
- Diminution Dopamine Flow Through Basal Ganglia →
  - Thalamic Underactivation →
    - Cortical Limb Motor Area Underactivation →
      - Reduced Slowed Limb Movements (Bradykinesia, Hypokinesia)
    - Cortical Face Motor Area Underactivation →
      - Reduced Slowed Orofacial, Laryngeal, Respiratory Movements (Hypokinetic Dysarthria, Dysphagia)

2002). These results certainly raise questions as to the underlying neuropathophysiologic similarities in speech and limb motor control in the BG motor circuit.

There are two other ways to determine whether the same underlying neuropathology is the cause of the limb motor and speech motor symptoms in PD (as hypothesized in the motor circuit model and by Darley and colleagues, 1969a, 1969b). One method is to determine whether the effects of surgical intervention are the same for limb symptoms as for speech and voice symptoms. Surgical procedures such as pallidotomy and STN deep brain stimulation (DBS) have produced mixed results regarding improvements in voice and speech symptoms (Putzer, Barry, & Moringlane, 2008; Santens, De Letter, Van Borsel, De Reuck, & Caemaert, 2003; Schulz, Greer, & Friedman, 2000) (see Chapter 3), whereas they consistently have positive effects on limb symptoms such as bradykinesia and rigidity (Ostergaard & Sunde, 2006). The typical explanation for this is that the surgical sites are targeted to the "arm" and "leg" projections and not to the "face" projections (Schulz et al., 2000; Schulz, Peterson, Sapienza, Greer, & Friedman, 1999), or that these areas could well be differentially affected in individuals with PD and thus give rise to differences observed between limb and speech symptoms. In addition, depletion of DA may be differentially affected across various basal ganglia-thalamus-cortex motor loops, resulting in observed differences within limb and speech motor systems.

The second way is to develop an animal model for vocalization and to experimentally alter dopamine levels. This method has obvious limitations; that is, animals do not speak. However, mammals and humans share many neural substrates for vocalization (Schulz, Varga, Jeffires, Ludlow, & Braun, 2005) so the notion of determining the effects of altering dopamine on vocalization is not quite as farfetched as it originally sounds. Inducing short- or long-term dopamine deficiency produces qualitative changes in the ultrasonic vocalizations in rats (Ciucci et al., 2007). In particular there was a diminished modulation of the vocal trill structure in dopamine deficient rats which the authors likened to the reduction in pitch variation in human PD (Ciucci et al., 2007).

In addition to the differences in limb versus speech response to treatment in PD, there are some obvious and not so obvious differences in the neurologic motor control for limb versus speech, voice, and swallowing. Speech and swallowing are, as alluded to above, performed in the midline and as such are axial movements which differ from limb movements. The muscles used in voice, speech, and swallowing are under the control of the cranial nerves which for the most part are themselves under bilateral control from upper motor neurons. Additionally, many voice, speech, and swallowing muscles do not have the same composition as limb muscles; there are no obvious agonist/antagonist pairs (except for jaw opening and closing); and speech muscles do not have muscle spindles that provide the nervous system with information on length changes that help to determine position of limbs in space, and in regulating muscle contraction. One large difference between motor control for speech and that for limb movement is that for speech there must be multilayered interactions among language and motor systems (Smith, 2006). Therefore, a greater number, and more distinct parts of the central nervous system are involved in speech production than in limb movement.

In conclusion, it appears that the evidence is not in complete agreement with the theory that the same underlying neuropathologic processes cause voice, speech, and swallowing symptoms and limb motor symptoms in PD. Clearly, although there are similar effects on movement kinematics, there are differences in the neural architecture for limb versus voice/speech and perhaps swallowing, as well as differences in response to treatment.

The motor circuit model of PD, however, is somewhat more complicated than simply the hypoactivation of cortical motor areas as described (Akkal et al., 2007). Neuroimaging studies of PD and healthy participants have shown as predicted, increased activity in inhibitory BG output nuclei and underactivation of SMA, but contrary to prediction, hyperactivation of the primary motor cortex (Eggers, Hilker, Burghaus, Schumacher, & Heiss, 2009; Hosey, Thompson, Metman, van den Munckhof, & Braun, 2005). Imaging studies have also demonstrated increased activation of the cerebellum in PD (Hosey et al., 2005). The implication is that since cerebellar projections also terminate in the primary motor cortex (Akkal et al., 2007), the increased activity observed in the cerebellum may be a compensatory mechanism to offset the otherwise hypoactive primary motor cortex in PD (Akkal et al., 2007). This hypothesis is partially confirmed by neuroimaging studies that have shown a reduction in cerebellar activity with the administration of dopamine agonists (Hosey et al., 2005). Increased activity of the cerebellum, however, may not be sufficient to compensate for reduced SMA activity in PD due to the fact that SMA has three to four times more BG than cerebellar input (Akkal et al., 2007).

Such compensatory mechanisms in the motor circuit may account for the fact that the amount of DA depletion needed before PD symptoms become clinically noticeable is >80% (Bernheimer et al., 1973). An alternative, although not necessarily mutually exclusive, hypothesis is that it may take such a great loss of SNc cells before PD symptoms appear clinically because cell loss in SNc may not be the primary pathobiologic process in PD (Eriksen, Wszolek, & Petrucelli, 2005; Gupta, Dawson, & Dawson, 2008; van Rooden, Visser, Verbaan, Marinus, & van Hilten, 2009a). However, once the SNc is affected there are additional processes that affect DA neurons causing an accelerated cell loss in SNc sufficient for the clinical manifestation of symptoms (Lang, 2007). Candidates for primary pathobiologic processes include oxidative stress which will also cause cell death in SNc (Carrasco, Casper, & Werner, 2007; Danielson & Andersen, 2008).

Given either hypothesis above regarding the clinical onset of limb symptoms, and the fact that there is no direct relationship between length of PD symptoms and onset of hypokinetic dysarthria (Miller et al., 2007), it is not surprising that greater severity of PD (assessed by the motor scale of the UPDRS) is correlated with increased disability of voice, speech, and swallowing disorders (Midi et al., 2008). It could be that it takes a greater degree of SNc cell loss and/or additional pathobiologic processes such as oxidative stress in the "oral/face" motor pathway before clinical symptoms of hypokinetic dysarthria and dysphagia appear. Alternatively, it could be that speech, voice, and swallowing are really to be considered an "axial" feature of PD, like gait, posture, and rising from a chair, which are known to be less responsive to dopaminergic therapy (Bejjani et al., 2000). It also is possible that other corticobasal ganglia-thalamocortical circuits need to be affected as well before hypokinetic dysarthric and dysphagic symptoms become clinically apparent.

Other Motor Symptoms

Bradykinesia, although a primary sign of PD, is not the only cardinal sign of PD. Resting tremor and rigidity also are hallmarks of PD. How can the motor circuit hypothesis explain these PD symptoms? Rigidity is defined as increased resistance to passive stretch and is associated with increased tone in PD (Berardelli, Sabra, & Hallett, 1983). This symptom arises from a change of central nervous system reflex responsiveness (Cantello, Tarletti, Varrasi, Cecchin, & Monaco, 2007). In this regard, long latency reflex responses to stretch in PD are prominent, are higher in amplitude and longer in duration, and often merge with subsequent voluntary activity (Berardelli et al., 1983). Support for a central nervous system change that might be responsible for such prominent long latency reflex responses comes from a study that demonstrated that hyperactivation in the contralateral primary motor cortex was directly related to upper limb rigidity (Yu, Sternad, Corcos, & Vaillancourt, 2007).

Tremor is often an early sign in PD and may affect up to 70% of PD patients. Typically, it initially is unilateral affecting the upper limb (Marsden, 1994). PD tremor occurs at rest and attenuates with movement. Lesioning or stimulation of the thalamus has been shown to ameliorate resting tremor (Fishman, 2008). This finding has led to the theory that the thalamus is the locus of tremor in PD. However, STN DBS has also been shown to ameliorate tremor (Esselink et al., 2004) and there are several studies that implicate a role of the STN in the generation of PD resting tremor (Amtage et al., 2008).

Dyskinesia, or abnormal involuntary movements, often occur with long-term use of L-dopa (Marsden, 1994). Typically, after five or more years of L-dopa replacement therapy, PD patients exhibit fluctuations called the "on-off" phenomenon. When the effects of dopamine replacement are maximal the PD patient will experience dyskinesia and motor complications, whereas when the effects of dopamine replacement therapy are minimal, the patient may be nearly akinetic (Marsden, 1994). There are several theories as to why the continued use of L-dopa causes dyskinesias. One is that the BG have a reduced capacity to store and effectively use L-dopa (Caudle, Colebrooke, Emson, & Miller, 2008; Leenders et al., 1986). The other hypothesis relates to serotonin. There is seratonergic innervation of all BG nuclei and these terminals have synaptic connections with DA SNc neurons and their terminal areas in the striatum, GP and STN (Di Matteo et al., 2008). Dyskinesias may result from dysregulation of dopamine from serotonin terminals in the basal ganglia (Carta, Carlsson, Kirik, & Bjorklund, 2007). Dyskinesias can be treated effectively with amantadine and STN DBS (Pahwa et al., 2006) which argues for the serotonin-related hypothesis.

Circuits Involved in Nonmotor Symptoms of PD

Several additional BG-thalamocortical circuits have been postulated in addition to the motor circuit. The frequent nonmotor symptoms observed in PD have been associated with the existence of these other circuits (Middleton & Strick, 2000; Zgaljardic et al., 2006). Such symptoms include neuropsychological and cognitive/executive function impairments, autonomic symptoms, sleep disorders, sensory problems, and depression (Simuni & Sethi, 2008). In addition, symptoms often included in the "nonmotor" or "noncardinal" category are axial symptoms such as difficulty rising from a chair, difficulty with gait, postural instability, gait freezing, speech, and swallowing problems (van Rooden, Visser, Verbaan, Marinus, & van Hilten, 2009b).

These nonmotor symptoms frequently appear during the time course of PD when dopaminergic replacement therapy produces fluctuations in motor responsiveness, the "on-off" phenomenon (Marsden, 1994). The exception to this appears to be in tremor dominant PD where there is a reported clinical impression of a slower progression of disease severity, and greater preservation of cognitive function (Hoehn & Yahr, 1967; Jankovic & Kapadia, 2001; Poewe & Wenning, 1998). These findings are in agreement with reports demonstrating slower deterioration of the caudate than the putamen (Hilker et al., 2005), and lower neuronal density in the SNc in akinetic rigid dominant PD compared to tremor-dominant PD (Paulus & Jellinger, 1991).

The etiology of these nonmotor symptoms is multifactorial and evidence for the involvement of various systems has come from many lines of research. Increased abnormal activity in nondopaminergic areas has been implicated for noncardinal symptoms of PD such as gait disturbances, postural instability, and the emergence of dysarthria and dysphagia because these symptoms continue to deteriorate long after the cardinal symptoms of bradykinesia, rigidity, and tremor stabilize following dopaminergic therapy (Bonnet, Loria, Saint-Hilaire, Lhermitte, & Agid, 1987). Additionally, the presence of nonmotor neuropsychiatric symptoms often are correlated with the presence of Lewy body pathology which also occurs in several types of dementia (Chaudhuri & Schapira, 2009; Marsden, 1994). Finally, several researchers have noted that focal frontal lesions can cause similar cognitive and behavioral impairments as those exhibited by patients with PD (Taylor, Saint-Cyr, & Lang, 1986).

Cognitive Changes

Cognitive changes that occur in PD include poorer performance on tests of psychomotor speed, memory, attention, visuospatial functions, language, and executive function. However, deficits in attention, executive function and memory appear to be the most prominent features of cognitive dysfunction in patients with PD relative to other cognitive domains (Muslimovic, Post, Speelman, & Schmand, 2005) (see Chapter 5). These cognitive changes have been shown to occur in recently diagnosed PD patients (less than 2 years) (Muslimovic et al., 2005) but it is well established that nonmotor and cognitive symptoms are related to disease severity (van Rooden et al., 2009b) and duration of PD (Azuma, Cruz, Bayles, Tomoeda, & Montgomery, 2003; Steiger, Thompson, & Marsden, 1996). Even in the tremor dominant subtype of PD that has a slower progression (Jankovic & Kapadia, 2001), the clinical presentation does shift to include axial symptoms of postural instability and gait dysfunction, and this transition is associated with accelerated declines in cognitive function (Lim, Fox, & Lang, 2009). Many studies have demonstrated a clear relationship between axial motor symptoms (including speech impairments and swallowing disorders) and cognitive decline in PD (Gago et al., 2009; Manor et al., 2009; Miller et al., 2009; Muslimovic et al., 2005).

The fact that the degree of cognitive decline in PD is not related to the severity of the traditional cardinal motor signs of PD (tremor, bradykinesia, rigidity) implies that the neuropathologic changes that underlie these changes are distinct from those which underlie the motor symptoms (Muslimovic et al., 2005). It is now well established that the cognitive decline in PD is the result of dysfunction in prefrontal nonmotor cortical areas (Lin et al., 2008).

Nonmotor/Cognitive Circuits

Alexander, and colleagues proposed five BG-thalamocortical circuits that can be divided broadly into motor and nonmotor, or complex circuits (Alexander et al., 1990; Alexander et al., 1986). The motor circuit sends projections from cortex to putamen, whereas in the other four circuits, cortical projections are sent to the caudate (Alexander et al., 1990). Motor circuits include the motor circuit detailed above and the oculomotor circuit which controls eye gaze and fixation (Alexander et al., 1990). In part, this circuit may be responsible for the appearance of the masked face in PD in which there is a lack of normal saccadic eye movement and a fixed gaze (Alexander et al., 1990; Middleton & Strick, 2000). The three nonmotor/complex circuits originate in areas of the prefrontal cortex: (a) the dorsolateral prefrontal cortex (DLPFC), (b) the anterior cingulate cortex (ACC), and (c) the orbitofrontal cortex (OFC) (Alexander et al., 1990; Middleton & Strick, 2002). Each of these circuits like the motor circuit projects to the striatum topographically and remains segregated in their projections throughout the BG and thalamus before finally looping back to their respective cortical origin (Middleton & Strick, 2000, 2002). These circuits receive inputs from multiple neurotransmitter cell groups (dopaminergic, noradrenergic, serotonergic, and cholinergic) (Tekin & Cummings, 2002) which in part may explain why dopamine replacement therapy is much less effective in ameliorating nonmotor symptoms and why such symptoms often can predate the onset of clinical motor symptoms (Lim et al., 2009; Simuni & Sethi, 2008). Dysregulation in these prefrontal circuits are thought to underlie the cognitive and language changes in PD, particularly the poorer performance of verbal fluency, in PD patients (De Gaspari et al., 2006; Troster, Woods, & Fields, 2003).

Evidence for the contribution of BG circuits involving the DLPFC and the ACC in the speech motor, cognitive, and language disorders observed in PD comes from neuroimaging studies of nonbrain-damaged individuals, PD patients (Zgaljardic et al., 2006), patients with frontal lobe lesions (Cummings, 1993), as well as from anatomic pathway analyses (Middleton & Strick, 2002). The DLPFC has been shown to be involved in motor planning; in the preparation of action to speak in nonbrain-damaged individuals (Riecker et al., 2005); and when attending to action by establishing functional connections between various frontal motor areas (prefrontal, premotor and SMA) in nonbrain-damaged individuals. This pattern of activity was not observed in participants with PD (Rowe et al., 2002). Patients with damage to this area have particular difficulties with shifting sets as evidenced by difficulties with card sorting tasks and reduced verbal fluency when asked to produce phonologically related words (all beginning with the same letter) and/or semantically related words (all belonging to the same category, e.g., animals) (Cummings, 1993). Patients with PD have difficulty with verbal fluency tasks (Henry & Crawford, 2004) and these difficulties become more pronounced with pallidotomy (Troster et al., 2003) and DBS (De Gaspari et al., 2006) interventions. Additionally, the left DLPFC is also active in nonbrain-damaged individuals during syntactic processing in the comprehension of sentences (Hashimoto & Sakai, 2002) whereas the right DLPFC has been shown to be active during the selection of spatial representations (Cools, Stefanova, Barker, Robbins, & Owen, 2002; Rowe, Toni, Josephs, Frackowiak, & Passingham, 2000).

Damage to the ACC results in either transient or long-standing akinetic mutism depending upon whether the lesion is unilateral or bilateral, and generally, these patients lack initiation (Cummings, 1993). In nonhuman primate lesion studies, the ACC has been shown to be involved in linking actions to outcomes, both when outcomes are negative, that is, errors, and when outcomes are positive, that is, rewards (Hadland, Rushworth, Gaffan, & Passingham, 2003). Thus, the ACC is said to play a role in intentional, internally motivated behaviors. It is interesting to note that the ACC plays a well-recognized role in vocalization behavior in lower species, where lesion studies demonstrate that it participates in hierarchical regulation of periacqueductal grey (PAG) matter induced vocalizations (Jurgens, 2002; Jurgens & Lu, 1993). Such vocalizations are species specific calls that encode information about emotional status and behavioral arousal, for example, calls made to warn others of an impending danger that are intended to alert others to action. This behavior reflects the linking of outcomes (danger) to actions (moving away from such danger) in the vocal modality. In neuroimaging studies, the ACC has been shown to be active during speech (Paus, Petrides, Evans, & Meyer, 1993; Schulz et al., 2005) and functionally coupled to the PAG (Schulz et al., 2005) thus providing evidence that, as in lower mammalian species, these midline regions may operate as an integrated system during human vocalization. Finally, a recent study investigating the Bereitschaftspotential (BP), an electrophysiological index of voluntary movement, found that it is modulated by tasks that differ purely in terms of cognitive-linguistic operations (McArdle, Mari, Pursley, Schulz, & Braun, 2009). In particular, tasks that involve lexical search and selection (that is, verbal fluency tasks) elicited the greatest amplitude BP in the left frontolateral recording sites; that is, pre-SMA, DLPFC, and possibly ACC. Thus, there is collaborating evidence that these areas play an active role in language and vocalization and indicate how these areas affected in PD could account for the cognitive linguistic deficits observed.

Oscillatory Models of Basal Ganglia Function

The traditional model of the pathophysiology of PD detailed above is based on changes in the discharge rates of various BG nuclei. Indeed, there are such changes, but not all experimental findings fit with the rate model and more recent work suggests that changes in discharge *patterns* (oscillatory and synchrony) in these nuclei and circuits underlie PD symptoms (Wichmann & DeLong, 2006). This more recent emphasis on discharge patterns potentially could unify many disparate findings and observations regarding the differences in limb versus speech, voice, swallowing, and language symptoms, and patient responses to various treatments.

The resurgence of functional neurosurgery, especially DBS implantation to ameliorate the movement disorders in patients with PD, has made recordings from BG nuclei possible in a large number of individuals. Both single unit recordings and recordings of local field potentials (LFP) are possible intraoperatively. In addition, LFPs can be recorded from DBS electrodes for several days postoperatively prior to the connection of those leads to the subcutaneous stimulator (Brown & Williams, 2005). Local field potentials represent the synchronized current changes in local populations of neurons (Brown & Williams, 2005). For example, LFP oscillations have been shown to be synchronized with neuronal activity in BG nuclei in both primates (Goldberg, Rokni, Boraud, Vaadia, & Bergman, 2004) and alert PD patients (Kühn et al., 2005).

There appear to be three frequency bands that characterize LFP activity in BG structures; below 8 to 10 Hz, 8/10 to 30 Hz, and above 30 Hz. LFP activity in the 8/10 to 30-Hz band has been documented in human striatum (Sochurkova & Rektor, 2003), STN (Brown et al., 2001; Kühn et al., 2005), and GPi (Brown et al., 2001; Silberstein et al., 2005). Of particular significance is the finding that in PD, synchronized activity in a 8/10 to 30-Hz frequency band (the "beta-band") has been demonstrated in BG-thalamocortical circuits and that such activity is reduced with dopaminergic treatment (Brown et al., 2001; Gatev & Wichmann, 2009). The implication is that entrainment in this frequency band somehow disrupts normal processing which leads to bradykinesia, and perhaps tremor (Gatev & Wichmann, 2009).

However, coherent oscillations between various components in the nervous system have been shown to occur in healthy nonbrain-damaged individuals during movement (Brown & Marsden, 1998). For example, coherent oscillations between contralateral motor cortex electroencephalogram (EEG) and electromyographic (EMG) recordings from muscles in humans making voluntary muscle contractions have been reported in the 15 to 30-Hz range (Halliday, Conway, Farmer, & Rosenberg, 1998). Additionally, functionally active cortical areas oscillate coherently in the 30 to 50-Hz frequency band (the gamma band) during voluntary movement (Murthy & Fetz, 1996). Higher frequency oscillations also may occur in normal BG function (Gatev, Darbin, & Wichmann, 2006).

Although not completely understood such oscillations in the gamma band may provide a mechanism in the nondamaged brain to synchronize activity in distinct and distant parts of the central nervous system (Marsden, Limousin-Dowsey, Ashby, Pollak, & Brown, 2001). An interesting and potentially unifying hypothesis about the role of the BG is to "facilitate coherence" in various cortical motor areas by synchronizing some of them over others, thereby focusing attention on what is relevant among numerous activities at any one time (Brown & Marsden, 1998). This focused attention " . . . provides the automatic link between voluntary effort, sensory input, and the calling up and operation of a sequence of motor programmes or thoughts." (Brown & Marsden, 1998). The physiologic basis for this attentional mechanism may lie in the tendency of distributed, but related, cortical activities to synchronize in the gamma (30 to 50-Hz) band.

The cardinal sign of PD, bradykinesia, would then be the result of the inability to focus (motor) attention or the inability to "favor certain channels of activity over others" resulting in increased time required to process motor events (Brown & Marsden, 1998). Indeed the available evidence points to coherent oscillatory activity in the beta band (8 to 30 Hz) being essentially antikinetic in character and inversely related to motor processing (Degardin et al., 2009; Sharott et al., 2005). Such activity therefore may contribute to the bradykinesia of PD (Brown & Williams, 2005; Devos et al., 2006).

It is not difficult to extrapolate similar mechanisms behind the cognitive and other nonmotor symptoms of PD. The inability to draw various cortical and subcortical areas together over others in synchrony, or the inability to selectively facilitate particular processes, easily could lead to deficits in attention, executive function and memory common in PD (McAuley, 2003). As further evidence for the BG 's potential role in "selective facilitation" of particular processes, it is interesting to note that dopamine is involved not only in the pathophysiology of the motor disorder in PD but also in schizophrenia and attention deficit hyperactivity disorder (Marsden, 2006). In each of these disorders there are clinical manifestations of the inability to selectively attend in various domains.

Both dopaminergic therapy and DBS are effective in improving the motor symptoms of PD and both have been shown to disrupt or reduce low-frequency (beta band) oscillations associated with the parkinsonian state (Chang, Shi, Luo, Zhang, & Woodward, 2007). It is clear, therefore, how each of these therapies might have a similar net effect on the limb motor system even though they are quite different in their underlying neurophysiologic mechanisms of action.

Synchronization and Speech

To date there has been only one study that has assessed coherence patterns during speech in PD patients and in healthy age-matched participants (Caviness, Liss, Adler, & Evidente, 2006). In this study the coherence between cortical EEG and obicularis oris (OO) muscles during tonic and phasic nonspeech oral movements, sustained vowel production, syllable repetition, and reading tasks was measured. For the healthy participants, significant corticomuscular coherence (8 to 50-Hz band) was found between sensorimotor cortex and OO muscles for the tonic oral task (sustained pucker) but not for the phasic oral task or for any speech task.

Significant corticomuscular coherence (8 to 50-Hz band) was found between SMA and OO muscles for all tasks with greater coherence for speech than nonspeech tasks and greater coherence for syllable repetition than for reading tasks. No hemispheric lateralization for any tasks was observed in either the sensorimotor or SMA fields for the healthy participants. The authors interpreted these findings as reflecting corticomuscular coherence for different functional reasons; sensorimotor cortex coherence reflected primary muscle activation whereas SMA coherence reflected the production of more complex muscle activations.

This same study found two coherence abnormalities in the PD group in the form of elevated coherence for sustained pucker at sensorimotor cortex, and reduced coherence at SMA for all other tasks (Caviness et al., 2006). The authors suggested that the elevated coherence indicated a pathologic synchronization of sensorimotor neurons and motor unit firing that would effectively reduce modulation flexibility and may be implicated in the inability of PD patients to reach normal spatial and temporal oral movement excursions observed in healthy participants (Forrest et al., 1989). In addition, the authors found a 20 to 25-Hz band peak in both corticomuscular and muscle-muscle coherence in PD which supported the robust finding of excessive coupling that could be the underlying pathophysiology of abnormal OO control in PD. The reduced coherence found at SMA for all tasks in PD patients is consistent with the decreased/abnormal input to the SMA from the BG (GPi). This finding implies that the SMA is not providing a normal contribution to the production of more complex oral movements involved in nonspeech and speech tasks.

The first coherence abnormality noted above for the PD group (elevated coherence for sustained pucker at sensorimotor cortex) is corroborated by evidence from a study investigating non-invasive stimulation of sensorimotor cortex. Repeated transcranial magnetic stimulation (rTMS) in the mouth area of the sensorimotor cortex was shown to improve vocal intensity and fundamental frequency in PD (Dias et al., 2006). These changes were most likely due to rTMS disrupting the abnormal oscillatory/synchronous activity between M1 (primary motor cortex) and peripheral muscles and/or between M1 and BG nuclei. The authors did not record any muscle activity so these two potential explanations cannot be distinguished. However, in a meta-analysis of (r)TMS studies, a modest positive effect on motor function in PD patients (as measured by UPDRS) was found as well (Fregni, Simon, Wu, & Pascual, 2005). The authors discuss two possible pathophysiologic mechanisms for such improvements and provide evidence from the literature for each. One possible mechanism is that rTMS induces network changes that indirectly and positively affect BG, whereas the other suggests that cortical rTMS compensates for the abnormal cortical activity associated with PD. In support of the former are studies demonstrating network changes following rTMS utilizing neuroimaging (Fuggetta, Pavone, Fiaschi, & Manganotti, 2008), and those that have demonstrated greater dopamine release in BG in rats following frontal stimulation (Keck et al., 2002). In support of the latter mechanism are studies that implicate modulation of cortical excitability to "normalize" otherwise abnormal cortical excitability associated with PD (Lefaucheur, 2005).

The second coherence abnormality in PD patients, reduced coherence between SMA and OO, noted by Caviness et al. (2006) is corroborated by the BP findings of McArdle et al. (2009) noted above. They demonstrated that left frontolateral mesial premotor areas had a higher BP amplitude for verbal fluency tasks, and that these "motor" areas may also be involved in word search and retrieval. Reduced coherence between cortical premotor areas (SMA) and articulatory muscles (OO) might be a consequence of faulty activation of premotor areas (as per the traditional network model of PD) or might be a consequence of faulty network synchrony (according to the oscillatory model of BG function).

Taken together these studies provide a potentially unifying model for the various behavioral symptoms and abnormal neurophysiological findings in PD. However, further investigation with larger participant pools with varying degrees of severity (both limb and speech) need to be completed both to elucidate the oscillatory model more completely, and to validate and extend the clinical therapeutic utility of rTMS. For example, there are no studies to date of the efficacy of rTMS on dysphagia in PD, although the technique appears promising for dyphagia secondary to stroke (Khedr, Abo-Elfetoh, & Rothwell, 2009).

Summary

A great deal of knowledge regarding the neurophysiological bases for Parkinson disease has been gained in the nearly 200 years since James Parkinson first described the motor, and speech and swallowing symptoms, common to the disorder. Parkinson incorrectly attributed these symptoms to impairments in the cervical spine and the medulla. We now understand PD to be the result of disturbances to a group of subcortical nuclei, the basal ganglia, which in turn affects cortical and brainstem areas. The degeneration of dopaminergic neurons in the substantia nigra is considered to be the cause of these disruptions. The develop-

Oscillatory Network Pattern Model of Basal Ganglia Function

Normal Basal Ganglia Function
- Basal Ganglia Synchronize Various Cortical and Subcortical Areas Together →
  - Accomplish Particular Motor, Speech, Language, Cognitive Processes

Basal Ganglia Function in PD:
- Abnormal (Synchronous or Dys-synchronous) Basal Ganglia Neuronal Oscillatory Activity →
  - Disruption of Particular Motor, Speech, Language, Cognitive Processes

Unifies Disparate Findings:
- Differences in Limb Versus Speech, Voice, Swallowing, and Language Symptoms
- Patient Responses to Treatment

Explanatory Power in New Treatment rTMS (repetitive transcranial magnetic stimulation):
- Beneficial in Attenuating the Limb Symptoms
- Beneficial in Attenuating the Speech, Voice, Swallowing, Cognitive Symptoms

ment of an animal model for PD led to many advances in the development of the highly explanatory circuit model. Several motor and nonmotor circuits were traced through the basal ganglia; each circuit originates in the cortex and sends pathways to the basal ganglia which then connect to the thalamus and the circuit is completed by pathways back to the area of cortex from which the circuit originated.

By far, the most studied of these circuits is the motor circuit which originates in the primary sensorimotor cortex which sends topographically segregated ("leg," "arm," "face") excitatory input to the striatum (mainly the putamen). There then are direct inhibitory and indirect excitatory pathways through to the basal ganglia output nuclei which in turn send inhibitory signals to the motor areas of the thalamus from where excitatory signals are sent back to the primary sensorimotor cortex. The net result of the depletion of dopamine in the motor circuit is the underactivation of the sensorimotor cortex which in this model is thought to be the basis of the bradykinesia and hypokinesia in limb movements. By extension, as the movement abnormalities are similar in speech and swallowing, the same neurophysiologic dysregulation in the motor circuit traditionally has been invoked, albeit for the topographically segregated "face" projections in this pathway.

The explanatory power of this model has been significant, and medical interventions based on this model (dopaminergic replacement and surgical techniques including pallidotomy and subthalamic nucleus deep brain stimulation) have proven invaluable for ameliorating PD limb motor symptoms (bradykinesia, rigidity, tremor). The fact that speech and voice disorders (along with other "axial" symptoms) do not respond in the same positive manner to such medical interventions poses some problems and requires adjustment to the simple interpretation that the underlying neurophysiologic deficits that cause limb and speech motor symptoms are the same.

There are several nonmotor circuits identified that form corticostriatal-thalamocortical loops that have been linked to the nonmotor cognitive symptoms in PD. Among the many cognitive disorders (attention, memory, and executive function) that typically occur later in the course of PD are language symptoms such as difficulty with verbal fluency tasks, and difficulty producing and comprehending complex syntax. Dysregulation in the prefrontal nonmotor circuits are thought to underlie the cognitive and language changes in PD. In particular, two of the prefrontal cortical circuits, the dorsolateral prefrontal cortex and the anterior cingulate cortex, have been shown to be involved in these cognitive and language functions.

With the incorporation of in vivo electrophysiologic data, the traditional circuit anatomy model of PD that emphasized altered neuronal firing has developed into a new network model. PD is now viewed as a complex network disorder in which abnormal oscillatory activity of neurons in the basal ganglia affects electrophysiologic activity (synchronous or dys-synchronous). Such activity involves neuronal firing in various, cortical, subcortical, and thalamic areas involved in motor, executive, limbic, and sensory processing. One specific interpretation of electrophysiologic data that emphasizes discharge patterns is that it appears to unify many disparate findings and observations regarding the differences in limb versus speech, voice, swallowing, and language symptoms, and patient responses to treatment. With this view, the basal ganglia act to draw various cortical and subcortical areas together over others in synchrony to accomplish particular motor or cognitive processes. Therefore, the basal ganglia act rather like a symphony conductor variously highlighting certain instruments over others during the course of the program such that the acoustic output of the instruments is coherent and true to the composer in terms of both the tempo and intensity of the score. The scant evidence to date in relation to speech appears to be in line with this new oscillatory pattern model. In addition, there is some evidence that a potential treatment that interrupts the abnormal patterns of firing in the various networks, (repetitive transcranial magnetic stimulation) is beneficial in attenuating the limb symptoms of PD. Further research, however, is needed to elucidate the oscillatory model and determine the potential benefits of other therapies such as rTMS.

References

Ackermann, H., & Ziegler, W. (1991). Articulatory deficits in parkinsonian dysarthria: An acoustic analysis. *Journal of Neurology, Neurosurgery, and Psychiatry, 54*, 1093–1098.

Akkal, D., Dum, R. P., & Strick, P. L. (2007). Supplementary motor area and presupplementary motor area: Targets of basal ganglia and cerebellar output. *Journal of Neuroscience, 27*, 10659–10673.

Alexander, G. E., Crutcher, M. D., & DeLong, M. R. (1990). Basal ganglia-thalamocortical circuits: parallel substrates for motor, oculomotor, "prefrontal" and "limbic" functions. *Progress in Brain Research, 85*, 119–146.

Alexander, G. E., DeLong, M. R., & Strick, P. L. (1986). Parellel organization of functionally segregated circuits linking basal Ganglia and cortex. *Annual Review of Neuroscience, 9*, 357–381.

Amtage, F., Henschel, K., Schelter, B., Vesper, J., Timmer, J., & Lucking, C. H. (2008). Tremor-correlated neuronal activity in the subthalamic nucleus of parkinsonian patients. *Neuroscience Letters, 442*, 195–199.

Azuma, T., Cruz, R. F., Bayles, K. A., Tomoeda, C. K., & Montgomery, E. B., Jr. (2003). A longitudinal study of neuropsychological change in individuals with Parkinson's disease. *International Journal of Geriatric Psychiatry, 18*, 1043–1049.

Bejjani, B.-P., Gervais, D., Arnulf, I., Papadopoulos, S., Demeret, S., & Bonnet, A.-M. (2000). Axial parkinsonian symptoms can be improved: The role of levodopa and bilateral subthalamic stimulation. *Journal of Neurology, Neurosurgery and Psychiatry, 68*, 595–600.

Berardelli, A., Rothwell, J. C., Thompson, P. D., & Hallett, M. (2001). Pathophysiology of bradykinesia in Parkinson's disease. *Brain, 124*, 2131–2146.

Berardelli, A., Sabra, A. F., & Hallett, M. (1983). Physiological mechanisms of rigidity in Parkinson's disease. *Journal of Neurology, Neurosurgery, and Psychiatry, 46*, 45–53.

Bernheimer, H., Birkmayer, W., Hornykiewicz, O., Jellinger, K., & Seitelberger, F. (1973). Brain dopamine and the syndromes of Parkinson and Huntington:

Clinical, morphological and neurochemical correlations. *Journal of Neurological Science, 20*, 415–455.

Blumin, J. H., Pcolinsky, D. E., & Atkins, J. P. (2004). Laryngeal findings in advanced Parkinson's disease. *Annals of Otology Rhinology and Laryngology, 113*, 253–258.

Bonnet, A. M., Loria, Y., Saint-Hilaire, M. H., Lhermitte, F., & Agid, Y. (1987). Does long-term aggravation of Parkinson's disease result from nondopaminergic lesions? *Neurology, 37*, 1539–1542.

Brown, P., & Marsden, C. D. (1998). What do the basal ganglia do? *Lancet, 351*, 1801–1804.

Brown, P., Oliviero, A., Mazzone, P., Insola, A., Tonali, P., & Di Lazzaro, V. (2001). Dopamine dependency of oscillations between subthalamic nucleus and pallidum in Parkinson disease. *Journal of Neuroscience, 21*, 1033–1038.

Brown, P., & Williams, D. (2005). Basal ganglia local field potential activity: Character and functional significance in the human. *Clinical Neurophysiology, 116*, 2510–2519.

Burns, R. S., Chiueh, C. C., Markey, S. P., Ebert, M. H., Jacobowitz, D. M., & Kopin, I. J. (1983). A primate model of parkinsonism: selective destruction of dopaminergic neurons in the pars compacta of the substantia nigra by N-methyl-4-phenyl-1,2,3,6-tetrahydropyridine. *Proceedings of the National Academy of Sciences, USA, 80*, 4546–4550.

Bushmann, M., Dobmeyer, S. M., Leeker, L., & Perlmutter, J. S. (1989). Swallowing abnormalities and their response to treatment in Parkinson's disease. *Neurology, 39*, 1309–1314.

Cahill, L. M., Murdoch, B. E., Theodoros, D. G., Triggs, E. J., Charles, B. G., & Yao, A. A. (1998). Effect of oral levodopa treatment on articulatory function in Parkinson's disease: Preliminary results. *Motor Control, 2*, 161–172.

Cantello, R., Tarletti, R., Varrasi, C., Cecchin, M., & Monaco, F. (2007). Cortical inhibition in Parkinson's disease: New insights from early, untreated patients. *Neuroscience, 150*, 64.

Carrasco, E., Casper, D., & Werner, P. (2007). PGE2 receptor EP1 renders dopaminergic neurons selectively vulnerable to low-level oxidative stress and direct PGE2 neurotoxicity. *Journal of Neuroscience Research, 85*, 3109.

Carta, M., Carlsson, T., Kirik, D., & Bjorklund, A. (2007). Dopamine released from 5-HT terminals is the cause of L-Dopa-induced dyskinesia in parkinsonian rats. *Brain, 130*, 1819–1833.

Caudle, W. M., Colebrooke, R. E., Emson, P. C., & Miller, G. W. (2008). Altered vesicular dopamine storage in Parkinson's disease: A premature demise. *Trends in Neurosciences, 31*, 303.

Caviness, J. N., Liss, J. M., Adler, C., & Evidente, V. (2006). Analysis of high-frequency electroencephalographic-electromyographic coherence elicited by speech and oral nonspeech tasks in Parkinson's disease. *Journal of Speech Language and Hearing Research, 49*, 424–438.

Chang, J. Y., Shi, L. H., Luo, F., Zhang, W. M., & Woodward, D. J. (2007). Studies of the neural mechanisms of deep brain stimulation in rodent models of Parkinson disease. *Neuroscience and Biobehavioral Reviews, 31*, 643.

Chaudhuri, K. R., & Schapira, A. H. (2009). Nonmotor symptoms of Parkinson's disease: Dopaminergic pathophysiology and treatment. *Lancet Neurology, 8,* 464–474.

Ciucci, M. R., Ma, S. T., Fox, C., Kane, J. R., Ramig, L. O., & Schallert, T. (2007). Qualitative changes in ultrasonic vocalization in rats after unilateral dopamine depletion or haloperidol: A preliminary study. *Behavioral Brain Research, 182,* 284–289.

Coates, C., & Bakheit, A. M. (1997). Dysphagia in Parkinson disease. *European Neurology, 38,* 49–52.

Cools, R., Stefanova, E., Barker, R. A., Robbins, T. W., & Owen, A. M. (2002). Dopaminergic modulation of high-level cognition in Parkinson's disease: The role of the prefrontal cortex revealed by PET. *Brain, 125,* 584–594.

Cummings, J. L. (1993). Frontal-subcortical circuits and human behavior. *Archives of Neurology, 50,* 873–880.

Danielson, S. R., & Andersen, J. K. (2008). Oxidative and nitrative protein modifications in Parkinson's disease. *Free Radicals in Biologic Medicine, 44,* 1787–1794.

Darley, F. L., Aronson, A. E., & Brown, J. R. (1969a). Clusters of deviant speech dimensions in the dysarthrias. *Journal of Speech and Hearing Research, 12,* 462–496.

Darley, F. L., Aronson, A. E., & Brown, J. R. (1969b). Differential diagnostic patterns of dysarthria. *Journal of Speech and Hearing Research, 12,* 246–269.

Degardin, A., Houdayer, E., Bourriez, J. L., Destee, A., Defebvre, L., & Derambure, P. (2009). Deficient "sensory" beta synchronization in Parkinson's disease. *Clinical Neurophysiology, 120,* 636–642.

De Gaspari, D., Siri, C., Di Gioia, M., Antonini, A., Isella, V., & Pizzolato, A. (2006). Clinical correlates and cognitive underpinnings of verbal fluency impairment after chronic subthalamic stimulation in Parkinson's disease. *Parkinsonism and Related Disorder, 12,* 289–295.

De Letter, M., Santens, P., De Bodt, M., Van Maele, G., Van Borsel, J., & Boon, P. (2007). The effect of levodopa on respiration and word intelligibility in people with advanced Parkinson's disease. *Clinical Neurology and Neurosurgery, 109,* 495.

DeLong, M. R. (1990). Primate models of movement disorders of basal ganglia origin. *Trends in Neurosciences, 13,* 281.

DeLong, M. R., & Wichmann, T. (2007). Circuits and circuit disorders of the basal ganglia. *Archives of Neurology, 64,* 20–24.

Devos, D., Szurhaj, W., Reyns, N., Labyt, E., Houdayer, E., & Bourriez, J. L. (2006). Predominance of the contralateral movement-related activity in the subthalamo-cortical loop. *Clinical Neurophysiology, 117,* 2315–2327.

Dias, A. E., Barbosa, E. R., Coracini, K., Maia, F., Marcolin, M. A., & Fregni, F. (2006). Effects of repetitive transcranial magnetic stimulation on voice and speech in Parkinson's disease. *Acta Neurologica Scandinavica, 113,* 92–99.

Di Matteo, V., Pierucci, M., Esposito, E., Crescimanno, G., Benigno, A., & Di Giovanni, G. (2008). Serotonin modulation of the basal ganglia circuitry: Therapeutic implication for Parkinson's disease and other motor disorders. *Progress in Brain Research, 172,* 423–463.

Eggers, C., Hilker, R., Burghaus, L., Schumacher, B., & Heiss, W. D. (2009). High resolution positron emission tomography demonstrates basal ganglia dysfunction in early Parkinson's disease. *Journal of the Neurological Sciences, 276*, 27–30.

Eriksen, J. L., Wszolek, Z., & Petrucelli, L. (2005). Molecular pathogenesis of Parkinson disease. *Archives of Neurology, 62*, 353–357.

Esselink, R. A. J., de Bie, R. M. A., de Haan, R. J., Lenders, M. W. P. M., Nijssen, P. C. G., & Staal, M. J. (2004). Unilateral pallidotomy versus bilateral subthalamic nucleus stimulation in PD: A randomized trial. *Neurology, 62*, 201–207.

Fishman, P. S. (2008). Paradoxical aspects of parkinsonian tremor. *Movement Disorders, 23*, 168–173.

Forrest, K., Weismer, G., & Turner, G. S. (1989). Kinematic, acoustic, and perceptual analyses of connected speech produced by parkinsonian and normal geriatric adults. *Journal of the Acoustical Society of America, 85*, 2608–2622.

Fregni, F., Simon, D. K., Wu, A., & Pascual, A. P. (2005). Noninvasive brain stimulation for Parkinson's disease: A systematic review and meta-analysis of the literature. *Journal of Neurology, Neurosurgery, and Psychiatry, 76*, 1614–1623.

Fuggetta, G., Pavone, E. F., Fiaschi, A., & Manganotti, P. (2008). Acute modulation of cortical oscillatory activities during short trains of high-frequency repetitive transcranial magnetic stimulation of the human motor cortex: A combined EEG and TMS study. *Human Brain Mapping, 29*, 1–13.

Gago, M., Garrett, M., Fonseca, M., Rosas, M., Simões, M., & Vieira, S. (2009). How do cognitive and axial motor signs correlate in Parkinson's disease? A 6-year prospective study. *Journal of Neurology, 256*, 1655–1662.

Galvan, A., & Wichmann, T. (2008). Pathophysiology of parkinsonism. *Clinical Neurophysiology, 119*, 1459–1474.

Gatev, P., Darbin, O., & Wichmann, T. (2006). Oscillations in the basal ganglia under normal conditions and in movement disorders. *Movement Disorders, 21*, 1566–1577.

Gatev, P. & Wichmann, T. (2009). Interactions between cortical rhythms and spiking activity of single basal ganglia neurons in the normal and parkinsonian state. *Cerebral Cortex, 19*, 1330–1344.

Goberman, A., Coelho, C., & Robb, M. (2002). Phonatory characteristics of parkinsonian speech before and after morning medication: The ON and OFF states. *Journal of Communication Disorders, 35*, 217–239.

Goldberg, J. A., Rokni, U., Boraud, T., Vaadia, E., & Bergman, H. (2004). Spike synchronization in the cortex-basal ganglia networks of parkinsonian primates reflects global dynamics of the local field potentials. *Journal of Neuroscience, 24*, 6003–6010.

Grafton, S. T. (2004). Contributions of functional imaging to understanding parkinsonian symptoms. *Current Opinion in Neurobiology, 14*, 715–719.

Grewel, F. (1957). Classification of dysarthrias. *Acta Psychiatrica Scandinavica, 39*, 325–337.

Gupta, A., Dawson, V. L., & Dawson, T. M. (2008). What causes cell death in Parkinson's disease? *Annals of Neurology, 64*(Suppl.), S3–S15.

Hadland, K. A., Rushworth, M. F. S., Gaffan, D., & Passingham, R. E. (2003). The anterior cingulate and reward-guided selection of actions. *Journal of Neurophysiology, 89*, 1161–1164.

Halliday, D. M., Conway, B. A., Farmer, S. F., & Rosenberg, J. R. (1998). Using electroencephalography to study functional coupling between cortical activity and electromyograms during voluntary contractions in humans. *Neuroscience Letters, 241*, 5–8.

Hashimoto, R., & Sakai, K. L. (2002). Specialization in the left prefrontal cortex for sentence comprehension. *Neuron, 35*, 589–597.

Henry, J. D., & Crawford, J. R. (2004). Verbal fluency deficits in Parkinson's disease: A meta-analysis. *Journal of the International Neuropsychological Society, 10*, 608–622.

Hilker, R., Schweitzer, K., Coburger, S., Ghaemi, M., Weisenbach, S., & Jacobs, A. H. (2005). Nonlinear progression of Parkinson disease as determined by serial positron emission tomographic imaging of striatal fluorodopa F-18 activity. *Archives of Neurology, 62*, 378–382.

Hirose, H., Kiritani, S., Ushijima, T., Yoshioka, H., & Sawashima, M. (1981). Patterns of dysarthric movements in patients with parkinsonism. *Folia Phoniatrica, 33*, 204–215.

Ho, A., Bradshaw, J., & Iansek, R. (2008). For better or worse: The effect of levodopa on speech in Parkinson's disease. *Movement Disorders, 23*, 574–580.

Hoehn, M. M., & Yahr, M. D. (1967). Parkinsonism: Onset, progression and mortality. *Neurology, 17*, 427–442.

Hoover, J. E., & Strick, P. L. (1993). Multiple output channels in the basal ganglia. *Science, 259*, 819.

Hoover, J. E. & Strick, P. L. (1999). The organization of cerebellar and basal ganglia outputs to primary motor cortex as revealed by retrograde transneuronal transport of herpes simplex virus type 1. *Journal of Neuroscience, 19*, 1446–1463.

Hosey, L. A., Thompson, J. L., Metman, L. V., van den Munckhof, P., & Braun, A. R. (2005). Temporal dynamics of cortical and subcortical responses to apomorphine in Parkinson disease: An H2(15)O PET study. *Clinical Neuropharmacology, 28*, 18–27.

Jankovic, J., & Kapadia, A. S. (2001). Functional decline in Parkinson disease. *Archives of Neurology, 58*, 1611–1615.

Jurgens, U. (2002). Neural pathways underlying vocal control. *Neuroscience and Biobehavioral Reviews, 26*, 235–258.

Jurgens, U., & Lu, C. L. (1993). The effects of periaqueductally injected transmitter antagonists on forebrain-elicited vocalization in the squirrel monkey. *European Journal of Neuroscience, 5*, 735–741.

Keck, M. E., Welt, T., Muller, M. B., Erhardt, A., Ohl, F., & Toschi, N. (2002). Repetitive transcranial magnetic stimulation increases the release of dopamine in the mesolimbic and mesostriatal system. *Neuropharmacology, 43*(1), 101–109.

Khedr, E. M., Abo-Elfetoh, N., & Rothwell, J. C. (2009). Treatment of post-stroke dysphagia with repetitive transcranial magnetic stimulation. *Acta Neurologica Scandinavica, 119*, 155–161.

Kish, S. J., Shannak, K., & Hornykiewicz, O. (1988). Uneven pattern of dopamine loss in the striatum of patients with idiopathic Parkinson's disease: Pathophysiologic and clinical implications. *New England Journal of Medicine, 318,* 876–880.

Kühn, A. A., Trottenberg, T., Kivi, A., Kupsch, A., Schneider, G.-H., & Brown, P. (2005). The relationship between local field potential and neuronal discharge in the subthalamic nucleus of patients with Parkinson's disease. *Experimental Neurology, 194,* 212–220.

Lang, A. E. (2007). The progression of Parkinson disease: A hypothesis. *Neurology, 68,* 948–952.

Leenders, K. L., Palmer, A. J., Quinn, N., Clark, J. C., Firnau, G., & Garnett, E. S. (1986). Brain dopamine metabolism in patients with Parkinson's disease measured with positron emission tomography. *Journal of Neurology, Neurosurgery, and Psychiatry, 49,* 853–860.

Lefaucheur, J. P. (2005). Motor cortex dysfunction revealed by cortical excitability studies in Parkinson's disease: Influence of antiparkinsonian treatment and cortical stimulation. *Clinical Neurophysiology, 116,* 244–253.

Leopold, N. A.,& Kagel, M. C. (1997). Laryngeal deglutition movement in Parkinson's disease. *Neurology, 48,* 373–375.

Li, X. Y., Zhuang, P., & Li, Y. J. (2008). Patterns of neuronal activity in the basal ganglia nucleus in parkinsonian patients with levodopa-induced dyskinesia. *National Medical Journal of China, 88,* 1607.

Lim, S.-Y., Fox, S. H., & Lang, A. E. (2009). Overview of the extranigral aspects of Parkinson Disease. *Archives of Neurology, 66,* 167–172.

Lin, T. P., Carbon, M., Tang, C., Mogilner, A. Y., Sterio, D., & Beric, A. (2008). Metabolic correlates of subthalamic nucleus activity in Parkinson's disease. *Brain: A Journal of Neurology, 131,* 1373.

Logemann, J. A., Blonsky, E. R., & Boshes, B. (1975). Dysphagia in Parkinsonism. *Journal of American Medical Association,* 231, 69-70.

Manor, Y., Balas, M., Giladi, N., Mootanah, R., & Cohen, J. T. (2009). Anxiety, depression and swallowing disorders in patients with Parkinson's disease. *Parkinsonism and Related Disorders, 15,* 453.

Marsden, C. A. (2006). Dopamine: The rewarding years. *British Journal of Pharmacology, 147,* S136.

Marsden, C. D. (1994). Parkinson's disease. *Journal of Neurology, Neurosurgery, and Psychiatry, 57,* 672–681.

Marsden, J. F., Limousin-Dowsey, P., Ashby, P., Pollak, P., & Brown, P. (2001). Subthalamic nucleus, sensorimotor cortex and muscle interrelationships in Parkinson's disease. *Brain, 124,* 378–388.

McArdle, J. J., Mari, Z., Pursley, R. H., Schulz, G. M., & Braun, A. R. (2009). Electrophysiological evidence of functional integration between the language and motor systems in the brain: A study of the speech Bereitschaftspotential. *Clinical Neurophysiology, 120,* 275–284.

McAuley, J. H. (2003). The physiological basis of clinical deficits in Parkinson's disease. *Progress in Neurobiology, 69,* 27–48.

Middleton, F. A., & Strick, P. L. (2000). Basal ganglia and cerebellar loops: Motor and cognitive circuits. *Brain Research Reviews, 31*(2–3), 236.

Middleton, F. A. & Strick, P. L. (2002). Basal-ganglia "projections" to the prefrontal cortex of the primate. *Cerebral Cortex, 12*, 926–935.

Midi, I., Dogan, M., Koseoglu, M., Can, G., Sehitoglu, M. A., & Gunal, D. I. (2008). Voice abnormalities and their relation with motor dysfunction in Parkinson's disease. *Acta Neurologica Scandinavica, 117*, 26–34.

Miller, N., Allcock, L., Hildreth, A. J., Jones, D., Noble, E., & Burn, D. J. (2009). Swallowing problems in Parkinson disease: Frequency and clinical correlates. *Journal of Neurology, Neurosurgery, and Psychiatry, 80*, 1047–1049.

Miller, N., Allcock, L., Jones, D., Noble, E., Hildreth, A. J., & Burn, D. J. (2007). Prevalence and pattern of perceived intelligibility changes in Parkinson's disease. *Journal of Neurology, Neurosurgery, and Psychiatry, 78*, 1188–1190.

Montgomery, E. B. (2007). Basal ganglia physiology and pathophysiology: A reappraisal. *Parkinsonism and Related Disorders, 13*, 455.

Murthy, V. N. & Fetz, E. E. (1996). Oscillatory activity in sensorimotor cortex of awake monkeys: Synchronization of local field potentials and relation to behaviour. *Journal of Neurophysiology, 76*, 3949–3967.

Muslimovic, D., Post, B., Speelman, J. D., & Schmand, B. (2005). Cognitive profile of patients with newly diagnosed Parkinson disease. *Neurology, 65*, 1239–1245.

Ostergaard, K. & Sunde, N. (2006). Evolution of Parkinson's disease during 4 years of bilateral deep brain stimulation of the subthalamic nucleus. *Movement Disorders, 21*, 624–631.

Pahwa, R., Factor, S. A., Lyons, K. E., Ondo, W. G., Gronseth, G., & Bronte-Stewart, H. (2006). Practice parameter: Treatment of Parkinson disease with motor fluctuations and dyskinesia (an evidence-based review): Report of the Quality Standards Subcommittee of the American Academy of Neurology. *Neurology, 66*, 983–995.

Parkinson, J. (2002). An essay on the shaking palsy. *Journal of Neuropsychiatry and Clinical Neurosciences, 14*, 223–236.

Paulus, W., & Jellinger, K. (1991). The neuropathologic basis of different clinical subgroups of Parkinson's disease. *Journal of Neuropathology and Experimental Neurology, 50*, 743–755.

Paus, T., Petrides, M., Evans, A. C., & Meyer, E. (1993). Role of the human anterior cingulated cortex in the control of oculomotor, manual, and speech responses: A positron emission tomography study. *Journal of Neurophysiology, 70*, 453–469.

Poewe, W. H., & Wenning, G. K. (1998). The natural history of Parkinson's disease. *Annals of Neurology, 44*, S1–S9.

Putzer, M., Barry, W. J., & Moringlane, J. R. (2008). Effect of bilateral stimulation of the subthalamic nucleus on different speech subsystems in patients with Parkinson's disease. *Clinical Linguistics Phonetics, 22*, 957–973.

Riecker, A., Mathiak, K., Wildgruber, D., Erb, M., Hertrich, I., & Grodd, W. (2005). fMRI reveals two distinct cerebral networks subserving speech motor control. *Neurology, 64*, 700–706.

Rowe, J., Stephan, K. E., Friston, K., Frackowiak, R., Lees, A., & Passingham, R. (2002). Attention to action in Parkinson's disease: Impaired effective connectivity among frontal cortical regions. *Brain, 125*, 276–289.

Rowe, J. B., Toni, I., Josephs, O., Frackowiak, R. S., & Passingham, R. E. (2000). The prefrontal cortex: response selection or maintenance within working memory? *Science, 288*, 1656–1660.

Santens, P., De Letter, M., Van Borsel, J., De Reuck, J., & Caemaert, J. (2003). Lateralized effects of subthalamic nucleus stimulation on different aspects of speech in Parkinson's disease. *Brain and Language, 87*, 253–258.

Schulz, G. M., & Grant, M. K. (2000). Effects of speech therapy and pharmacologic and surgical treatments on voice and speech in Parkinson's disease: A review of the literature. *Journal of Communication Disorders, 33*, 59–88.

Schulz, G. M., Greer, M., & Friedman, W. (2000). Changes in vocal intensity in Parkinson's disease following pallidotomy surgery. *Journal of Voice, 14*, 589–606.

Schulz, G. M., Peterson, T., Sapienza, C. M., Greer, M., & Friedman, W. (1999). Voice and speech characteristics of persons with Parkinson's disease pre- and post-pallidotomy surgery: preliminary findings. *Journal of Speech Language and Hearing Research, 42*, 1176–1194.

Schulz, G. M., Varga, M., Jeffires, K., Ludlow, C. L., & Braun, A. R. (2005). Functional neuroanatomy of human vocalization: An H2(15)O PET study. *Cerebral Cortex, 15*, 1835–1847.

Sharott, A., Magill, P. J., Harnack, D., Kupsch, A., Meissner, W., & Brown, P. (2005). Dopamine depletion increases the power and coherence of beta (15–30 Hz) oscillations in the cerebral cortex and subthalamic nucleus of the awake rat. *European Journal of Neuroscience, 21*, 1413–1422.

Silberstein, P., Pogosyan, A., Kuhn, A. A., Hotton, G., Tisch, S., & Kupsch, A. (2005). Cortico-cortical coupling in Parkinson's disease and its modulation by therapy. *Brain, 128*, 1277–1291.

Simuni, T., & Sethi, K. (2008). Nonmotor manifestations of Parkinson's disease. *Annals of Neurology, 64*, S65–S80.

Smith, A. (2006). Speech motor development: Integrating muscles, movements, and linguistic units. *Journal of Communication Disorders, 39*, 331–349.

Sochurkova, D., & Rektor, I. (2003). Event-related desynchronization/synchronization in the putamen. An SEEG case study. *Experimental Brain Research, 149*, 401–404.

Solomon, N. P., & Hixon, T. J. (1993). Speech breathing in Parkinson's disease. *Journal of Speech and Hearing Research, 36*, 294–310.

Spencer, K. A., Morgan, K. W., & Blond, E. (2009). Dopaminergic medication effects on the speech of individuals with Parkinson's disease. *Journal of Medical Speech-Language Pathology, 17*, 125–144.

Steiger, M. J., Thompson, P. D., & Marsden, C. D. (1996). Disordered axial movement in Parkinson's disease. *Journal of Neurology, Neurosurgery, and Psychiatry, 61*, 645–648.

Stoffers, D., Bosboom, J. L. W., Deijen, J. B., Wolters, E. C., Berendse, H. W., & Stam, C. J. (2007). Slowing of oscillatory brain activity is a stable characteristic of Parkinson's disease without dementia. *Brain, 130*, 1847–1860.

Taylor, A. E., Saint-Cyr, J. A., & Lang, A. E. (1986). Frontal lobe dysfunction in Parkinson's disease. *Brain, 109*, 845–883.

Tekin, S., & Cummings, J. L. (2002). Frontal-subcortical neuronal circuits and clinical neuropsychiatry: An update. *Journal of Psychosomatic Research, 53*, 647–654.

Troster, A. I., Woods, S. P., & Fields, J. A. (2003). Verbal fluency declines after pallidotomy: An interaction between task and lesion laterality. *Applied Neuropsychology, 10*, 69–75.

van Rooden, S. M., Visser, M., Verbaan, D., Marinus, J., & van Hilten, J. J. (2009a). Motor patterns in Parkinson's disease: A data-driven approach. *Movement Disorders, 24*, 1042–1047.

van Rooden, S. M., Visser, M., Verbaan, D., Marinus, J., & van Hilten, J. J. (2009b). Patterns of motor and nonmotor features in Parkinson's disease. *Journal of Neurology, Neurosurgery, and Psychiatry, 80*, 846–850.

Wichmann, T., & DeLong, M. R. (2006). Basal ganglia discharge abnormalities in Parkinson's disease. *Journal of Neural Transmission* (Suppl. 70), 21–25.

Yu, H., Sternad, D., Corcos, D. M., & Vaillancourt, D. E. (2007). Role of hyperactive cerebellum and motor cortex in Parkinson's disease. *NeuroImage, 35*, 222.

Zgaljardic, D. J., Borod, J. C., Foldi, N. S., Mattis, P. J., Gordon, M. F., & Feigin, A. (2006). An examination of executive dysfunction associated with frontostriatal circuitry in Parkinson's disease. *Journal of Clinical and Experimental Neuropsychology, 28*, 1127–1144.

3

Speech Disorder in Parkinson Disease

DEBORAH THEODOROS

Speech disturbance is a hallmark of Parkinson disease (PD) and has been identified in up to 90% of people, with the severity of the disorder generally increasing over time (Hartelius & Svensson, 1994; Logemann, Fisher, Boshes, & Blonsky, 1978). The decline in communication skills has a significant impact on the quality of life of the person with PD, and their families. Considerable personal effort and healthcare resources are required to manage this speech disorder in order to maintain communication throughout the course of the disease. The speech disturbance, known as hypokinetic dysarthria, has been studied extensively to acquire a greater understanding of the prevalence and nature of the disorder, the effects of medical and surgical interventions on speech, and the impact of this communication impairment on the social interactions and quality of life of people with PD.

Onset and Prevalence

The onset of the speech disorder is insidious with a slow progression of impairment throughout the course of the disease. Clinically, the onset of speech difficulties varies widely, and is not consistently related to the duration and/or severity of the disease. Although the speech disorder usually is evident on referral to a speech-language pathologist (SLP), research suggests that subtle changes in speech may affect a person's capacity to communicate long before obvious impairment in speech intelligibility is apparent (Miller, Noble, Jones, & Burn, 2006; Miller, Noble, Jones, Allcock, & Burn, 2008). To date, detailed information about the development of the speech disorder in PD is unavailable due to a lack of longitudinal studies on this topic.

Although the onset of the speech disorder is variable, the prevalence of abnormal speech and voice features has been found to be reasonably predictable in people with PD. Changes in speech and voice have been identified in 70 to 90% of people with PD during assessment, and from self-report surveys. An early study by Logemann et al. (1978) found that approximately 90% of 200 speakers had a speech impairment with 89% demonstrating voice disorders, and 45% exhibiting difficulties with articulation. Similarly, Ho, Iansek, Marigliani, Bradshaw, and Gates (1998) determined that 74% of their 200 patients with PD exhibited voice impairments. Speech intelligibility has been found to be reduced compared to a control group in 69.6% of people with PD, with over half of these speakers more than one standard deviation below the control group mean (Miller et al., 2007). For those people with PD who perceived changes in speech intelligibility, 38% reported that their speech difficulty was one of their top four major concerns (Miller et al., 2007). These findings concurred with an earlier survey conducted in Sweden in which 70% of people with PD considered that their speech had worsened since their diagnosis (Hartelius & Svensson, 1994). The high prevalence of speech disturbances in people with PD, the variable onset of the disorder, and the slow progression of the disease highlights the need for long-term management strategies to address the communication impairment.

Characteristics of the Speech Disorder

Hypokinetic dysarthria, a motor speech disorder, is one of the most tenacious symptoms of PD. This speech disturbance initially was identified and described by Darley, Aronson, and Brown (1969a, 1969b) based on observations of people with PD, and on the known anatomical and pathophysiology of the disease. The distinct features of the speech disturbance have been attributed to the effects of muscle rigidity, slowness of movement, reduced force and range of movement and, on occasion, rapid repetitive movements evident in people with PD (Duffy, 2005). More recently, several studies have suggested that the speech disorder may be due to multiple factors, including deficits in sensory processing, scaling and maintenance of movement amplitude or force, internal cuing, automaticity, vocal vigilance, and temporal mechanisms (Ho, Bradshaw, Iansek, & Alfredson, 1999a; Ho, Iansek, & Bradshaw, 2001; Merchant, Luciana, Hooper, Majestic, & Tuite, 2008). Several of these factors are discussed in detail in Chapter 4.

Since the initial description of hypokinetic dysarthria, numerous studies have examined the perceptual, physiologic, and acoustic features of this speech disorder. Parkinson disease has been shown to impact on all aspects of speech production including respiration, phonation, resonance, articulation, and prosody, to varying degrees. The variable presentation of the speech disturbance in individuals with PD is a prominent feature of the disorder. The major speech impairments occur in the prosodic, phonatory, and articulatory aspects of speech production. Common abnormal speech characteristics include: monopitch and monoloudness, reduced stress/intonation, reduced loudness, imprecise consonants, inappropriate silences, a harsh and breathy voice, high or low pitch levels, variable speech rate (either too fast or too slow), short rushes of speech or "accelerated speech," repetition of phonemes (sounds), and difficulty with the initiation of speech (Adams & Dykstra, 2009; Darley et al., 1969a, 1969b; Ludlow & Bassich, 1983, 1984).

Prosody

Prosodic disturbances are the most prominent features of hypokinetic dysarthria (Chenery, Murdoch, & Ingram, 1988; Darley et al., 1975; Ludlow & Bassich, 1984; Plowman-Prine et al., 2009). Monopitch, monoloudness, and reduced stress pattern were identified as the most frequently occurring speech features in hypokinetic dysarthria by Darley et al. (1975) and subsequently confirmed by other investigators (Chenery et al., 1988; Ludlow & Bassich, 1984; Plowman-Prine et al., 2009).

Acoustic analyses of fundamental frequency (F_0) variation (acoustic correlate of pitch variation) in the speech of persons with PD strongly support the perception of monopitch. Numerous studies have consistently documented a reduced range of F_0 in various speech samples and on maximum F_0 range tasks performed by persons with PD compared to normal speakers (Bunton, Kent, Kent, & Duffy, 2001; Gamboa et al., 1997; Kent, Vorperian, Kent, & Duffy, 2003; Ludlow & Bassich, 1984). Reduction in F_0 variation would appear to be a robust indicator of parkinsonian speech and has the potential to be a diagnostic marker prior to the manifestation of other typical signs. In a unique case study, Harel, Cannizzaro, and Snyder (2004) were able to identify and document changes in F_0 variability in the speech of a newsreader as early as five years prior to clinical presentation and diagnosis of the disease. During this prodromal period, F_0 variability in this person's speech was found to be significantly less than that of a matched control speaker. Monoloudness in the speech of a person with PD is thought to be associated with a reduction in vocal intensity (Fox & Ramig, 1997) and impaired perception of loudness (Ho, Iansek, & Bradshaw, 1999b) as discussed below.

Disturbances of speech rate are a distinguishing feature of this speech disorder. Primarily, these rate disturbances include short rushes of speech or "accelerated speech," increased or decreased rate overall, increased rate of speech segments, or a variable rate of speech (Chenery et al., 1988; Darley et al., 1975; Duffy, 2005; Plowman-Prine et al., 2009; Scott, Caird, & Williams, 1985; Skodda & Schlegel, 2008; Zwirner & Barnes, 1992). The majority of perceptual studies support the presence of varying speaking rates in this population (Ludlow & Bassich, 1984; Plowman-Prine et al., 2009; Scott et al., 1985). It has been observed that only 6 to 13% of people with PD are likely to exhibit an overall increase in speech rate (Canter, 1963; Darley et al., 1975; Logemann et al., 1978; Ludlow & Bassich, 1984) with the majority of people exhibiting a slow rate of speech (Canter, 1963; Darley et al., 1975). Plowman-Prine et al. (2009) found that all types of rate disturbances (rapid, slow, variable, increased segment rate, short rushes, increased overall rate) were identified perceptually in their study of 16 speakers, although only to a minor degree. Perceived disturbances in rate reflect the heterogeneity of speech production in this population.

To date, acoustic and physiologic investigations of speech rate have identified variable rate disturbances, although these findings remain inconsistent. There is evidence that speech rate can be normal (Skodda & Schlegel, 2008; Weismer, Jeng, Laures, Kent, & Kent, 2001), reduced (Dworkin & Aronson, 1986; Kruel, 1972; Ludlow, Connor & Bassich, 1987), or increased or accelerated (Adams, 1994; Hammen, Yorkston, & Beukelman, 1989; Metter & Hanson, 1986). In a large study in which the speech rate in patients with PD was found to be comparable to normal, Skodda and Schlegel (2008) also identified a greater acceleration of articulation rate, and a significant reduction in the total number of pauses during speech.

Although different rates of speech have been identified in people with PD, the capacity of any one individual to vary their speech rate by altering sentence and phrase durations has been found to be problematic (Ludlow et al, 1987). Research has also shown that there can be a marked mismatch between perceptual and acoustic findings for speech rate. For example, a listener may perceive a fast rate of speech in a person with PD compared to a normal speaker even though actual speaking rates may be equivalent. This difference may be due to articulatory imprecision and continuous voicing that blur the acoustic contrasts of the speech signal (Kent & Rosenbek, 1982; Weismer, 1984). It is important, therefore, that clinicians pay particular attention to validating their perceptual assessment of speech rate by comparison with other raters, and through acoustic analyses.

Dysfluent speech is another prosodic disturbance apparent in hypokinetic dysarthria. Dysfluency may manifest in the form of initiation difficulties, inappropriate silences, phoneme and/or syllable repetition or, less commonly, palilalia (Chenery et al., 1988; Darley et al., 1975; Duffy, 2005; Ludlow & Bassich, 1983). Phoneme or single sound repetition has been observed in 16 to 44% of people with PD to a mild degree (Darley et al., 1975; Logemann, Boshes, & Fisher, 1973). Palilalia, which is the compulsive, effortless repetition of words and phrases, occurs against a background of increasing rate and decreasing loudness. Word and phrase repetitions tend to occur at the end of an utterance in palilalia as opposed to phoneme repetition which occurs at the beginning of words (Duffy, 2005; LaPointe & Horner, 1981). Adams and Dykstra (2009) suggested that moderate-severe dysfluency is less common in people with PD, occurring in fewer than 5% of those with disordered speech. In the case of individuals who have a history of stuttering in childhood, dysfluency may reemerge following the onset of PD, and present as similar to the childhood stutter but in a more severe form (Shahed & Jankovic, 2001).

Phonation

Disordered phonation or voice may be the initial sign of an impending speech disturbance in a person with PD, and in some cases, may herald the onset of the disease itself (Duffy, 2005; Logemann et al., 1978). In a group of 200 people with PD studied by Logemann et al. (1978), voice disorders occurred in 89% of the sample with 45% of these participants exhibiting a problem with their voice as the only symptom of hypokinetic dysarthria. Features of the voice disorder commonly include reduced loudness, a harsh/hoarse and breathy voice, vocal tremor, and either an increased or decreased pitch level (Darley et al., 1969a, 1969b; Logemann et al., 1978; Ludlow & Bassich, 1984).

For many people with PD, reduced loudness associated with generalized laryngeal weakness (hypophonia) is one of the most frustrating and debilitating symptoms of the disease due to its impact on a person's ability to communicate in everyday situations against background noise. Decreased loudness may vary from mild to severe and is considered to be one of the major underlying causes of reduced speech intelligibility in people with PD (Fox, Morrison, Ramig, & Sapir, 2002; Ramig, 1992). Interestingly, not all people with PD will demonstrate reduced loudness at the time of diagnosis or the speech assessment. This may be due to the nature or stage of development of the speech disorder, the individual's capacity to increase loudness when performing during assessment, the speech task itself, or to the context/environment in which the assessment takes place (Adams & Dykstra, 2009).

Early acoustic measurement of vocal sound pressure level (SPL) did not consistently demonstrate reduced vocal volume in people with PD compared to normal control speakers (Ludlow & Bassich, 1983, 1984; Metter & Hanson, 1986). In contrast, Fox and Ramig (1997) found that the average vocal SPL in their group of 29 people with PD was 2 to 4 dB less than a control group across several speech tasks performed within a research laboratory. These authors have suggested that this reduction in SPL is equivalent to a 40% perceptual change in the loudness of the voice, and therefore is likely to impact on the person's speech intelligibility and ability to be understood. These findings generally have been supported by other investigators (Adams, Haralabous, Dykstra, Abrams, & Jog, 2005; Ho et al., 1999b).

The speech task may also influence loudness levels in a person with PD. Moon, Adams, and Jog (2006) found that a greater reduction in loudness occurred during conversational speech as opposed to reading or rehearsed speech materials. It is likely that reduced loudness during conversation may be partly due to the attentional demands of this speech activity in people with PD (Ho, Iansek, & Bradshaw, 2002). The capacity of people with PD to maintain vocal loudness has also been shown to be impaired with a much faster rate of loudness decay evident during the prolongation of vowels and reading (Ho et al., 2001), and during diadochokinetic tasks (Rosen, Kent, & Duffy, 2005), compared to normal healthy control speakers. However, further research is needed to fully understand the effects of the type of speech activity on loudness (Rosen et al., 2005).

Studies investigating the effects of differing speech contexts or environments on vocal loudness have shown that people with PD will systematically increase their vocal loudness in response to increasing background noise and interlocutor distance but remain consistently lower (2 to 4 dB) than normal speakers in the same environments (Adams et al., 2005; Ho et al., 2001). Although the general assumption is that the majority of people with PD will present with reduced loudness, many factors impact on the assessment of this aspect of speech production. In order to obtain a reliable and functional measure of loudness, it is important that assessment should include perceptual and instrumental assessment of vocal loudness across several different tasks and contexts within the clinic, and in real-world environments.

Despite variations in loudness level, changes in vocal quality have been consistently identified in the speech of people with PD. Although the terminology used to describe vocal quality varies across studies, dysphonic voices are clearly evident in people with PD. Logemann et al. (1978) identified breathiness, hoarseness, roughness, and vocal tremor in 89% of their 200 participants whereas Darley et al. (1975) reported the presence of both harshness and breathiness as prominent vocal qualities. Harsh vocal quality has been identified in 77 to 84% of people with PD (Chenery et al., 1988; Ludlow & Bassich, 1984; Zwirner & Barnes, 1992) and was identified as the fifth most severely deviant vocal feature in the study by Plowman-Prine et al. (2009). Similarly, hoarseness has been perceived in the voices of 33 to 100% of cases studied (Chenery et al., 1988; Logemann et al., 1978; Ludlow & Bassich, 1984; Murdoch, Manning, Theodoros, & Thompson, 1997). More recent research has found that breathiness and hoarseness tend to co-occur in the speech of people with PD (Baumgartner, Sapir, & Ramig, 2001). Acoustic studies of vocal quality in PD have identified irregular vocal fold vibration reflected in abnormally high jitter and shimmer values compared to normal voices (Holmes, Oates, Phyland, & Hughes, 2000; Kent et al., 2003; Ludlow & Bassich, 1984). The high shimmer values seen in people with PD have been correlated with perceived breathiness in the voice and are most likely associated with vocal fold bowing (Ludlow & Bassich, 1984).

Vocal tremor occurs less frequently in PD with only 14% of 200 people being identified perceptually with true vocal tremor (Logemann et al., 1978). It is possible that vocal tremor may be incorrectly perceived to be present as a result of associated head and body tremors in some people, and is more likely to be present in later stages of the disease (Duffy, 2005; Holmes et al., 2000). In concert with perceptual findings, acoustic signs of vocal tremor are not distinctive features of the acoustic voice profile in PD. However, voice tremor in the range of 4 Hz to 7 Hz has been identified in some speakers with PD (Jiang, Lin, & Hanson, 2000). Similarly, physiologic evidence of vocal tremor is limited, although Perez, Ramig, Smith, and Dromey (1996) identified vertical laryngeal tremor or tremor of the arytenoids cartilages in over half of their 29 cases with PD or Parkinson-plus syndrome.

For a person with PD, the pitch level of the voice may be heard as either too high or too low compared to normal (Darley et al, 1975; Ludlow

& Bassich, 1983, 1984). Acoustic studies, however, have mostly confirmed the presence of either a normal or an increased overall F_0 level rather than a reduction (Ludlow & Bassich, 1983, 1984). An increase in F_0 has been noted to occur with increasing disease severity (Metter & Hanson, 1986).

The phonatory disturbances observed in people with PD have been supported by physiologic findings of laryngeal dysfunction such as vocal fold bowing and laryngeal asymmetry (Hanson, Gerratt & Ward, 1984; Perez et al., 1996), as well as abnormal laryngeal muscle activity (Baker, Ramig, Luschei, & Smith, 1998; Gallena, Smith, Zeffiro, & Ludlow, 2001; Hirose, 1986; Luschei, Ramig, Baker, & Smith, 1999), vocal fold vibratory patterns (Jiang, Lin, Wang, & Hanson, 1999), and laryngeal aerodynamics (Vincken et al., 1984). Bowing of the vocal folds or incomplete vocal fold adduction have been observed laryngoscopically as prominent features of laryngeal dysfunction in persons with PD (Blumin, Pcolinsky, & Atkins, 2004; Gallena et al., 2001; Hanson et al., 1984; Perez et al., 1996). Hanson et al. (1984) found that, during phonation, patients exhibited a significant glottal gap with tightly approximated vocal processes. These findings were noted to co-occur with perceived breathiness and reduced vocal loudness. It has been postulated that the vocal fold bowing observed in PD is due to either underactivation (reduced muscular effort and activation) (Baker et al., 1998; Fox et al., 2002) or overactivation (muscle rigidity and excessive laryngeal muscle activation) (Gallena et al., 2001) of the laryngeal musculature. In addition to vocal fold bowing, Hanson et al. (1984) identified laryngeal asymmetries in 26 patients with PD relating to the contraction of the vocal fold, and the posterior positioning of the vocal process and apex of the arytenoids on one side. Electroglottography (EEG) has provided additional evidence to support poor glottal closure with the presence of a weakly defined closing period suggesting slower than normal opening of the folds in the glottal cycle, followed by inadequate closure (Jiang et al, 1999). In addition to dysfunction at vocal fold level, abnormal airflow patterns and increased aerodynamic variability have been identified in persons with PD resulting in inadequate subglottal pressure for voice production (Vincken et al., 1984).

Articulation

Consonant imprecision is the most prominent articulatory disturbance seen in PD (Darley et al., 1975; Logemann et al., 1978; Plowman-Prine et al., 2009). The imprecision is due to distortion of speech sounds such as stops /p/, affricatives /tʃ/, and fricatives /s, z/, as a result of incomplete closure of the vocal tract for the production of stops, and to only partial constriction for fricatives (Logemann & Fisher, 1981). Stops tend to be perceived as fricatives due to incomplete closure and ongoing air emission, whereas fricatives are reduced in sharpness due to poor constriction of the vocal tract (Logemann & Fisher, 1981). It has been suggested that there is a relationship between the location of the articulation errors and the severity of the articulation disorder (Logemann & Fisher, 1981). A milder articulation disorder tends to be associated with errors in the production of phonemes requiring placement of the dorsum of the tongue (/k/, /g/), whereas a more severe articulatory disturbance is associated with errors in the production of phonemes requiring the tongue blade and tip, and the lips (Logemann & Fisher, 1981).

Numerous acoustic and physiologic studies have been conducted to investigate the articulatory imprecision in hypokinetic dysarthria. Many of these studies appear to support the notion of articulatory "undershoot" where speakers fail to reach articulatory targets or maintain sufficient contact to effect precise articulation of a speech sound, as a possible basis for the impaired articulation associated with PD. In support of this concept, acoustic studies have identified a "fused" acoustic speech signal lacking distinction between sounds and syllables (Kent & Rosenbek, 1982), reduced articulatory occlusion for stop production (Ackermann & Ziegler, 1991), reduced formant transitions (Forrest, Weismer, & Turner, 1989), restricted vowel space (consistent with reduced range of movement of the articulators) (Weismer et al., 2001), reduced F2i/F2u ratio (Sapir, Spielman, Ramig, Story, & Fox, 2007), increased formant centralization ratio (FCR) (Sapir, Ramig, Spielman, & Fox, 2010), reduced vowel articulation index (VAI), the inverse of FCR, (Skodda, Visser, & Schlegel, 2010a), and spirantization in the speech signal (Kent & Rosenbek, 1982; Weismer, 1984). Spirantization, where stop gaps are replaced with low-intensity frication, is a common feature in hypokinetic dysarthria representing the failure of complete oral closure for stop production. In addition to evidence supporting articulatory undershooting in PD, articulatory imprecision has been attributed to continuous or inappropriate voicing of consonants, a prominent feature of the speech of people with PD (Ludlow & Bassich, 1983; Weismer, 1984).

The failure to reach and maintain articulatory targets may also be due to physiologic changes in the speech mechanism associated with PD such as abnormal patterns of orofacial muscle activity, reduced amplitude and velocity of articulatory movements, impaired muscle strength, endurance and control, and tremor of the orofacial structures. Abnormal patterns of orofacial muscle activity such as increased levels of tonic resting and background electromyographic (EMG) activity in the lip and jaw muscles (Hirose, 1986; Hunker, Abbs & Barlow, 1982; Leanderson, Meyerson, & Persson, 1971; Moore & Scudder, 1989) and loss of reciprocity of opposing muscle groups in the orofacial structures (Hirose, 1986; Moore & Scudder, 1989) have been identified. It has been suggested that these patterns of muscle activity may reflect rigidity of the orofacial muscles and contribute to articulatory imprecision. Reductions in the amplitude and velocity of movement of the articulators in PD have been shown to occur in the lips (Caligiuri, 1989; Forrest & Weismer, 1995; Forrest et al., 1989; Hunker et al., 1982) and jaw (Connor, Ludlow, & Schulz, 1989; Forrest et al., 1989; Svensson, Henningson, & Karlsson, 1993) lending support to the "undershoot" hypothesis. Although a reduction in the velocity of articulatory movements is the most common finding in persons with PD, increases in the rate of repetitive movements of the articulators may occur in some people with PD who present with oral festination (OF) (Moreau et al., 2007). Interestingly, in this study, OF was found to be highly correlated with gait festination but not with the severity of the dysarthria.

Studies using nonspeech measures of the strength, endurance, and control of orofacial musculature in people with PD have identified reduced maximum lip and tongue strength (Solomon, Robin, & Luschei, 2000; Solomon, Lorell, Robin, Rodnitzky, & Luschei, 1995; Ward, Theodoros, Murdoch, & Cahill, 1999), greater instability of force control of lips, tongue, and jaw (Abbs, Hartman & Vishwanat, 1987; Barlow & Abbs, 1983; Gentil, Tournier, Pollak, & Benabid, 1999), and slower rates of development of lip and tongue forces (Gentil, Perrin, Tournier, & Pollak, 1999). Differential impairment of force stability has been identified across the articulators with the tongue demonstrating the greatest degree of force instability compared to the lips, and the jaw (Abbs et al., 1987; Barlow & Abbs, 1983). Although there is evidence to suggest that reduced strength, endurance, and control of orofacial muscles in people with PD may contribute to articulatory imprecision, no consistent relationship has been found to exist between these parameters and perceived speech impairment. In that only 10 to 25% of maximum strength of the articulators is used for speech, it is likely that there is a specific level at which the level of impairment must reach before a speech deficit becomes apparent (Duffy, 2005). This concept may explain the findings of McAuliffe, Ward, Murdoch, and Farrell (2005) who failed to demonstrate any significant differences between 14 people with PD and 11 control participants on measures of tongue strength, rate of repetitive movements, and tongue strength endurance. Furthermore, no relationship between nonspeech measures and the severity of consonant imprecision was identified in this study.

Orofacial tremors evident in people with PD may also have an impact on articulation by interfering with speech initiation and quality of performance. Hunker and Abbs (1984) were able to identify distinct pathological tremors in the lips, tongue, and jaw when at rest, postured, and actively or passively moved. These authors concluded that different forms of tremor may be present simultaneously in different articulators, affecting precision and initiation of speech.

Resonance

Clinically, impaired resonance in the form of hypernasal speech is not a hallmark feature of hypokinetic dysarthria. Some studies have reported a low level of severity (Plowman-Prine et al., 2009) and a low incidence (10 to 25%) of mild hypernasality in people with PD (Darley et al., 1975; Logemann et al., 1978) whereas others have suggested that hypernasality is a prominent deviant speech feature in some individuals (Hoodin & Gilbert, 1989a, 1989b; Ludlow & Bassich, 1983).

Findings from acoustic and physiologic studies, on the other hand, have provided objective evidence to support impairment of velopharyngeal dysfunction in persons with PD. Studies have identified a decrease in velar displacement and elevation during speech (Robbins, Logemann & Kirshner, 1986), increased nasal pressures (Netsell, Daniel, & Celesia, 1975) and airflows (Hoodin & Gilbert, 1989a, 1989b), retentive and anticipatory opening of the velopharyngeal valve (Hoodin & Gilbert, 1989a, 1989b), increased nasality during speech (Theodoros, Murdoch, & Thompson, 1995), and nasalization of sounds (Kent & Rosenbek, 1982). The disparity between perceptual and instrumental findings may reflect the greater sensitivity of instrumentation compared to perceptual judgements in the identification of velopharyngeal dysfunction and hypernasal speech. Although hypernasality typically does not occur in the speech of people with hypokinetic dysarthria, individual variations may occur.

Respiration

Impaired respiratory support for speech has been identified perceptually and physiologically in people with PD (Bunton, 2005; Chenery et al., 1988; Murdoch, Chenery, Bowler, & Ingram, 1989; Solomon & Hixon, 1993). The respiratory dysfunction is thought to contribute to specific speech features such as reduced loudness and phrase length, loudness decay, variable rate of speech, and short rushes of speech (Darley et al., 1975).

Physiologic abnormalities in respiratory function that may affect speech production in people with PD include: reduced respiratory muscle strength and endurance, vital capacity, and amplitude of chest wall movement; breath pattern irregularities; paradoxic movements of the rib cage and abdomen during speech; and impaired respiratory-phonatory control (e.g., inflexible breathing patterns, delays in exhalation and in initiating phonation, and impaired breath grouping) (Bunton, 2005; Murdoch et al., 1989; Solomon & Hixon, 1993). These abnormal respiratory features are likely to underlie impaired speech performance on measures such as duration of vowel phonation, and the number of syllables per breath and breath groups (Huber, Stathopolous, Ramig, & Lancaster, 2003; Mueller, 1971). It has been proposed that the respiratory abnormalities in PD are a result of muscle rigidity and reduced muscle activation patterns which limit the movement of the chest wall, affecting respiratory capacity, and the coordination of the rib cage and abdomen (Darley et al., 1975; Estenne, Hubert, & Troyer, 1984; Murdoch et al., 1989; Solomon & Hixon, 1993).

Role of Sensory and Perceptual Impairments

Although the basis of the speech disorder in PD generally is assumed to be related to the motor disturbances associated with the disease, there is increasing evidence to support a role for sensory and perceptual deficits

Speech Characteristics of Hypokinetic Dysarthria

Prosody

- monopitch
- monoloudness
- reduced stress
- variable speech rate (fast and slow)
- short rushes of speech/"accelerated speech"
- inappropriate silences
- difficulty initiating speech
- phoneme repetition
- palilalia

Phonation

- reduced loudness
- harsh/hoarse and breathy voice
- high or low pitch
- vocal tremor

Articulation

- imprecise consonants

Resonance

- variable hypernasality

Respiration

- impaired respiratory support

in the development of the speech impairment (Fox et al., 2002). Sensorimotor deficits have been recognized for some time in people with PD (Jobst, Melnick, Byl, Dowling, & Aminoff, 1997; Koller, 1984). Research has identified both sensorimotor deficits in the speech mechanism per se (Diamond, Schneider, & Markham, 1987; Schneider, Diamond, & Markham, 1986; Schneider & Lidsky, 1987), as well as abnormal speech perception (Ackermann, Konczak, & Hertrich, 1997; Breitenstein, Van Lancker, Daum, & Waters, 2001; Graber, Hertrich, Daum, Spieker, & Ackermann, 2002; Ho et al., 1999a; Ho, Bradshaw, & Iansek, 2000; Kiran & Larson, 2001; Pell & Leonard, 2003).

At present, the mechanisms underlying the sensory impairments observed in people with PD are not clearly understood. With respect to sensorimotor integration, researchers have suggested that the motor dysfunction observed in PD is linked to impaired processing of sensory inputs required for the development and execution of movement (Schneider et al, 1986). Schneider proposed that poor integration of sensory input may be a result of abnormal sensory gating or filtering associated with basal ganglia dysfunction. It also has been postulated that the impaired perception and modulation of speech volume may be related to the influence of a motor-sensory inhibitory mechanism on auditory cortical activity during self-produced vocalization (Ho et al., 2000; Sapir, Ramig, & Fox, 2008). A PET study conducted by Liotti et al. (2003) has provided preliminary evidence to support this concept. Compared to controls, people with PD were found to demonstrate an overactivation of the auditory cortex during speech motor activity, suggestive of impaired audiovocal gating. Further research is required to explore the interplay between sensory and motor components of the speech disturbance. In the meantime, sensory and perceptual impairments in individuals with PD must be recognized by speech clinicians and duly considered in the management of the speech disorder (see Chapter 4).

Effects of Medical and Surgical Intervention on Speech

Advances in medical and surgical interventions for the management of people with PD have been substantial, resulting in significant improvements in motor function. Pharmacologic intervention predominantly using levopdopa (L-dopa) and other anticholinergic agents remains the most efficacious therapy for the management of the movement disorders seen in PD (Rascol et al., 2003). Although providing effective relief for many of the abnormal motor symptoms, drug therapy does not provide complete and enduring amelioration of motor disturbances. Indeed, the side effects of the medication may pose major challenges to people with PD in their attempts to maintain an acceptable quality of life.

A resurgence of interest in surgical procedures for the treatment of movement disorders in PD has occurred in order to provide additional and more effective relief of motor symptoms that cannot be achieved with medication alone. The increased effectiveness and safety of neurosurgical procedures, and a greater understanding of the neuropathologic bases for PD has led to major advances in this form of treatment. Surgical interventions such as pallidotomy, thalamotomy, and deep brain stimulation have been found to have dramatic and beneficial effects on the limb motor system, and on general motor function in people with PD (Benabid, Deuschl, Lang, Lyons, & Rezai, 2006; Gan et al., 2007; Iacono, Lonser, & Kuniyoshi, 1995a; Kleiner-Fisman et al., 2006; Schrag et al., 1999; Tasker, Lang, & Lozano, 1997). Despite the positive impact of combined medical and surgical interventions on motor function, these treatments have failed to effect concomitant improvements in the motor speech system. Studies to date have revealed equivocal perceptual, acoustic, and physiologic findings, without definitive improvements in functional everyday speech.

Effects of Levodopa on Speech

The definitive effects of levodopa on speech remain unconfirmed with studies reporting improvements in certain aspects of speech function, while other studies have found either no improvement, or a worsening of speech, associated with levodopa therapy (Plowman-Prine et al., 2009; Schulz & Grant, 2000). Improvements in speech intelligibility (Adelman, Hoel, & Lassman, 1970; Nakano, Zubick, & Tyler, 1973), vocal quality, articulation, and pitch variation (Wolfe, Garvin, Bacon, & Waldrop, 1975) have been identified perceptually following levodopa treatment. Similarly, more recent perceptual studies have supported these findings with reports of improvements in word intelligibility, pitch and loudness variation, and comprehensibility of speech following medication (De Letter, Santens, & van Borsel, 2005; De Letter et al., 2007). Other studies have reported changes in acoustic properties of speech associated with medication including increases in sound pressure level and decreases in jitter, shimmer, and frequency tremor (Jiang et al., 1999; Sanabria et al., 2001).

Positive physiologic changes in the speech mechanism associated with levodopa have also been documented. Electromyographic studies have revealed improved muscle activation in the mandible (Svensson et al., 1993), lips (De Letter, Santens, & van Borsel, 2003; Leanderson et al., 1971; Nakano et al., 1973; Sandyk & Brennan, 1982), and larynx (Gallena et al., 2001). In the latter study, significant improvements in vocal fold gestures and voice onset and offset control were found to occur as a result of medication. Furthermore, Cahill et al. (1998) found that labial pressures in speech and nonspeech tasks tended to improve following levodopa.

In contrast, several studies have reported either no improvement, or deterioration in speech with medication (Daniels, Oates, Phyland, Feiglin, & Hughes, 1996; Goberman, Coelho, & Robb, 2002; Kompoliti, Wang, Goetz, Leurgans, & Raman, 2000; Plowman-Prine et al., 2009; Poluha, Teulings, & Brookshire, 1998; Wang, Kompoliti, Jiang, & Goetz, 2000). In a recent comprehensive study of the effects of levodopa on specific speech features, Plowman-Prine et al. (2009) failed to identify any significant difference between "on" and "off" medicated states for any of the 35 speech dimensions, or clusters of speech features studied. Furthermore, medication has not been shown to alter spirometric measures of speech-breathing function (Solomon & Hixon, 1993). Speech rate has been shown to be negatively affected by medication with an increase in variability during the "on" state and poor response to change (De Letter, Santens, DeBodt, Boon, & Van Borsel, 2006; De Letter et al., 2007). A common negative effect of levodopa reported in the literature is the exacerbation of dysfluency in people with PD (Anderson, Hughes, Rothi, Crucian, Heilman, 1999; Benke, Hohenstein, Poewe, & Butterworth, 2000; Louis, Winfield, Fahn, & Ford, 2001).

It should be noted that, although as a group, individuals with PD may not show effects of dopamine treatment on voice and speech, such effects (improvement or deterioration) might be present in some individuals within the group (Skodda, Visser, & Schlegel, 2010b; Spencer, Morgan, & Blond, 2009). The differential effects of levodopa on speech were highlighted in a study by Ho, Bradshaw, and Iansek (2008) in which levodopa was found to significantly increase vocal loudness and speech rate, but failed to facilitate the maintenance of speech intensity over successive speech segments. Although the changes in vocal loudness and rate were small but consistent, the findings suggested that dopaminergic medication did have some influence on the speech mechanism. However, Ho et al. (2008) proposed that persons with different speech patterns are likely to demonstrate different responses to levodopa depending on their specific speech profiles. For example, these researchers suggested that a person with dysfluency may only improve with medication if the speech rate is below a particular level for that individual. Similarly, a person with impaired intelligibility may improve with an increase in loudness but may have no perceptible net improvement if festinant speech coexists.

To date, the findings concerning the effects of levodopa on speech remain equivocal. Although it is possible that these results may reflect the inherent variability of performance observed in people with PD across various outcome measures, further large scale investigations are required to determine the effects of levodopa on speech. Clinically, however, the fact remains that levodopa fails to effect an obvious improvement in speech compared to the therapeutic response seen in general motor function.

Effects of Surgical Intervention on Speech

Surgical interventions such as thalamotomy, pallidotomy, and deep brain stimulation (DBS) have been shown to have varying effects on speech. The general consensus from the evidence to date, however, is that these procedures do not result in significant functional improvements in speech that are consistent with those observed in limb and general motor function.

Pallidotomy

Studies involving pallidotomy have reported marked improvements (Iacono et al., 1995b; Laitinen, Bergenheim, & Hariz, 1992), negative changes (Kumar, Lozano, Montgomery, & Lang, 1998; Schrag et al., 1999; Scott et al., 1998; Theodoros, Ward, Murdoch, Silburn, & Lethlean, 2000; Uitti et al., 2000), minimal improvement, or mixed outcomes (Barlow, Iacono, Paseman, Biswas, & D'Antonio, 1998; Baron et al., 1996; Schulz & Grant, 2000; Schulz, Peterson, Sapienza, Greer, & Friedman, 1999). Iacono et al. (1995b) reported a significant improvement in speech following pallidotomy based on postoperative decline in the UPDRS speech rating, while Barlow et al. (1998) observed evidence of improved orofacial motor control and speech aerodynamics after bilateral pallidotomy in many of their 11 participants with PD.

Some studies have identified a substantial risk for the development of persisting speech impairments following unilateral pallidotomy (Kumar et al., 1998), with an even greater risk after bilateral pallidotomy (Scott et al., 1998). Theodoros et al. (2000) noted negative changes in speech following bilateral pallidotomy with a decrease in speech intelligibility in 10 out of 12 PD participants following surgery. Similarly, Uitti et al. (2000) recorded a mild decline of speech intelligibility in one-third of their PD participants following unilateral pallidotomy.

Other studies have reported variable changes in speech following pallidotomy. Schulz et al. (1999) found that only four out of six PD participants demonstrated positive changes in either phonatory or both phonatory and articulatory acoustic parameters following unilateral pallidotomy. Similarly, a further study of vocal intensity postpallidotomy by Schulz, Greer, and Friedman (2000) demonstrated high interparticipant variability. Although postoperative improvements in vocal intensity were noted for many participants with mild speech impairment, negative changes were observed for most of the moderate-severely dysarthric speakers. These findings suggest that pallidotomy may pose a particular risk for speech for persons with PD who present with marked dysarthria initially.

Thalamotomy

Reports of the negative effects of thalamotomy on speech have appeared in the literature for over several decades. Early studies identified postoperative impairments in respiratory support for speech, pitch, volume, and articulation following this procedure (Allan, Turner, & Gadea-Ciria, 1966; Canter & Van Lancker, 1985; Jenkins, 1968; Petrovici, 1980). It also has been suggested that the negative effects on speech are more likely to occur when the thalamotomy is performed on the person's dominant hemisphere as opposed to the nondominant hemisphere (Allan et al., 1966; Jenkins, 1968). In contrast to these reports of negative change in speech following unilateral thalamotomy, more recent investigations have suggested that speech remains largely unchanged in most participants with PD following surgery (Fox, Ahlskog, & Kelly, 1991; Linhares & Tasker, 2000; Schuurman et al., 2000). Schuurman et al. (2000) found only 14% of 34 participants demonstrated persistent speech change following unilateral thalamotomy, whereas Linhares and Tasker (2000) reported neutral outcomes for speech and gait for 40 PD participants following thalamotomy. These findings may reflect recent improvements in surgical and imaging procedures.

Research has indicated that bilateral thalamotomy is more likely to have negative effects on speech than a unilateral procedure (Allan et al., 1966; Matsumoto, Asano, Baba, Miyamoto, & Ohmoto, 1976; Selby, 1967). Indeed, a very early study by Selby (1967) found that thalamotomy resulted in speech deterioration in 8.9% of participants following unilateral thalamotomy, and in 23.8% of participants following bilateral thalamotomy. As in the case of pallidotomy, these investigators postulated that the presence of a preoperative speech impairment created a higher risk for negative speech changes following bilateral thalamotomy. Findings from these earlier studies have been supported by investigations of contemporary bilateral thalamotomy procedures suggesting deterioration in speech postsurgery (Tasker, DeCarvalho, Li, & Kestle, 1996).

Deep Brain Stimulation

Although effective for many people with PD, ablative procedures such as pallidotomy and thalamotomy have now been surpassed, to a large extent, by bilateral subthalamic nucleus deep brain stimulation (STN-DBS) as the surgical treatment of choice. The advantages of deep brain stimulation include the capacity to reverse, adjust, and fine tune the stimulation to achieve optimal motor function outcomes (Moro, Poon, Lozano, Saint-Cyr, & Lang, 2006). It has been estimated that over 35,000 people with PD worldwide have had this procedure (Benabid et al., 2006; Kleiner-Fisman et al., 2006).

The impact of STN-DBS on speech, however, has been less than encouraging with most studies reporting either no response to the stimulation, or a negative effect on speech production (D'Alatri et al., 2008; Klostermann et al., 2008; Ostergaard & Sunde, 2006; Pinto et al., 2005; Pinto et al., 2004). Indeed, the most common finding is an increase in the severity of the speech disturbance (Narayana et al., 2009). The incidence of dysarthria developing or worsening following implantation has been reported to range from 5 to 61% of cases (Gan et al., 2007; Guehl et al., 2006; Krack et al., 2003; Rodriguez-Oroz et al., 2005). These negative effects of STN-DBS on speech have included decreases in speech intelligibility and vocal volume (Klostermann et al, 2008; Rousseaux et al., 2004); Santens, De Letter, Van Borsel, De Reuck, & Caemaert, 2003), greater impairment of articulation and prosody (Santens et al., 2003), and difficulty with the initiation of speech (Moretti et al., 2003).

Despite the reports of neutral or negative effects of STN-DBS on speech, a few studies have reported varying degrees of improvement in speech, vowel duration, pitch variation, oral force measures (Gentil et al., 1999; Gentil, Pinto, Pollak, & Benabid, 2003), lip movements, pitch and loudness variation (Rousseaux et al., 2004), vocal function (Gentil, Chauvin, Pinto, Pollak, & Benabid, 2001; Lee, Zhou, Rahn, Wang, & Jiang, 2008), and vocal tremor (D'Alatri et al., 2008). Putzer, Barry, and Moringlane (2008) identified differential effects of STN-DBS on the motor speech subsystem in that the precision of glottal and supraglottal articulation, and phonation were reduced in some patients but not others. Some researchers have attempted to explain the variable effects of STN-DBS on the speech mechanism by proposing that this procedure may improve some motor speech functions attributable to inherent motor disturbances such as rigidity, tremor, and bradykinesia, but not those less closely aligned to these motor disturbances (Klostermann et al., 2008; Rousseaux et al., 2004).

The lack of change, or worsening of speech following STN-DBS, has been attributed to diffusion of the current from the stimulator site to the surrounding corticobulbar fibres involved in speech production (Pinto et al., 2005). As a result, researchers have begun to investigate the effects of different stimulator locations and parameters on speech (Tornqvist, Schalen, & Rehncrona, 2004; Tripoliti et al., 2008). Tornqvist et al. (2004) found that high frequency or increased amplitude stimulator settings resulted in significantly decreased speech intelligibility. Similarly, Tripoliti et al. (2008) noted significant deterioration in speech intelligibility with high voltage stimulation both inside and outside the STN. Other studies have demonstrated a laterality effect where stimulation of the STN on the left side of the brain resulted in a decrease in articulatory accuracy and syllable rates, whereas stimulation on the right side resulted in either no change or an improvement in these speech features (Wang, Metman, Bakay, Arzbaecher, & Bernard, 2003; Wang et al., 2006). Further investigation of the effects of stimulator location and varying parameters on speech is required to optimize speech outcome with STN-DBS.

The difference in the effects of levodopa therapy and surgical interventions on speech compared to motor disturbance in PD is remarkable, and remains unexplained. Several hypotheses have been proposed regarding the neural mechanisms underlying these outcomes. One such hypothesis suggests that the speech disorder in PD is nondopaminergic in origin and therefore may not be responsive to the levodopa and surgical interventions that target the dopaminergic pathways (D'Alatri et al., 2008; Farrell, Theodoros, Ward, Hall, & Silburn, 2005). Another hypothesis proposes that the motor programs for speech and limbs differ in their neural innervations, organization, and motor planning (Farrell et al., 2005; Pinto et al., 2004), and therefore respond differently to medical and surgical intervention. It also has been postulated that, based on the somatotopic organization of the basal ganglia (Alexander, Crutcher, & DeLong, 1990; Alexander, DeLong, & Strick, 1986) , surgical interventions target only the neural substrates for limb functions and not those specific to speech (Farrell et al., 2005).

Although the speech disorder in PD has not been found to demonstrate significant functional improvements in response to medication and surgical procedures, studies in this area have provided a greater understanding of the nature of this speech disorder, and its management. It clearly is evident that behavioral speech treatment remains the primary intervention of choice in the management of the speech disorder.

Impact on Quality of Life

As communication is an integral component of social functioning, it is not surprising that deterioration in speech and other aspects of communication will impact significantly on the quality of life of people with PD. Not surprisingly, studies conducted to date have identified the negative impact of the speech disorder on a person's everyday activities and interactions, their self-esteem, and on the perception of others. People with PD have reported a greater reduction in quality of life than the general population (Schrag, Jahanshahi, & Quinn, 2000) with impaired physical and social functioning having the greatest effect. Although significant research has been devoted to defining the characteristics and effects of various interventions on the speech disorder in PD, there has been limited investigation of the impact of the speech disturbance and other aspects of communication on the quality of life of individuals and their families.

In the early stages of the disease, people with PD may begin to experience subtle changes in their ability to communicate, for example, difficulty being heard on the telephone and in conversations involving more than one or two people. Over time, the person may experience an increasing number of requests for repetition, difficulty in recalling words (see Chapter 5), and increasing frustration when attempting to communicate (DePippo, 1994; Stewart, 2000). In addition to these communication changes, PD is frequently associated with reduced facial expression which affects the person's ability to appropriately convey their feelings and to signal engagement in social interactions (DePippo, 1994; Stewart, 2000). As a result, the dynamics of the interaction are affected and often altered in such a way as to invoke discomfort in both the person with PD and the communication partner (Miller et al., 2006; Stewart, 2000). Early studies lend support to these findings in that impaired facial expression and even subtle changes in speech have been found to negatively impact on the perception of others (Pentland, 1987; Pitcairn, Clemie, Gray, & Pentland, 1990). Slowness of movement, lack of spontaneous gesture, and, at times, poor eye contact due to a stooped posture may further compromise the communication process (Robertson, 1988).

When interviewed about communication changes associated with PD and the impact of these changes on quality of life, people with PD reported four main areas of concern (Miller et al., 2006). These included changes to their interaction with others, problems with conversation, and issues and feelings about speech intelligibility and voice. When interacting with others, people with PD felt that listeners were impatient, failing to allow then to complete what they wished to say, talking over them, or, in some cases, answering for them. As a result, these interactions directly impacted on the person's socialization to the point that some people consciously avoided contact with others. Participants reported that changes in speech and voice made it difficult for them to engage and maintain conversations due to the physical and mental effort involved in overcoming these impairments. However, it was clear that study participants were less concerned about the changes to their speech and voice per se but more about the impact of these changes on their self-concept, family dynamics, and their ability to participate in everyday activities. They reported that concomitant changes in language and cognition contributed to these difficulties. It was evident that participants did not identify any one specific change in communication that impacted more than others on their quality of life, but rather that different factors may have an impact at various times depending on the situation. Interestingly, almost all participants reported being aware of the negative impact of speech and other communicative changes on quality of life well before a significant reduction in speech intelligibility had occurred (Miller et al., 2006).

These qualitative findings were supported by a recent study by Miller et al. (2008) who investigated the psychosocial impact of perceived changes in communication of 104 people with PD and 45 carers. The study found that the PD group perceived a significant deterioration in communication after the onset of the disease. The most prominent perceptions relating to changes in communication included a feeling of not being in control, not feeling confident, having difficulty getting the message across to listeners, a lack of enjoyment in speaking, a sense of inadequacy, and a sense of loss of independence. These perceived communication changes were found to occur irrespective of age and gender and were only weakly correlated with disease severity and duration, level of speech intelligibility, and cognitive status. Despite these negative perceptions of communication changes, people with PD reported that they continued to feel valued, and that they conveyed a sense of caring and friendliness. Caregivers' perception of change in communication tended to be more optimistic with no significant differences in their ratings before and after the onset of the disease. This finding suggested that carers may underestimate the impact of communication changes on people with PD, highlighting the need to improve the level and extent of information provided to carers and family members (Miller et al., 2008).

People with PD have reported a variety of strategies to cope with their altered communication abilities (Miller et al., 2006). They have indicated that helping others to understand PD and its symptoms, monitoring their physical and mental resources to ensure optimal communication, occasionally adopting a nonengaging approach to communication, or using alternative means of communication (e.g., gesture, writing, e-mail) have been beneficial in reducing the impact of communication changes. When absolutely necessary, a common strategy is to maximize physical effort and concentration to achieve effective communication (Miller et al., 2006). People with PD tend to use these strategies in various ways at different times according to their physical and emotional states, and the specific social situation (Miller et al., 2006).

The finding that communication changes are perceived to occur prior to an obvious reduction in speech intelligibility highlights the need for early referral to the SLP. Delayed referral until an obvious speech disturbance is apparent may lead to the development of maladaptive coping strategies and, ultimately, reduced quality of life (Miller et al., 2006). Currently, the Lee Silverman Voice Treatment (LSVT LOUD) is the most efficacious speech treatment for individuals with Parkinson disease with Level 1 evidence documenting short and long-term success (Ramig et al., 2001). LSVT LOUD addresses the underlying motor, sensory and cognitive bases for the speech and voice disorder observed in PD (see Chapter 4).

Furthermore, there is a need to address cognitive-linguistic dysfunction (see Chapter 5), the role of communication partners in the management of people with PD, and the use of strategies to facilitate and maintain communication for as long as possible throughout the course of the disease (Miller et al., 2006; Robertson, 2006). A critical component of the management of the communication disorders in PD involves optimizing the sequencing and staging of intervention to address communication needs and maintain quality of life (Yorkston, 2007).

Accessing Speech Treatment

Despite the impact of the speech disorder on people with PD, the obvious need for early intervention and ongoing maintenance of communication, and the existence of an efficacious speech treatment, access to SLP services for people with PD is less than adequate worldwide. Studies conducted in the United Kingdom, Sweden, and the Netherlands have found that only 3 to 20% of people with PD and a speech disorder make

Effects of Parkinson Disease on Everyday Communication and Quality of Life

- Increased requests for repetition
- Difficulty being heard on telephone and in conversation
- Difficulty recalling words
- Reduced ability to convey feelings and signal social interaction due to:
  - impaired facial expression
  - poor eye contact
  - impaired spontaneous gesture
  - stooped posture
- Negative responses from listeners
- Reduced confidence and sense of inadequacy
- Loss of independence
- Decreased enjoyment in conversation

contact with a SLP (Hartelius & Svensson, 1994; Nijkrake et al., 2008; Noble, Jones, Miller, & Burn, 2006). Limited access to speech-language services may be due not only to restricted levels of health service, but also to the tyranny of distance, and the mobility issues experienced by people with PD.

For some people with PD, the unavailability of speech treatment close to home, particularly in rural settings, is an unfortunate reality. As a result, a person may need to travel long distances to access treatment from a SLP experienced in the management of this disorder. The movement disorders associated with PD, and the need for assistance may preclude or impede repeat attendance at a health care facility. Mobility issues not only impact on people living in rural communities, but also may directly affect those living in urban areas.

Improving access to speech-language services for people with PD is a challenge, and one that requires alternative and innovative models of service delivery. Rapid advances in technology and telecommunications, however, have provided the means by which these challenges may be overcome. One solution for the management of the speech disorder in

PD is the use of telerehabilitation or telepractice (American Speech and Hearing Association, 2010) whereby treatment is delivered via telecommunications technology to supplement, or in some cases, substitute, for face-to-face intervention. Such technology has the capacity to enable reliable and valid assessment and treatment of communication disorders across the Internet via videoconferencing (Theodoros & Russell, 2008). Studies conducted at the Telerehabilitation Research Unit at the University of Queensland have shown that the speech disorder in PD can be validly and reliably assessed and treated via the Internet using a customized multimedia videoconferencing system within a laboratory and home-based setting (Constantinescu et al., 2010a, 2010b, 2010c; Theodoros et al., 2006). Treatment outcomes following the online delivery of LSVT LOUD were found to be comparable to face-to-face intervention in these studies. Larger scale studies involving home-based treatment are now being conducted to establish the ecological validity and cost benefit of telerehabilitation as an alternate mode of service delivery for people with PD. Other platforms for delivering speech treatment at a distance such as interactive Web sites, speech training software (Halpern, Matos, Ramig, Petska, & Spielman, 2005), mobile technologies (e.g., Smartphones), and virtual therapists have the potential to address the need for ongoing maintenance and self-management of the speech disorder. The ubiquity of technology-based service delivery has the potential to alleviate many of the access issues facing people with PD, and may ultimately provide a way to ensure more effective management of the communication disorders associated with this disease.

Summary

The speech disorder associated with PD is a common and distinctive symptom of the disease. The dysarthric speech disturbance is characterized by reduced volume, monoloudness, monopitch, imprecise articulation, dysfluency, and changes to speech rate and vocal quality.

Although the basis of the speech disorder is assumed to be related to the motor disturbances associated with PD, considerable evidence, based on the limited effects of medication and surgical procedures on speech performance, now exists to challenge this assumption. The impact of other factors, such as sensory and perceptual impairment, is now being considered as contributing to the speech disorder. The slow and progressive deterioration in speech has a significant impact on social functioning and the quality of life of people with PD and their families. The need to initiate speech intervention early in the course of the disease to maintain communication is clear, despite this being an uncommon practice worldwide. Although an efficacious speech treatment for people with PD does exist, ready access to speech services remains limited. Rapid advancements and innovations in technology, however, have now provided the tools by which people with PD can gain access to speech treatment. Telerehabilitation or telepractice holds great promise as an alternate method of service delivery for providing initial treatment, and for facilitating speech maintenance throughout the course of the disease.

References

Abbs, J. H., Hartman, D. E., & Vishwanat, B. (1987). Orofacial motor control impairment in Parkinson's disease. *Neurology, 37*, 394–398.

Ackermann, H., Konczak, J., & Hertrich, I. (1997). The temporal control of repetitive articulatory movements in Parkinson's disease. *Brain and Language, 56*, 312–319.

Ackermann, H., & Ziegler, W. (1991). Articulatory deficits in Parkinson's dysarthria: An acoustic analysis. *Journal of Neurology, Neurosurgery, and Psychiatry, 54*, 1093–1098.

Adams, S. G. (1994). Accelerating speech in a case of hypokinetic dysarthria: Descriptions and treatment. In J. A. Till, K. M. Yorkston, & D. R. Beukelman (Eds.), *Motor speech disorders: Advances in assessment and treatment*. (pp. 213–228). Baltimore, MD: Brookes.

Adams, S. G., & Dykstra, A. (2009). Hypokinetic dysarthria. In M. R. McNeil (Ed.), *Clinical management of sensorimotor speech disorders* (2nd ed., pp. 166–186). New York, NY: Thieme.

Adams, S. G., Haralabous, O., Dykstra, A., Abrams, K., & Jog, M. S. (2005). Effects of multitalker background noise on the intensity of spoken sentences in Parkinson's disease. *Canadian Acoustics, 33*, 94–95.

Adelman, J., Hoel, R., & Lassman, M. (1970). The effect of L- dopa treatment on speech in Parkinson's disease. *Journal of Neurology, Neurosurgery, and Psychiatry, 20*, 410–411.

Alexander, G. E., Crutcher, M. D., & DeLong, M. R. (1990). Basal ganglia-thalamocortical circuits: Parallel substrates for motor, oculomotor, "prefrontal" and "limbic" functions. *Progress in Brain Research, 85*, 119–146.

Alexander, G. E., DeLong, M. R., & Strick, P. L. (1986). Parallel organization of functionally segregated circuits linking basal ganglia and cortex. *Annual Review of Neuroscience, 9*, 357–381.

Allan, C. M., Turner, J. W., & Gadea Ciria, M. (1966). Investigations into speech disturbances following stereotaxic surgery for parkinsonism. *British Journal of Disorders of Communication, 1*, 55–59.

American Speech-Language-Hearing Association. (2010). *Professional issues in telepractice for speech-language pathologists* [Professional issues statement]. Available from http://www.asha.org/policy

Anderson, J. M., Hughes, J. D., Rothi, L. J., Crucian, G. P., & Heilman, K. M. (1999). Developmental stuttering and Parkinson's disease: The effects of levodopa treatment. *Journal of Neurology, Neurosurgery, and Psychiatry, 66*, 776–778.

Baker, K. K., Ramig, L. O., Luschei, E. S., & Smith, M. E. (1998). Thyroarytenoid muscle activity associated with hypophonia in Parkinson disease and aging. *Neurology, 51*, 1592–1598.

Barlow, S. M., & Abbs, J. H. (1983). Force transducers for the evaluation of labial, lingual, and mandibular motor impairments. *Journal of Speech and Hearing Research, 26*, 616–621.

Barlow, S. M., Iacono, R. P., Paseman, L. A., Biswas, A., & D'Antonio, L. (1998). The effects of posteroventral pallidotomy on force and speech aerodynamics in Parkinson's disease. In M. Cannito, K. M. Yorkston, & D. R. Beukelman (Eds.), *Neuromotor speech disorders: Nature, assessment, and management* (pp. 117–155). Baltimore, MD: Brookes.

Baron, M. S., Vitek, J. L., Green, J., Kaneoke, Y., Hashimoto, T., Turner, R. S., . . . McDonald, W. M. (1996). Treatment of advanced Parkinson's disease by posterior GPi pallidotomy: One-year results of a pilot study. *Annals of Neurology, 40*, 335–366.

Baumgartner, C. A., Sapir, S., & Ramig, L. O. (2001). Voice quality changes following phonatory-respiratory effort treatment (LSVT) versus respiratory effort treatment for individuals with Parkinson disease. *Journal of Voice, 15*, 105–114.

Benabid, A. L., Deuschl, G., Lang, A. E., Lyons, K. E., & Rezai, A. R. (2006). Deep brain stimulation for Parkinson's disease. *Movement Disorders, 21*(Suppl. 14), S168–S170.

Benke, T., Hohenstein, C., Poewe, W., & Butterworth, B. (2000). Repetitive speech phenomena in Parkinson's disease. *Journal of Neurology, Neurosurgery, and Psychiatry, 69*, 319–324.

Blumin, J. H., Pcolinsky, D. E., & Atkins, J. P. (2004). Laryngeal findings in advanced Parkinson's disease. *Annals of Otology, Rhinology, and Laryngology, 113*, 253–258.

Breitenstein, C., Van Lacker, D., Daum, I., & Waters, C. H. (2001). Impaired perception of vocal emotions in Parkinson's disease: Influence of speech time processing and executive functioning. *Brain and Cognition, 45*, 277–314.

Bunton, K. (2005). Patterns of lung volume use during an extemporaneous speech task in persons with Parkinson disease. *Journal of Communication Disorders, 38*, 331–348.

Bunton, K., Kent, R. D., Kent, J. F., & Duffy, J. R. (2001). Effects of flattening fundamental frequency contours on sentence intelligibility in speakers with dysarthria. *Clinical Linguistics and Phonetics, 15*, 181–193.

Cahill, L. M., Murdoch, B. E., Theodoros, D. G., Triggs, E. J., Charles, B. G., & Yao, A. A. (1998). Effect of oral levodopa treatment on articulatory function in Parkinson's disease: Preliminary results. *Motor Control, 2*, 161–172.

Caligiuri, M. P. (1989). The influence of speaking rate on articulatory hypokinesia in Parkinsonian dysarthria. *Brain and Language, 36*, 493–502.

Canter, G. J. (1963). Speech characteristics of patients with Parkinson's disease: I. Intensity, pitch, and duration. *Journal of Speech and Hearing Disorders, 28*, 221–229.

Canter, G. J., & van Lancker, D. R. (1985). Disturbances of the temporal organization of speech following bilateral thalamic surgery in a patient with Parkinson's disease. *Journal of Communication Disorders, 18*, 329–349.

Chenery, H. J., Murdoch, B. E., & Ingram, J. C. L. (1988). Studies in Parkinson's disease: I. Perceptual speech analyses. *Australian Journal of Human Communication Disorders, 16*, 17–29.

Connor, N. P., Ludlow, C. L., & Schulz, G. M. (1989). Stop consonant production in isolated and repeated syllables in Parkinson's disease. *Neuropsychologia, 27*, 829–838.

Constantinescu, G., Theodoros, D. G., Russell, T., Ward, E. C., Wilson, S. J., & Wootton, R. (2010a). Home-based speech treatment for Parkinson's disease delivered remotely: A case report. *Journal of Telemedicine and Telecare, 16*, 100–104.

Constantinescu, G., Theodoros, D. G., Russell, T., Ward, E. C., Wilson, S., & Wootton, R. (2010b). Assessing disordered speech and voice in Parkinson's disease: A telerehabilitation application. *International Journal of Language and Communication Disorders*. Elub ahead of print.

Constantinescu, G., Theodoros, D. G., Russell, T., Ward, E. C., Wilson, S., & Wootton, R. (2010c). Treating disordered speech and voice in Parkinson's disease online: A randomised controlled noninferiority trial. *International Journal of Language and Communication Disorders.* Epub ahead of print

D'Alatri, L., Paludetti, G., Contarino, M. F., Galla, S., Marchese, M. R., & Bentivoglio, A. R. (2008). Effects of bilateral subthalamic nucleus stimulation and medication on Parkinsonian speech impairment. *Journal of Voice, 22*, 365–372.

Daniels, N., Oates, J., Phyland, D., Feiglin, A., & Hughes, A. (1996). Vocal characteristics and response to levodopa in parkinson's disease. *Movement Disorders, 11*, 117.

Darley, F. L., Aronson, A. E., & Brown, J. R. (1969a). Differential diagnostic patterns of dysarthria. *Journal of Speech and Hearing Research, 12*, 246–269.

Darley, F. L., Aronson, A. E., & Brown, J. R. (1969b). Clusters of deviant speech dimensions in the dysarthrias. *Journal of Speech and Hearing Research, 12*, 462–496.

Darley, F. L., Aronson, A. E., & Brown, J. R. (1975). *Motor speech disorders*. Philadelphia, PA: W. B. Saunders.

De Letter, M., Santens, P., & Van Borsel, J. (2003). The effects of levodopa on tongue strength and endurance in patients with Parkinson's disease. *Acta Neurologica Belgium, 103*, 35–38.

De Letter, M., Santens, P., & Van Borsel, J. (2005). The effects of levodopa on word intelligibility in Parkinson's disease. *Journal of Communication Disorders, 38,* 187–196.

De Letter, M., Santens, P., De Bodt, M., Boon, P., & Van Borsel, J. (2006). Levodopa-induced alterations in speech rate in advanced Parkinson's disease. *Acta Neurologica Belgium, 106,* 19–22.

De Letter, M., Santens, P., Estercam, I., Van Maele, G., De Bodt, M., Boon, P., & Van Borsel, J. (2007). Levodopa-induced modifications of prosody and comprehensibility in advanced Parkinson's disease as perceived by professional listeners. *Clinical Linguistics and Phonetics, 21,* 783–791.

DePippo, K. L. (1994). Management of communication dysfunction. In A. M. Cohen & W. J. Weiner (Eds.), *The comprehensive management of Parkinson's disease* (pp. 75–88). New York, NY: Demos.

Diamond, S. G., Schneider, J. S., & Markham, C. H. (1987). Oral sensorimotor defects in patients with Parkinson's disease. *Advances in Neurology, 45,* 335–338.

Duffy, J. F. (2005). Hypokinetic dysarthria. In J. R. Duffy, *Motor speech disorders: Substrates, differential diagnosis, and management* (2nd ed., pp. 187–215). St. Louis, MO: Elsevier Mosby.

Dworkin, J. P., & Aronson, A. E. (1986). Tongue strength and alternate motion rates in normal and dysarthric speakers. *Journal of Communication Disorders, 19,* 115–132.

Estenne, M., Hubert, M., & Troyer, A. D. (1984). Respiratory-muscle involvement in Parkinson's disease. *New England Journal of Medicine, 311,* 1516–1517.

Farrell, A., Theodoros, D., Ward, E., Hall, B., & Silburn, P. (2005). Effects of neurosurgical management of Parkinson's disease on speech characteristics and oromotor function. *Journal of Speech, Language, and Hearing Research, 48,* 5–20.

Forrest, K., & Weismer, G. (1995). Dynamic aspects of lower lip movement in parkinsonian and neurologically normal geriatric speakers' production of stress. *Journal of Speech and Hearing Research, 38,* 260–272.

Forrest, K., Weismer, G., & Turner, G. S. (1989). Kinematic, acoustic, and perceptual analyses of connected speech produced by parkinsonian and normal geriatric adults. *Journal of Acoustical Society of America, 85,* 2608–2622.

Fox, C., & Ramig, L. O. (1997). Vocal sound pressure level and self-perception of speech and voice in men and women with idiopathic Parkinson disease. *American Journal of Speech-Language Pathology, 39,* 85–94.

Fox, C. M., Morrison, C. E., Ramig, L. O., & Sapir, S. (2002). Current perspectives on the Lee Silverman Voice Treatment (LSVT) for individuals with idiopathic Parkinson disease. *American Journal of Speech-Language Pathology, 11,* 111–123.

Fox, M. W., Ahlskog, J. E., & Kelly, P. J. (1991). Stereotactic ventrolateralis thalamotomy for medically refractory tremor in post-levodopa era Parkinson's disease patients. *Journal of Neurosurgery, 75,* 723–730.

Gallena, S., Smith, P. J., Zeffiro, T., & Ludlow, C. L. (2001). Effects of levodopa on laryngeal muscle activity for voice onset and offset in Parkinson's disease. *Journal of Speech, Language, and Hearing Research, 44,* 1284–1299.

Gamboa, J., Jimenez, F. J., Nieto, A., Montojo, J., Orti Pareja, M., Molina, J. A., . . . Cobeta, I. (1997). Acoustic voice analysis in patients with Parkinson's disease treated with dopaminergic drugs. *Journal of Voice*, *11*, 314–320.

Gan, J., Xie-Brustolin, J., Mertens, P., Polo, G., Klinger, H., Mollion, H., . . . Thobois, S.(2007). Bilateral subthalamic nucleus stimulation in advanced Parkinson's disease: Three years follow-up. *Journal of Neurology*, *254*, 99–106.

Gentil, M., Chauvin, P., Pinto, S., Pollak, P., & Benabid, A. L. (2001). Effect of bilateral stimulation of the subthalamic nucleus on Parkinsonian voice. *Brain and Language*, *78*, 233–240.

Gentil, M., Perrin, S., Tournier, C. L., & Pollack, P. (1999). Lip, tongue and forefinger force control in Parkinson's disease. *Clinical Linguistics and Phonetics*, *13*, 45–54.

Gentil, M., Pinto, S., Pollak, P., & Benabid, A. L. (2003). Effect of bilateral stimulation of the subthalamic nucleus on parkinsonian dysarthria. *Brain and Language*, *85*, 190–196.

Gentil, M., Tournier, C.-L., Pollak, P., & Benabid, A.-L. (1999). Effect of bilateral subthalamic nucleus stimulation and dopatherapy on oral control in Parkinson's disease. *European Neurology*, *42*, 136–140.

Goberman, A., Coelho, C., & Robb, M. (2002). Phonatory characteristics of parkinsonian speech before and after morning medication: The "on" and "off" states. *Journal of Communication Disorders*, *35*, 217–239.

Graber, S., Hertrich, I., Daum, I., Spieker, S., & Ackermann, H. (2002). Speech perception deficits in Parkinson's disease: Underestimation of time intervals compromises indentification of durational phonetic contrasts. *Brain and Language*, *82*, 65–74.

Guehl, D., Cuny, E., Benazzouz, A., Rougier, A., Tison, F., Machado, S., . . . Burbaud, P. (2006). Side-effects of subthalamic stimulation in Parkinson's disease: Clinical evolution and predictive factors. *European Journal of Neurology*, *13*, 963–971.

Halpern, A., Matos, C., Ramig, L., Petska, J., & Spielman, J. (2005). *LSVTC—A PDA supported speech treatment for Parkinson's disease.* Presented at the 9th International Congress of Parkinson's Disease and Movement Disorders. New Orleans, LA, USA.

Hammen, V. L., Yorkston, K. M., & Beukelman, D. R. (1989). Pausal and speech duration characteristics as a function of speaking rate in normal and parkinsonian dysarthric individuals. In K. M. Yorkston & D. R. Beukelman (Eds.), *Recent advances in clinical dysarthria* (pp. 213–224). Boston, MA: College-Hill.

Hanson, D. G., Gerratt, B. R., & Ward, P. (1984). Cinegraphic observations of laryngeal function in Parkinson's disease. *Laryngoscope*, *94*, 348.

Harel, B., Cannizzaro, M., & Snyder, P. J. (2004). Variability in fundamental frequency during speech in prodromal and incipient Parkinson's disease: A longitudinal case study. *Brain and Cognition*, *56*, 24–29.

Hartelius, L., & Svensson, P. (1994). Speech and swallowing symptoms associated with Parkinson's disease and multiple sclerosis—a survey. *Folia Phoniatrica Logopedia*, *46*, 9–17.

Hirose, H. (1986). Pathophysiology of motor speech disorders (dysarthria). *Folia Phoniatrica, 38,* 61–88.

Ho, A. K., Bradshaw, J. L., & Iansek, I. (2000). Volume perception in parkinsonian speech. *Movement Disorders, 15,* 1125–1131.

Ho, A. K., Bradshaw, J. L., & Iansek, I. (2008). For better or worse: The effect of levodopa on speech in Parkinson's disease. *Movement Disorders, 23,* 574–580.

Ho, A. K., Bradshaw, J. L., Iansek, R., & Alfredson, R. (1999a). Speech volume regulation in Parkinson's disease: Effects of implicit cues and explicit instructions. *Neuropsychologia, 37,* 1453–1460.

Ho, A. K., Iansek, R., & Bradshaw, J. L. (1999b). Regulation of parkinsonian speech volume: The effect of interlocutor distance. *Journal of Neurology, Neurosurgery, and Psychiatry, 67,* 199–202.

Ho, A. K., Iansek, R., & Bradshaw, J. L. (2001). Motor instability in parkinsonian speech intensity. *Neuropsychiatry, Neuropsychology, and Behavioural Neurology, 14,* 109–116.

Ho, A. K., Iansek, R., & Bradshaw, J. L. (2002). The effect of a concurrent task on parkinsonian speech. *Journal of Clinical Experimental Neuropsychology, 24,* 36–47.

Ho, A. K., Iansek, R., Marigliani, C., Bradshaw, J. L., & Gates, S. (1998). Speech impairment in a large sample of patients with Parkinson's disease. *Behavioral Neurology, 11,* 131–137.

Holmes, R. J., Oates, J. M., Phyland, D. J., & Hughes, A. J. (2000). Voice characteristics in the progression of Parkinson's disease. *International Journal of Language and Communication Disorders, 35,* 407–418.

Hoodin, R. B., & Gilbert, H. R. (1989a). Nasal airflows in parkinsonian speakers. *Journal of Communication Disorders, 22,* 169–180.

Hoodin, R. B., & Gilbert, H. R. (1989b). Parkinsonian dysarthria: An aerodynamic and perceptual description of velopharyngeal closure for speech. *Folia Phoniatrica, 41,* 249–258.

Huber, J. E., Stathopolous, E. T., Ramig, L. O., & Lancaster, S. L. (2003). Respiratory function and variability in individuals with Parkinson disease: Pre- and post-Lee Silverman Voice Treatment. *Journal of Medical Speech-Language Pathology, 11,* 185–201.

Hunker, C. J., & Abbs, J. H. (1984). Physiological analyses of parkinsonian tremors in the orofacial system. In M. R. McNeil, J. C. Rosenbek, & A. E. Aronson (Eds.), *The dysarthrias: Physiology, acoustics, perception, management* (pp. 69–100). San Diego, CA: College-Hill Press.

Hunker, C. J., Abbs, J. H., & Barlow, S. M. (1982). The relationship between parkinsonian rigidity and hypokinesia in the orofacial system: A quantitative analysis. *Neurology, 32,* 755–761.

Iacono, R. P., Lonser, R., & Kuniyoshi, S. (1995a). Unilateral versus bilateral simultaneous posteroventral pallidotomy in subgroups of patients with Parkinson's disease. *Stereotactic Functional Neurosurgery, 65,* 6–9.

Iacono, R. P., Shima, F., Lonser, R., Kuniyoshi, S., Maeda, G., & Yamada, S. (1995b). The results, indications, and physiology of posteroventral pallidotomy for patients with Parkinson's disease. *Neurosurgery, 3,* 1118–1125.

Jenkins, A. C. (1968). Speech defects following stereotaxic operations for the relief of tremor and rigidity in parkinsonism. *Medical Journal of Australia, 1,* 585–588.

Jiang, J., Lin, E., & Hanson, D. G. (2000). Acoustic and airflow spectral analysis of voice tremor. *Journal of Speech, Language and Hearing Research, 43,* 191–204.

Jiang, J., Lin, E., Wang, J., & Hanson, D. G. (1999). Glottographic measures before and after levodopa treatment in Parkinson's disease. *Laryngoscope, 109,* 1287–1294.

Jobst, E. E., Melnick, M. E., Byl, N. N., Dowling, G. A., & Aminoff, M. J. (1997). Sensory perception in Parkinson's disease. *Archives of Neurology, 54,* 450–454.

Kent, R. D., & Rosenbek, J. C. (1982). Prosodic disturbance and neurological lesion. *Brain and Language, 15,* 259–291.

Kent, R. D., Vorperian, H. K., Kent, J. F., & Duffy, J. R. (2003). Voice dysfunction in dysarthria: Application of the multidimensional voice program. *Journal of Communication Disorders, 36,* 281–306.

Kiran, S., & Larson, C. R. (2001). Effect of duration of pitch-shifted feedback on vocal responses in patients with Parkinson's disease. *Journal of Speech, Language, and Hearing Research, 44,* 975–987.

Kleiner-Fisman, G., Herzog, L., Fisman, D. N., Tamma, F., Lyons, K. E., Pahwa, R., Lang, A., & Deuschl, G. (2006). Subthalamic nucleus deep brain stimulation: Summary and meta-analysis of outcomes. *Movement Disorders, 21*(Suppl. 14), S290–S304.

Klostermann, F., Ehlen, F., Vesper, J., Nubel, K., Gross, M., Marzinzik, F., Curio, G., & Tanja, S. (2008). Effects of subthalamic deep brain stimulation on dysarthrophonia in Parkinson's disease. *Journal of Neurology, Neurosurgery, and Psychiatry, 79,* 522–529.

Koller, W. C. (1984). Sensory symptoms in PD. *Neurology, 43,* 957–959.

Kompoliti, K., Wang, Q. E., Goetz, C. G., Leurgans, S., & Raman, R. (2000). Effects of central dopaminergic stimulation by apomorphine on speech in Parkinson's disease. *Neurology, 54,* 458–462.

Krack, P., Batir, A., Van Blercom, N., Chabardes, S., Fraix, V., Ardouin, C., . . . Pollak, P. (2003). Five-year follow-up of bilateral stimulation of the subthalamic nucleus in advanced Parkinson's disease. *New England Journal of Medicine, 349,* 1925–1934.

Kruel, E. J. (1972). Neuromuscular control examination (NMC) for parkinsonism: Vowel prolongations and diadochokinetic and reading rates. *Journal of Speech and Hearing Research, 15,* 72–83.

Kumar, R., Lozano, A. M., Montgomery, E., & Lang, A. E. (1998). Pallidotomy and deep brain stimulation of the pallidum and subthalamic nucleus in advanced Parkinson's disease. *Movement Disorders, 13* (Suppl. 1), 73–82.

Laitinen, L. V., Bergenheim, A. T., & Hariz, M. I. (1992). Ventroposterolateral pallidotomy can abolish all parkinsonian symptoms. *Stereotactic Functional Neurosurgery, 58,* 14–21.

LaPointe, L. L., & Horner, J. (1981). Palilalia: A descriptive study of pathological reiterative utterances. *Journal of Speech and Hearing Research, 46,* 34–38.

Leanderson, R., Meyerson, B. A., & Persson, A. (1971). Effect of levodopa on speech in parkinsonism. An EMG study of labial articulatory function. *Journal of Neurology, Neurosurgery and Psychiatry, 34,* 679–681.

Lee, V. S., Zhou, X. P., Rahn, D. A., Wang, E. Q., & Jiang, J. J. (2008). Perturbation and nonlinear dynamic analysis of acoustic phonatory signal in parkinsonian patients receiving deep brain stimulation. *Journal of Communication Disorders, 41,* 485–500.

Linhares, M. N., & Tasker, R. R. (2000). Microelectrode-guided thalamotomy for Parkinson's disease. *Neurosurgery, 46,* 390–395.

Liotti, M., Ramig, L. O., Vogel, D., New, P., Cook, C. I., Ingham, R. J., . . . Fox, P. T. (2003). Hypophonia in Parkinson's disease: Neural correlates of voice treatment revealed by PET. *Neurology, 60,* 432–440.

Logemann, J. A., Boshes, B., & Fisher, H. B. (1973). The steps in the degeneration of speech and voice control in Parkinson's disease. In J. Siegfried (Ed.), *Parkinson's disease: Rigidity, akinesia, behavior* (pp. 101–112). Vienna, Austria: Hans Huber.

Logemann, J. A., & Fisher, H. B. (1981). Vocal tract control in Parkinson's disease: Phonetic feature analysis of misarticulations. *Journal of Speech and Hearing Disorders, 46,* 348–352.

Logemann, J. A., Fisher, H. B., Boshes, B., & Blonsky, E. R. (1978). Frequency and cooccurrence of vocal tract dysfunctions in the speech of a large sample of Parkinson patients. *Journal of Speech and Hearing Disorders, 43,* 47–57.

Louis, E. D., Winfield, L., Fahn, S., & Ford, B. (2001). Speech dysfluency exacerbated by levodopa in Parkinson's disease. *Movement Disorders, 16,* 562–565.

Ludlow, C. L., & Bassich, C. J. (1983). The results of acoustic and perceptual assessment of two types of dysarthria. In W. R. Berry (Ed.), *Clinical dysarthria* (pp. 121–153). San Diego, CA: College-Hill Press.

Ludlow, C. L., & Bassich, C. J. (1984). Relationships between perceptual ratings and acoustic measures of hypokinetic speech. In M. R. McNeil, J. C. Rosenbek, & A. E. Aronson (Eds.), *The dysarthrias: Physiology, acoustics, perception, management* (pp. 163–195). San Diego, CA: College-Hill Press.

Ludlow, C. L., Connor, N. P., & Bassich, C. J. (1987). Speech timing in Parkinson's and Huntington's disease. *Brain and Language, 32,* 195–214.

Luschei, E. S., Ramig, L. O., Baker, K. L., & Smith, M. E. (1999). Discharge characteristics of laryngeal single motor units during phonation in young and older adults and in persons with Parkinson's disease. *Journal of Neurophysiology, 81,* 2131–2139.

Matsumoto, K., Asano, T., Baba, T., Miyamoto, T., & Ohmoto, T. (1976). Long-term follow-up results of bilateral thalamotomy for parkinsonism. *Applied Neurophysiology, 39,* 257–260.

McAuliffe, M. J., Ward, E. C., Murdoch, B. E., & Farrell, A. M. (2005). A nonspeech investigation of tongue function in Parkinson's disease. *Journal of Gerontology, 60,* 667–674.

Merchant, H., Luciana, M., Hooper, C., Majestic, S., & Tuite, P. (2008). Interval timing and Parkinson's disease: Heterogeneity in temporal performance. *Experimental Brain Research, 184,* 233–248.

Metter, J. E., & Hanson, W. R. (1986). Clinical and acoustical variability in hypokinetic dysarthria. *Journal of Communication Disorders, 19*, 347–366.

Miller, N., Allcock, L., Jones, D., Noble, E., Hildreth, A. J., & Burn, D. J. (2007). Prevalence and pattern of perceived intelligibility changes in Parkinson's disease. *Journal of Neurology, Neurosurgery, and Psychiatry, 78*, 1188–1190.

Miller, N., Noble, E., Jones, D., Allcock, L., & Burn, D. J. (2008). How do I sound to me? Perceived changes in communication in Parkinson's disease. *Clinical Rehabilitation, 22*, 14–22.

Miller, N., Noble, E., Jones, D., & Burn, D. (2006). Life with communication changes in Parkinson's disease. *Age and Ageing, 35*, 235–239.

Moon, B., Adams, S. G., & Jog, M. (2006). Effects of background noise, listener context, speech task, and requests for clarification of on speech intensity in Parkinson's disease. *Stem-Sprak-en Taalpathologie, 14*, 84.

Moore, C. A., & Scudder, R. R. (1989). Coordination of jaw muscle activity parkinsonian movement: Description and response to traditional treatment. In K. M. Yorkston & D. R. Beukelman (Eds.), *Recent advances in clinical dysarthria* (pp. 147–163). Boston, MA: College-Hill.

Moreau, C., Ozsancak, C., Blatt, J-L., Derambure, P., Destee, A., & Defebvre, L. (2007). Oral festination in Parkinson's disease: Biomechanical analysis and correlation with festination and freezing of gait. *Movement Disorders, 22*, 1503–1506.

Moretti, R., Torre, P., Antonello, R. M., Capus, L., Gioulis, M., Zambito Marsala, S., Cazzato, G., & Bava, A. (2003). "Speech initiation hesitation" following subthalamic nucleus stimulation in a patient with Parkinson's disease. *European Neurology, 49*, 251–253.

Moro, E., Poon, Y. Y. W., Lozano, A.M., Saint-Cyr, J. A., & Lang, A. E. (2006). Subthalamic nucleus stimulation: Improvements in outcome with reprogramming. *Archives of Neurology, 63*, 1266–1272.

Mueller, P. B. (1971). Parkinson's disease: Motor-speech behaviour in a selected group of patients. *Folia Phoniatrica, 23*, 333–346.

Murdoch, B. E., Chenery, H. J., Bowler, S., & Ingram, J. C. (1989). Respiratory function in Parkinson's subjects exhibiting a perceptible speech deficit: A kinematic and spirometric analysis. *Journal of Speech and Hearing Disorders, 54*, 610–626.

Murdoch, B. E., Manning, C. Y., Theodoros, D. G., & Thompson, E. C. (1997). Laryngeal and phonatory dysfunction in Parkinson's disease. *Clinical Linguistics and Phonetics, 11*, 245–266.

Nakano, K. K., Zubick, H., & Tyler, H. R. (1973). Speech defects of parkinsonian patients: Effects of levodopa therapy on speech intelligibility. *Neurology, 23*, 865–870.

Narayana, S., Jacks, A., Robin, D. A., Poizner, H., Zhang, W., Franklin, C., . . . Fox, P. T. (2009). A non-invasive imaging approach to understanding speech changes following deep brain stimulation in Parkinson's disease. *American Journal of Speech-Language Pathology, 18*, 146–161.

Netsell, R., Daniel, B., & Celesia, G. G. (1975). Acceleration and weakness in parkinsonian dysarthria. *Journal of Speech and Hearing Disorders, 40*, 170–178.

Nijkrake, M. J., Keus, S. H. J., Oostendorp, R. A. B., Overeem, S., Mulleners, W., Bloem, B. R., & Munneke, M. (2008). Allied health care in Parkinson's disease: Referral, consultation, and professional expertise. *Movement Disorders, 24,* 282–286.

Noble, E., Jones, D., Miller, N., & Burn, D. (2006). Speech and language therapy provision for people with Parkinson's disease. *International Journal of Therapy and Rehabilitation, 13,* 323–327.

Ostergaard, K., & Sunde, N. A. (2006). Evolution of Parkinson's disease during 4 years of bilateral deep brain stimulation of the subthalamic nucleus. *Movement Disorders, 21,* 624–631.

Pell, M. D., & Leonard, C. L. (2003). Processing emotional tone from speech in Parkinson's disease: A role for the basal ganglia. *Cognitive, Affective, and Behavioral Neuroscience, 3,* 275–288.

Pentland, B (1987). The effects of reduced expression in Parkinson's disease on impression formation by health professionals. *Clinical Rehabilitation, 1,* 307–313.

Perez, K. S., Ramig, L. O., Smith, M. E., & Dromey, C. (1996). The Parkinson larynx: Tremor and videostroboscopic findings. *Journal of Voice, 10,* 354–361.

Petrovici, J. N. (1980). Speech disturbances following stereotaxic surgery in ventrolateral thalamus. *Neurosurgical Review, 3,* 189–195.

Pinto, S., Gentil, M., Krack, P., Sauleau, P., Fraix, V., Benabid, A-L., & Pollak, P. (2005). Changes induced by levodopa and subthalamic nucleus stimulation on parkinsonian speech. *Movement Disorders, 20,* 1507–1515.

Pinto, S., Ozsancak, C., Tripoliti, E., Thobois, S., Limousin-Dowsey, P., & Azou, P. (2004). Treatments for dysarthria in Parkinson's disease. *Lancet Neurology, 3,* 547–556.

Pitcairn, T. K., Clemie, S., Gray, J. M., & Pentland, B. (1990). Impressions of parkinsonian patients from their recorded voices. *British Journal of Disorders of Communication, 25,* 85–92.

Plowman-Prine, E. K., Okun, M. S., Sapienza, C. M., Shrivastav, R., Fernandez, H. H., Foote, K. D., . . . Rosenbek, J. C. (2009). Perceptual characteristics of Parkinsonian speech: A comparison of the pharmacological effects of levodopa across speech and non-speech motor systems. *NeuroRehabilitation, 24,* 131–144.

Poluha, P. C., Teulings, H. L., & Brookshire, R. H. (1998). Handwriting and speech changes across the levodopa cycle in Parkinson's disease. *Acta Psychologica, 100,* 71–84.

Putzer, M., Barry, W. J., & Moringlane, J. R. (2008). Effect of bilateral stimulation of the subthalmic nucleus on different speech subsystems in patients with Parkinson's disease. *Clinical Linguistics and Phonetics, 22,* 957–973.

Ramig, L. O. (1992). The role of phonation in speech intelligibility: A review and preliminary data from patients with Parkinson's disease. In R. Kent (Ed.), *Intelligibility in speech disorders: Theory, measurement, and management* (pp. 119–155). Amsterdam, the Netherlands: John Benjamin.

Ramig, L. O., Sapir, S., Countryman, S., Pawlas, A. A., O'Brien, C., Hoehn, M., & Thompson, L.L. (2001). Intensive voice treatment (LSVT) for patients with

Parkinson's disease: A 2-year follow-up. *Journal of Neurology, Neurosurgery and Psychiatry, 71*, 493–498.
Rascol, O., Payoux, P., Ory, F., Ferreira, J. J., Brefel-Courbon, C., & Montastruc, J. L. (2003). Limitations of current Parkinson's disease therapy. *Annals of Neurology, 53* (Suppl. 3), S3–S12.
Robbins, J. A., Logemann, J. A., & Kirshner, H. S. (1986). Swallowing and speech production in Parkinson's disease. *Annals of Neurology, 19*, 283–287.
Robertson, D. (1988). Parkinson's disease: Does speech therapy work and defining the problems. *Speech Therapy in Practice, 4*, 18–19.
Robertson, D. (2006). Maintaining the art of conversation in Parkinson's disease. *Age and Ageing, 35*, 211.
Rodriguez-Oroz, M. C., Obeso, J. A., Lang, A. E., Houeto, J. L., Pollak, P., Rehncrona, S., & Van Blercom, N. (2005). Bilateral deep brain stimulation in Parkinson's disease: A multicentre study with 4 years follow-up. *Brain, 128*, 2240–2249.
Rosen, K. M., Kent, R. D., & Duffy, J. R. (2005). Task-based profile of vocal intensity decline in Parkinson's disease. *Folia Phoniatrica et Logopaedica, 57*, 28–37.
Rousseaux, M., Krystkowiak, P., Kozlowski, O., Ozsancak, C., Blond, S., & Destee, A. (2004). Effects of subthalamic nucleus stimulation on parkinsonian dysarthria and speech intelligibility. *Journal of Neurology, 251*, 327–334.
Sanabria, J., Ruiz, P. G., Gutierrez, R., Marquez, F., Escobar, P., Gentil, M., & Cenjor, C. (2001). The effect of levodopa on vocal function in Parkinson's disease. *Clinical Neuropharmacology, 24*, 99–102.
Sandyk, R., & Brennan, M. J. (1982). Impairment of somatosensory feedback control of the tongue in Parkinson's disease: Effect of L-dopa therapy. *South African Journal of Communication Disorders, 29*, 49–54.
Santens, P., De Letter, M., Van Borsel, J., De Reuck, J., & Caemaert, J. (2003). Lateralized effects of subtnalamic nucleus stimulation on different aspects of speech in Parkinson's disease. *Brain and Language, 87*, 253–258.
Sapir, S., Ramig, L., & Fox, C. (2008). Speech and swallowing disorders in Parkinson's disease. *Current Opinion in Otolaryngology and Head and Neck Surgery, 16*, 205–210.
Sapir, S., Ramig, L. O., Spielman, J. L., & Fox, C. (2010). Formant Centralization Ratio (FCR): A proposal for a new acoustic measure of dysarthric speech. *Journal of Speech and Hearing Research*. Epub ahead of print.
Sapir, S., Spielman, J., Ramig, L., Story, B., & Fox, C. (2007).Effects of intensive voice treatment (LSVT®) on vowel articulation in dysarthric individuals with idiopathic Parkinson disease: Acoustic and perceptual findings. *Journal of Speech and Hearing Research, 50*, 889–912.
Schneider, J. S., Diamond, S. G., & Markham, C. H. (1986). Deficits in orofacial sensorimotor function in Parkinson's disease. *Annals of Neurology, 19*, 275–282.
Schneider, J. S., & Lidsky, T. I. (1987). *Basal ganglia and behavior: Sensory aspects of motor functioning*. Toronto, Canada: Hans Huber.
Schrag, A., Jahanshahi, M., & Quinn, N. (2000). What contributes to quality of life in patients with Parkinson's disease? *Journal of Neurology, Neurosurgery, and Psychiatry, 69*, 308–312.

Schrag, A., Samuel, M., Caputo, E., Scaravilli, T., Troyer, M., Marsden, C. D., . . . Quinn, N. (1999). Unilateral pallidotomy for Parkinson's disease: Results after more than 1 year. *Journal of Neurology, Neurosurgery and Psychiatry, 67,* 511–517.

Schulz, G. M., & Grant, M. K. (2000). Effects of speech therapy and pharmacologic and surgical treatments on voice and speech in Parkinson's disease: A review of the literature. *Journal of Communication Disorders, 33,* 59–88.

Schulz, G. M., Greer, M., & Friedman, W. (2000). Changes in vocal intensity in Parkinson's disease following pallidotomy surgery. *Journal of Voice, 14,* 589–606.

Schulz, G. M., Peterson, T., Sapienza, C. M., Greer, M., & Friedman, W. (1999). Voice and speech characteristics of persons with Parkinson's disease pre- and post-pallidotomy surgery: Preliminary findings. *Journal of Speech, Language, and Hearing Research, 42,* 1176–1194.

Schuurman, P. R., Bosch, A., Bossuyt, P. M., & Bonsel, G. J., . . . (2000). A comparison of continuous thalamic stimulation and thalamotomy for suppression of severe tremor. *New England Journal of Medicine, 342,* 461–468.

Scott, S., Caird, F. I., & Williams, B. O. (1985). *Communication in Parkinson's disease.* London, UK: Croom Helm.

Scott, R., Gregory, R., Hines, N., Carroll, C., Hyman, N., Papanasstasiou, V., . . . Aziz, T. (1998). Neuropsychological, neurological and functional outcome following pallidotomy for Parkinson's disease. A consecutive series of eight simultaneous bilateral and twelve unilateral procedures. *Brain, 121,* 659–675.

Selby, G. (1967). Stereotactic surgery for the relief of Parkinson's disease: A critical review. *Journal of the Neurological Sciences, 5,* 315–342.

Shahed, J., & Jankovic, J. (2001). Re-emergence of childhood stuttering in Parkinson's disease: A hypothesis. *Movement Disorders, 16,* 114–118.

Skodda, S., & Schlegel, U. (2008). Speech rate and rhythm in Parkinson's disease. *Movement Disorders, 23,* 985–992.

Skodda, S., Visser, W., & Schlegel, U. (2010a). Vowel articulation in Parkinson's disease. *Journal of Voice.* Epub ahead of print.

Skodda, S., Visser, W., & Schlegel, U. (2010b). Short- and long-term dopaminergic effects on dysarthria in early Parkinson's disease. *Journal of Neural Transmission.* Epub ahead of print.

Solomon, N. P., & Hixon, T. J. (1993). Speech breathing in Parkinson's disease. *Journal of Speech and Hearing Research, 36,* 294–310.

Solomon, N. P., Lorell, D. M., Robin, D. A., Rodnitzky, R. L., & Luschei, E. S. (1995). Tongue strength and endurance in mild to moderate Parkinson's disease. *Journal of Medical Speech-Language Pathology, 3,* 15–26.

Solomon, N. P., Robin, D. A., & Luschei, E. S. (2000). Strength, endurance, and stability of the tongue and hand in Parkinson's disease. *Journal of Speech, Language, and Hearing Research, 43,* 256–267.

Spencer, K., Morgan, K., & Blond, E. (2009). Dopaminergic medication effects on the speech of individuals with Parkinson's disease. *Journal of Medical Speech-Language Pathology, 17,* 125–144.

Stewart, C. (2000). Speech-language therapy for patients with Parkinson's disease. In L. Cote, L. L. Sprinzeles, R. Elliott, & A. H. Kutscher (Eds.), *Parkinson's disease and quality of life* (pp. 151–156). New York, NY: Haworth Press.

Svensson, P., Henningson, C., & Karlsson, S. (1993). Speech motor control in Parkinson's disease: A comparison between a clinical assessment protocol and a quantitative analysis of mandibular movements. *Folia Phoniatrica (Basel), 45*, 157–164.

Tasker, R. R., DeCarvalho, G. C., Li, C. S., & Kestle, J. R. (1996). Does thalamotomy alter the course of Parkinson's disease? *Advances in Neurology, 69*, 563–583.

Tasker, R. R., Lang, A. E., & Lozano, A. M. (1997). Pallidal and thalamic surgery for Parkinson's disease. *Experimental Neurology, 144*, 35–40.

Theodoros, D. G., Constantinescu, G., Russell, T., Ward, E. C., Wilson, S. J., & Wootton, R. (2006). Treating the speech disorder in Parkinson's disease online. *Journal of Telemedicine and Telecare, 12* (Suppl. 3), 88–91.

Theodoros, D. G., Murdoch, B. E., & Thompson, E. C. (1995). Hypernasality in Parkinson's disease: A perceptual and physiological analysis. *Journal of Medical Speech-Language Pathology, 3*, 73–84.

Theodoros, D., & Russell, T. (2008). Telerehabilitation: Current perspectives. In R. Lafiti (Ed.), *Current principles and practices of telemedicine and E-health* (pp. 191–209). Amsterdam, the Netherlands: IOS Publishing.

Theodoros, D. G., Ward, E. C., Murdoch, B. E., Silburn, P., & Lethlean, J. (2000). The impact of pallidotomy on motor speech function in Parkinson's disease. *Journal of Medical Speech-Language Pathology, 8*, 315–322.

Tornqvist, A. V., Schalen, L., & Rehncrona, S. (2004). Effects of different electrical parameter settings on the intelligibility of speech in patients with Parkinson's disease treated with subthalamic deep brain stimulation. *Movement Disorders, 20*, 416–423.

Tripoliti, E., Zrinzo, L., Martinez-Torres, I., Tisch, S., Frost, E., Borrell, E., . . . Limousin, P. (2008). Effects of contact location and voltage amplitude on speech and movement in bilateral subthalamic nucleus deep brain stimulation. *Movement Disorders, 23*, 2377–2383.

Uitti, R. J., Wharen, R. E., Duffy, J. R., Lucas, J. A., Schneider, S. L., Rippeth, J. D., & Atkinson, E.J. (2000). Unilateral pallidotomy for Parkinson's disease: Speech, motor, and neuropsychological outcome measurements. *Parkinsonism and Related Disorders, 6*, 133–143.

Vincken, W. G., Gauthier, S. G., Dollfus, R. E., Hanson, R. E., Daraway, C. M., & Cosio, M.G. (1984). Involvement in upper airway muscles in extrapyramidal disorders, a cause of airflow limitation. *New England Journal of Medicine, 311*, 438–442.

Wang, Q. E., Kompoliti, K., Jiang, J., & Goetz, C. (2000). An instrumental analysis of laryngeal response to apomorphine stimulation in Parkinson's disease. *Journal of Medical Speech-Language Pathology, 8*, 175–186.

Wang, E. Q., Metman, L. V., Bakay, R. A. E., Arzbaecher, J., & Bernard, B. (2003). The effect if unilateral electrostimulation of the subthalamic nucleus on respiratory/phonatory subsystems of speech production in Parkinson's disease—a preliminary report. *Clinical Linguistics and Phonetics, 17,* 283–289.

Wang, E. Q., Metman, L. V., Bakay, R. A. E., Arzbaecher, J., Bernard, B., & Corcos, D. M. (2006). Hemisphere-specific effects of subthalamic nucleus deep brain stimulation on speaking rate and articulatory accuracy of syllable repetitions in Parkinson' disease. *Journal of Medical Speech-Language Pathology, 14,* 323–334.

Ward, E. C., Theodoros, D. G., Murdoch, B. E., & Cahill, L. M. (1999). The use of a miniature lip transducer system in the assessment of patients with Parkinson's disease. *Journal of Medical Speech-Language Pathology, 7,* 175–179.

Weismer, G. (1984). Articulatory characteristics of parkinsonian dysarthria: Segmental and phrase-level timing, spirantization, and glottal-supraglottal coordination. In M. R. McNeil, J. C. Rosenbek, & A. E. Aronson (Eds.), *The dysarthrias: Physiology, acoustics, perception, management* (pp. 101–130). San Diego, CA: College-Hill.

Weismer, G., Jeng, J. Y., Laures, J. S., Kent, R. D., & Kent, J. F. (2001). Acoustic and intelligibility characteristics of sentence production in neurogenic speech disorders. *Folia Phoniatrica et Logopaedica, 53,* 1–18.

Wolfe, V. I., Garvin, J. S., Bacon, M., & Waldrop, W. (1975). Speech changes in Parkinson's disease during treatment with L-dopa. *Journal of Communication Disorders, 8,* 271–279.

Yorkston, K. M. (2007). The degenerative dysarthrias: A window into critical clinical and research issues. *Folia Phoniatrica et Logopaedica, 59,* 107–117.

Zwirner, P., & Barnes, G. J. (1992). Vocal tract steadiness: A measure of phonatory and upper airway motor control during phonation in dysarthria. *Journal of Speech and Hearing Research, 35,* 761–768.

4

Assessment and Treatment of the Speech Disorder in Parkinson Disease

SHIMON SAPIR
LORRAINE RAMIG
CYNTHIA FOX

As discussed in Chapter 3, speech disorders associated with PD may include: reduced vocal loudness (hypophonia), with a tendency for the voice to decay or fade out; reduced prosodic pitch inflection (monotone, hypoprosodia); breathy, harsh, or hoarse voice; imprecise articulation of consonants and vowels; and dysfluent, hesitant, or mumbled speech. Collectively, these speech abnormalities in PD have been termed *hypokinetic dysarthria* (Darley, Aronson, & Brown, 1969a, 1969b). Several studies have indicated that voice abnormalities may appear early in the course of the disease, whereas speech articulation and fluency problems may occur in more advanced stages of the disease (Cramer 1940; Ho, Iansek, Marigliani, Bradshaw, & Gates, 1998; Logemann, Boshes, & Fisher, 1973; Logemann, Fisher, Boshes, & Blonsky, 1978; Sapir, Pawlas, Ramig, Countryman, O'Brien, Hoehn, & Thompson, 2001; Stewart et al., 1995). However, recent studies suggest that speech articulation problems, although subtle or imperceptible to the listener, might also be present in early stages of the disease (Miller, Noble, Jones, Allcock, & Burn, 2008; Skodda, Visser, & Schlegel, 2010).

Assessment of the Speech Disorder

The diagnosis of hypokinetic dysarthria in PD is commonly made by a speech pathologist/clinician who routinely uses perceptual measures (Baumgartner, Sapir, & Ramig, 2001; Sapir, Ramig, Hoyt, O'Brien, & Hoehn, 2002) to assess the integrity and coordination of the speech production subsystems (respiration, phonation, articulation, velopharyngeal function). Perceptual analyses include a qualitative impression and rating of vocal loudness, pitch, and quality, prosodic variation, articulation, and rate and fluency of speech. The speech clinician assesses the impact of these percepts on speech clarity and/or intelligibility and their overall impact on functional and effective communication (Ramig, 1992). Acoustic analysis potentially can provide an objective, noninvasive, quantitative, reliable, and precise means to index the characteristics and severity of hypokinetic dysarthria in PD, and to monitor changes associated with treatment effects or progression of the disease (Sapir, Ramig, Spielman, & Fox, 2010; Sapir, Spielman, Ramig, Story, & Fox, 2007). Thus, for example, measures of vocal sound pressure level (vocSPL), voice fundamental frequency (F_0), phonatory stability (indexed by jitter, shimmer, harmonics-to-noise ratio), and various measures of articulatory acoustics (e.g., voice onset time, spirantization, formant frequencies, and transitions, and more complex indices such vowel space area, formant centralization ratio, vowel articulation index) are used to supplement the perceptual evaluation of the hypokinetic dysarthria in PD (Ackerman & Ziegler, 1991; Forrest, Weismer, & Turner, 1989; Fox & Ramig, 1997; King, Ramig, Lemke, & Horii, 1994; Ramig, Scherer, Titze, & Ringel, 1988; Sapir et al., 2007; Sapir, Ramig, Spielman, & Fox, 2010b; Winholtz & Ramig 1992).

Physiologic measures of speech have also been implemented to provide more specific information about the neurophysiologic and biomechanical abnormalities underlying the hypokinetic dysarthria. Such measures have been obtained using kinematic and/or electromyographic analyses of lips, jaw, tongue, velopharyngeal, and respiratory movements (Baker, Ramig, Johnson, & Freed, 1997; Baker, Ramig, Luschei, & Smith, 1998; Huber, Stathopoulos, Ramig, & Lancaster, 2003; Kleinow, Smith, & Ramig, 2001; Luschei, Ramig, Baker, Baker, & Smith, 1999; Solomon & Hixon, 1993), and videostroboscopic analyses of vocal fold vibrations and closure (Perez, Ramig, Smith, & Dromey, 1996; Smith, Ramig, Dromey, Perez, & Samandari, 1995;). When perceptual, acoustic, and physiologic measures of speech production are combined, they are likely to yield a detailed, comprehensive, quantitative and qualitative description of the speech disorder across the course of the disease and in response to treatment.

Brain imaging and neurophysiologic studies of sensorimotor, linguistic, and cognitive aspects of speech production in individuals with PD are also likely to improve diagnosis and treatment of the dysarthria (Liotti et al., 2003; Narayana et al., 2010; Rektorova, Barrett, Mikl, Rektor, & Paus, 2007). Outcomes following deep brain stimulation (DBS) may provide additional information about the neuropathology and neural mechanisms underlying the speech disorder in PD (Gentil, Chauvin, Pinto, Pollak, & Benabid 2001; Gentil, Garcia-Ruiz, Pollak, & Benabid, 2000; Gentil, Pinto, Pollak, & Benabid, 2003; Klosterman et al., 2008; Pinto, Gentil, Fraix, Benabid, & Pollak, 2003; Pitcairn, Clemie, Gray, & Pentland, 1990; Stewart et al., 1995; Tripoliti et al., 2008).

To assess the nature and severity of the dysarthria in individuals with PD, it is extremely important to employ a range of speech tasks because the speech abnormalities in PD tend to vary considerably as a function of the task being performed and the environment in which the communication interaction occurs (Ackerman & Ziegler 1991; Caligiuri, 1989; Kempler & Van Lankcer, 2002; Rosen, Kent, & Duffy, 2005). For example, the speech disorder in PD often is worse during conversational speech or rapid repetition of syllables, compared to when reading aloud a list of words or a paragraph, or when purposefully attempting to slow the rate of speech, or attempting to speak clearly (Ackerman & Ziegler, 1991; Caligiuri, 1989; Goberman & Elmer, 2005; Hammen, Yorkston, & Minifie, 1994; Hammen & Yorkston, 1996; Kempler & Van Lancker, 2002; Rosen et al., 2005). As for the communicative environment, individuals with PD may be heard and understood in the quiet medical examination room when answering short interview questions, but this situation often is not representative of their spontaneous speech production in daily living, where conversations tend to occur in noisy situations and under cognitively demanding tasks. Thus, optimal assessment of speech function in individuals with PD requires the testing of speech with different tasks that provide insight into breakdowns in the subsystems of speech production, simultaneously evaluating speech functions and intelligibility under the daily challenges of everyday communication. Specific speech tasks to be used include sustained vowel phonation; syllable repetition (diadochokinetic articulatory movements); reading words, sentences, or paragraphs aloud; describing a picture; and engaging in conversational speech. These speech tasks may be performed with dual cognitive or motor tasks, to simulate challenges of functional communication. These speech tasks may be tested at different levels of loudness and clarity to assess the severity of the speech impairment. Assessment should test the individual's speech performance when he or she is externally cued as well as when the speech system is maximally taxed (Ho, Bradshaw, Iansek, & Alfredson, 1999a; Tjaden & Wilding, 2004).

Assessment of the Speech Disorder in Parkinson Disease

PERCEPTUAL	ACOUSTIC
Ratings of:	
■ Vocal loudness	■ Vocal sound pressure level (vocSPL)
■ Pitch level	■ Voice fundamental frequency (F_0)
■ Vocal quality	■ Phonatory stability (jitter, shimmer, harmonic to noise ratio)
■ Prosodic variation	■ Standard deviation of SPL, F_0, vowel duration, and pauses
■ Articulation	■ Spirantization, voice onset time, formant centralization ratio, vowel articulation index, F2i/F2u ratio, formant transition, vowel space area
■ Fluency	■ Abnormally long pauses, repetition of vowels and consonants
■ Rate	■ Number of speech segments (phonemes, syllables, words) per minute
■ Intelligibility	■ Combination of the above
■ Overall functional communication level	
PHYSIOLOGIC	
■ Kinematic and electromyographic assessment of speech movements	■ Videostroboscopic analyses of vocal fold vibration and closure
BRAIN IMAGING AND NEUROPHYSIOLOGIC ASSESSMENT	
■ Sensorimotor, linguistic and cognitive aspects of speech	■ Positron Emision Tomography (PET) ■ Functional Magnetic Resonance Imaging (fMRI)

Treatment of the Speech Disorder

Effective treatment is likely to occur when it is theoretically driven and empirically based. Traditionally, hypokinetic dysarthria has been attributed to hypokinetic and bradykinetic movements, both associated with dopamine deficiency and muscle rigidity (Flint, Black, Campbell-Taylor, Gailey, & Levinton, 1993; Hanson, Gerratt, & Ward, 1984; Sanabria et al., 2001). However, as discussed in Chapter 3 and elsewhere (Ramig, Fox, & Sapir, 2008; Sapir, Ramig, & Fox, 2008a; 2008b), the role of dopamine and muscle rigidity in the etiology of hypokinetic dysarthria is far from clear (Kompoliti, Wang, Goetz, Leurgans, & Raman, 2000); also, many symptoms and signs of PD are likely to be related to nondopaminergic or special dopaminergic mechanisms (Ahlskog, 2007; Ramig, Fox, & Sapir, in press); thus, there is a need for alternative explanations to account for the speech abnormalities associated with PD.

As 89% of individuals with PD have a speech or voice disorder that may impact quality of life (Logemann et al., 1978; Miller, Noble, Jones & Burn, 2006b), the effects of behavioral treatment on the speech disorder in PD is of critical importance. It is well known that, when an individual with PD and hypokinetic dysarthria is instructed to speak loudly and clearly, his or her speech tends to improve considerably (Dromey & Ramig, 1998; Dromey, Ramig, & Johnson, 1995; Goberman & Elmer, 2005; Ho et al., 1999a). However, this improvement is likely to be short-lived and dependent on external cuing. Thus, for treatment of hypokinetic dysarthria to be considered efficacious, speech should be performed by the individual with PD at his or her optimal physiologic capacity, and this performance should be carried out consistently, by the individual's reliance on his or her own self-regulatory resources (internal cuing), rather than on instructions or other external cues. Such efficacious treatment is challenging, yet possible, when the treatment is directed to the disordered neurophysiologic mechanisms that are presumed to underlie the hypokinetic dysarthria and is based on principles of neural plasticity (Kleim & Jones, 2008).

In the following section, a model representing one perspective on the main aberrant neurophysiologic mechanisms that underlie hypokinetic dysarthria in PD is presented. The principles of neural plasticity and their relationship to LSVT LOUD are summarized in Table 4–1. This information will be integrated as a rationale for the treatment approach, the Lee Silverman Voice Treatment (LSVT LOUD). LSVT LOUD and its scientific efficacy will be reviewed. New computer and Internet technology to make the LSVT LOUD more accessible is described. The importance of early intervention for an effective treatment of hypokinetic dysarthria is emphasized.

Table 4–1. Translation of Principles of Neural Plasticity (Column 1) to Proposed Deficits in Parkinson Disease (Column 2) and the Corresponding Rationale and Task in LSVT LOUD (Column 3).

INTENSITY (Fisher et al, 2004; Pisani et al., 2005		
Principle	**Deficit Specific to PD**	**Speech Treatment**
Intensive practice is important for maximal plasticity. Intensity can be increased via frequency, repetitions, force/resistance, effort, and accuracy. Intensity increases activation of corticostriatal terminals inducing synaptic plasticity in striatum.	Intensive, high effort training can be difficult in PD due to sensory deficits, force control, fatigue, depression, and progressive loss of cardiac sympathetic innervation.	Train intensively 1-hour/day, 4 days/week, for 4 weeks; multiple repetitions (15 or more); increase resistance, amplitude (within healthy range) effort, accuracy; and daily homework exercises. Train maximum perceived effort.
USE IT OR LOSE IT/ USE IT AND IMPROVE IT (Jones et al., 1999; Kliem et al., 2003; Tillerson et al., 2002)		
Principle	**Deficit Specific to PD**	**Speech Treatment**
Spared, but compromised DA neurons highly vulnerable to bouts of inactivity/activity. Inactivity may accelerate deficits. Postexercise intervention, there may be a minimum use requirement to maintain positive effects.	Deficits are subtle—not "red flag" to seek speech therapy. Getting early PD to recognize need for exercise and then convincing them to continually exercise is challenging. Decreased physical activity may be a catalyst in degenerative process.	Educate people with PD on subtle deficits and improve motor function that directly impacts real life. Retrain a new way of speaking everyday life (HEALTHY LOUDNESS); normal activity offers continuous exercise.
SALIENCY (Alexander et al., 1990; Graybiel, 1998; Fox et al., 2002; Liotti et al., 2003)		
Principle	**Deficit Specific to PD**	**Speech Treatment**
Practicing rewarding tasks (success/emotionally salient) activates basal ganglia circuitry. Rewards are associated with phasic modulation of DA levels critical to induction of striatal plasticity and learning/relearning in PD.	People with early PD may experience lack of awareness of subtle motor deficits, depression, loss of motivation and a feeling of "helplessness." Thus, they do not feel they need, or would not benefit from speech therapy.	Train salient familiar movements (core patterns) of speech promoting success. Provide homework tasks that reinforce success of HEALTHY LOUDNESS in emotional social interactions. Provide extensive positive feedback.

COMPLEXITY (Brown & Marsden, 1991; Comery, 1995; Kleim et al., 1996; Plautz et al., 2000; Ramig et al., 1995)		
Principle	**Deficit Specific to PD**	**Speech Treatment**
Complex movements or environmental enrichment have been shown to promote greater structural plasticity (spine density, protein expression/ synapse number) in adjacent, and remote interconnected regions than simple movements	As basal ganglia pathology progresses, there is a loss in automaticity requiring greater conscious attention to task. When required to perform dual tasks, insufficient attentional resources results in the decrement in one or both of the concurrent tasks.	Train complexity of movement with single patient focus to multiple, motor tasks. Retrain automaticity of amplitude (HEALTHY LOUDNESS) in familiar movements. Progress complexity over 4 weeks by varying contexts, adding dual cognitive/motor loads, and increasing duration and difficulty of speech tasks (progress from words to conversation).
TIMING MATTERS (Faherty et al., 2005; Jones et al, 1999; Tillerson et al., 2001, 2003)		
Principle	**Deficit Specific to PD**	**Speech Treatment**
Early exercise has the potential to: rescue DA neurons, prevent chronic disuse, promote system-wide plasticity, and halt disease progression—particularly to the aymptomatic side.	People with early PD have subtle physical under activity (small movements/soft voice). This may be coupled with a lack of awareness or self-correction, leading to further inactivity.	Train people with early PD when they may not have deficits in all systems (laryngeal and orofacial). Train strategies to raise awareness/avoid neglect and increase muscle activation for normal effort/amplitude (HEALTHY LOUDNESS).

Major Deficits Underlying Hypokinetic Dysarthria in PD

Abnormal Scaling and Maintenance of Movement

There is evidence for reduced range (hypokinesia) of respiratory, laryngeal, and orofacial movements during speech sound production in dysarthric speakers with PD, with the tendency for the amplitude of the movements to decay (become more hypokinetic) within and across utterances (Ackermann & Ziegler, 1991; Caligiuri, 1989; Forrest et al., 1989; Ho, Iansek, & Bradshaw, 2001; Rosen et al., 2005). This reduction in amplitude may manifest as a systematic decrease and fading away of vocal loudness, reduced pitch intonation, and imprecision of vowels, consonants, and other sounds of speech (Forrest et al., 1989; Liss, Spitzer, Caviness, & Adler, 2002; Rosen et al., 2005; Sapir et al., 2007; Sapir et al., 2010b; Skodda, Rinsche, & Schlegel, 2009, Skodda et al., 2010). It has been suggested that these hypokinetic abnormalities in PD are related, at least partially, to the inability of the speaker to scale and/or maintain movement amplitude, force, or related parameters (Bartels, & Leenders, 2009; Demirci, Grill, McShane, & Hallett, 1995; Desmurget, Grafton, Vindras, Gréa, & Turner, 2003; Desmurget, Grafton, Vindras, Gréa, & Turner, 2004; Hallet, 1997; Ho et al., 2001; Morris, Iansek, Matyas, & Summers, 1998). Although the pathologic mechanisms underlying such underscaling and poor maintenance of movement amplitude or force in speech production are not clear, they likely share the same striatofrontal network mechanisms that underlie other motor dysfunctions, such as micrographia (abnormally small handwriting) and the small, shuffling gait characteristic of PD (Ho et al., 2001). As discussed below, underscaling movement amplitude may be secondary to abnormal processing of temporal and/or sensory information, and/or to deficits in internal cuing.

Abnormal Sensory Processing

In individuals with PD, there is evidence for sensorimotor deficits in the phonatory (Hammer & Barlow, 2010) and orofacial systems (Caligiuri & Abbs, 1987; Diamond, Schneider, & Markham, 1987; Schneider, Diamond, & Markham, 1986; Schneider & Lidsky, 1987) as well as abnormal sensory processing of voice and speech (Ackermann & Ziegler, 1991; Graber, Hertrich, Daum, Spieker, & Ackermann, 2002; Ho et al., 1999a; Ho, Bradshaw, & Iansek, 2000; Ho, Iansek, & Bradshaw, 1999b; Schneider et al., 1986; Schneider & Lidsky, 1987; Solomon, Robin, Lorell, Rodnitzky, & Luschei, 1994). Specifically, behavioral and physiologic studies of speech, oral, and head and neck functions in PD have demonstrated sensory abnormalities manifested as errors on tasks of kinesthesia (Demirci, Grill, McShane, & Hallett, 1997; Jobst, Melnick, Byl, Dowling, & Aminoff, 1997; Klockgether, Borutta, Rapp, Spieder, & Dichgans, 1997); difficulties with orofacial perception, including decreased jaw proprioception; tactile localization on tongue, gums, and teeth; and targeted and tracking head movements to perioral stimulation (Schneider et al., 1986); problems utilizing proprioceptive information for normal movement (Schneider et al., 1986; Jobst et al., 1997); and abnormal higher order processing of afferent information as demonstrated by abnormal reflex and voluntary motor responses to proprioceptive input (Rickards & Cody, 1997). There also is evidence for hypertonicity or hypotonicity in the phonatory (Baker et al., 1998; Gallena, Smith, Zeffiro, & Ludlow, 2001) and articulatory musculature (Caligiuri & Abbs, 1987), which suggests aberrant gating of sensory information. Collectively, these findings suggest that one aspect of disordered speech in PD might include complex deficits in the utilization of specific sensory inputs to organize and guide speech movements.

These deficits in sensory processing may account, at least partially, for deficits individuals with PD have in adequately scaling movement amplitude in speech and nonspeech functions. As argued by Demirci et al., (1995) and Hallet (1997), individuals with PD have problems with kinesthesia, and when these individuals attempt to match their effort to their kinesthetic feedback, they constantly underscale their movement, thus resulting in the hypokinetic movements. Albin, Young, and Penny (1989) and Penny and Young (1983) provided an alternative explanation for the underscaling of movement amplitude. They argued that the basal ganglia excitatory circuits inadequately activate cortical motor centers. Consequently, motor neuron pools are not provided with adequate activation, thus resulting in movements that are too small or too weak. Berardelli, Dick, Rothwell, Day, and Marsden (1986) have argued that the defect in motor cortex activation in PD is due to a perceptual failure to select the muscle commands that are needed to match the external force and speed requirements. Collectively, these explanations implicate deficits in sensorimotor processing associated with basal ganglia dysfunction as part of the mechanisms underlying hypokinetic movements.

One manifestation of sensory processing deficits in individuals with PD is their misperception of their own voice and vocal effort. When these soft-talking individuals with PD are asked to increase the loudness of their speech (i.e., increase amplitude of motor output) to a normal conversational level, they perceive this normal level to be "too loud." Furthermore, they often report that people in their environment who ask them to "speak up" must need hearing aids, rather than recognizing that their habitual speech loudness has become abnormally soft. Ho et al. (2000) studied this phenomenon when they contrasted the actual loudness level of speech production with perceived loudness in hypophonic individuals with PD and in age-matched healthy individuals with normal voice and speech. Ho and her colleagues found that, even though the individuals with PD spoke with a softer voice than the controls, they perceived their own speech to be louder than did the control subjects. Furthermore, individuals with PD overestimated the loudness of their speech during both reading and conversation. Ho et al. interpreted these findings to suggest that either the hypophonia in individuals with PD was the result of an abnormal perceptual mechanism, or their perceptual system was abnormal due to the generation of quiet speech. As discussed later, addressing problems of sensory processing deficits and misperception of vocal output and effort are important therapeutic goals for a successful treatment of speech disorders in individuals with PD (Fox, Morrison, Ramig, & Sapir, 2002).

Deficits in Internal Cuing

Perhaps the most puzzling and characteristic aspect of the speech disorder in individuals with PD is the fact that, when these individuals are instructed (externally cued) to speak loudly and clearly, their speech becomes much louder, articulatory movements increase in amplitude and precision (Dromey & Ramig, 1998), prosodic pitch inflection increases and becomes more normal and effective in imparting linguistic and emotive information, and pauses between words increase (Dromey & Ramig, 1998; Goberman & Elmer, 2005; Mobes, Joppich, Stiebritz, Dengler, & Schröder, 2008). With such changes, speech clarity and intelligibility often improve considerably. Cunnington, Iansek, Bradshaw, and Phillips (1995) have argued that reliance on external cuing is a compensatory mechanism to overcome or bypass deficits in internal cuing. In support of this argument, Ho and colleagues (1999a, 1999b) demonstrated, in a series of experiments, that people with PD failed to adequately increase or decrease vocal loudness in response to implicit cues such as changes in auditory feedback of their own voice or changes in background noise, yet they performed as well as healthy controls when given explicit cues (instructions) to increase loudness. These findings further suggest an impairment with online or autophonic scaling of loudness in people with PD; an impairment that can be overridden, in the short term, with explicit (external) cuing. The response of increased loudness by the person with PD when given an external cue to "be loud" may be analogous to the response of improved, larger handwriting by the person with micrographia when lines or the direction "write big" (external cues) are added to a paper. The handwriting, like the vocal loudness, improves dramatically, although typically transiently, in response to the cue (Oliveira, Gurd, Nixon, Marshall, & Passingham, 1997).

There is evidence for other factors that might affect voice and speech in individuals with PD. Among these factors are impairments in automaticity (Cunnington, Iansek, & Bradshaw, 1999), temporal processing (Ackerman, Konczak & Hertrich, 1997; Caligiuri, 1989; Liss et al., 2009), and vocal vigilance (Bohnen et al., 2006; McNamara, Obler, Au, Durso & Albert, 1992; Rowe et al., 2002). It is likely that ongoing research will continue to reveal additional factors that can be associated with disordered voice and speech in individuals with PD.

Summary of Deficits Underlying Hypokinetic Dysarthria in PD

The foregoing discussion indicates that the neural mechanisms underlying hypokinetic dysarthria in PD are likely to be highly complex yet interrelated. The treatment of hypokinetic dysarthria therefore should address these complex, aberrant mechanisms. Specifically, the treatment should train the person with PD to: (1) improve scaling and to maintain an optimal level of speech movement amplitude, (2) overcome the sensorimotor deficits, and (3) bypass or compensate for the problems associated with impaired internal cuing. It should be noted that addressing these aberrant neural mechanisms is insufficient in itself to improve speech and maintain treatment outcome for months or years. In order to best achieve these therapeutic goals, and to make the treatment most efficacious, it is of utmost importance to incorporate training methods that are based on principles of neural plasticity (Kleim & Jones, 2008; see Table 4–1).

Principles of Neural Plasticity

Neural plasticity, in the context of sensorimotor rehabilitation, refers to the fact that: (1) intensive training can result in learning and long-term improvement in sensorimotor functions, and (2) these behavioral changes are likely to be accompanied by structural, functional, or organizational changes in the nervous system (strengthening or weakening neural connections, compensatory responses, axonal sprouting, neural repair, modifying or adding new nerve cells, etc.). Neural plasticity may occur naturally, but also and more so with training. Moreover, it may result in recovery of functions even in the course of degenerative diseases such as PD. Neural plasticity in sensorimotor rehabilitation depends on the intensity of exercise and motor training, and the focus, saliency and relevance of the training to the specific function being rehabilitated. To be maximally effective, training should be applied early in the course of the disease, both because there are more neurons available for modification (plasticity), and because people at this early stage of the disease are more able, cognitively, physically, and emotionally, to benefit from the training regimen (Kleim & Jones, 2008).

Behavioral Speech and Voice Treatment for PD

In spite of high incidence of voice and speech disorders in individuals with PD (see Chapter 3), only a minority of these individuals (3 to 14%) are likely to receive speech therapy (Hartelius & Svensson, 1994; Mutch, Strucwick, Roy, & Downie, 1986; Nijkrake et al., 2009). This discrepancy might have to do with the fact that, in the past, carryover and long-term treatment outcomes for speech treatment in PD were disappointing, both in terms of magnitude and enduring maintenance of therapeutic gains (Allan, 1970; Greene, 1980; Sarno, 1968; Weiner & Lang, 1989). These disappointing outcomes have been observed in a variety of treatments, including training in speech rate control, prosody, loudness, articulation, respiration, or a combination of these (Adams, 1997; Yorkston, 1996). Devices such as delayed auditory feedback (DAF), voice amplifiers, and pacing boards, have been shown to improve speech only transiently (Adams, 1997; Downie, Low, & Lindsay, 1981; Helm 1979; Ludlow & Bassich 1984).

Reviews of evidence-based practice (EBP) for behavioral speech therapy for people with PD recently were summarized by Trail et al. (2005), and the Academy of Neurologic Communication Disorders and Sciences (ANCDS) has offered two additional reviews (Yorkston, Spencer, & Duffy, 2003; Yorkston, Hakel, Beukelman, & Fager, 2007). Conclusions from these reviews are that LSVT LOUD has the greatest number of outcome measures associated with any speech treatment examined. Furthermore, for the most part, outcomes of the LSVT LOUD are positive and can be interpreted with confidence (Yorkston et al., 2003). The second, more recent review concludes that the strongest evidence regarding treatment effectiveness is for modification of loudness, specifically the LSVT LOUD protocol, in people with PD. Since that review was published, there have been new acoustic and perceptual studies, that demonstrate improvement of speech articulation in individuals with PD following LSVT LOUD treatment (e.g., Sapir et al, 2007; Sapir et al., 2010b).

Intensive Voice Treatment (LSVT LOUD) for PD

Given the large research base supporting training-increased vocal loudness via LSVT LOUD, it is beneficial to examine this specific treatment protocol in more detail as it pertains to current and future speech treatment research (Pinto et al., 2004; Trail et al., 2005; Yorkston et al., 2003) as it provides insight into the underlying mechanism of the speech and voice disorders in PD as well.

In 1994, Ramig and colleagues introduced the Lee Silverman Voice Treatment (LSVT LOUD), a Parkinson-specific approach that trains amplitude (increased healthy vocal loudness) as a single motor control parameter, thereby targeting inadequate scaling of agonist muscle activation. LSVT LOUD also trains individuals with PD to "recalibrate" their motor and perceptual systems so that they are less inclined to underscale (reduce amplitude) speech movement parameters. LSVT LOUD takes advantage of the multisystemic effects of loud phonation on the entire vocal mechanism, namely, simultaneous amplification of respiratory, laryngeal, and orofacial agonist muscle activity. This multisystemic upscaling of motor output manifests itself as larger amplitude of speech movements that more closely resemble normal speech (Dromey et al., 1995; Sapir et al., 2001, Sapir et al., 2007, Sapir et al., 2010b). LSVT LOUD is geared toward addressing deficits in internal cuing and self-regulation of vocal effort during speech production. It trains individuals with PD to actively attend to the amount and effort and loudness required for a within normal limits voice.

Over the past 20 years, a series of studies have documented that LSVT LOUD increased movement amplitude of the respiratory-laryngeal system in individuals with PD (Huber et al., 2003; Smith et al., 1995) and generated a statistically significant and lasting positive impact on vocal SPL (Huber et al., 2003; Ramig & Dromey, 1996; Ramig et al., 2001a, 2001b; Smith et al., 1995). These findings were consistent with perceptual data demonstrating improved loudness and voice quality (Baumgartner et al., 2001). There was no evidence of vocal hyperfunction (i.e., vocal misuse) posttreatment; to the contrary, LSVT LOUD has been shown to reduce laryngeal hyperfunction (Countryman, Hicks, & Ramig, 1997) and improve voice quality (Baumgartner et al., 2001). It is critical to recognize that the loudness target in LSVT LOUD is healthy, normal vocal loudness. Patients are not trained to yell or scream or to use pressed voice. Indeed, videostroboscopic data indicate that the phonatory system becomes more efficient in the production of voice following LSVT LOUD, as reflected in the more adequate closure of the vocal folds, and larger and more symmetric movements of the vocal folds (Perez et al., 1996; Smith et al., 1995). Moreover, individuals with PD trained with the LSVT LOUD report that speaking is much easier than before treatment as far as vocal effort is considered.

In addition to the direct impact on the respiratory-laryngeal systems following LSVT LOUD, studies have documented distributed effects across the speech production system. Dromey et al., (1995) reported posttreatment improvements in articulation reflected in measures of transition duration, rate, and extent. More recently Sapir and colleagues (2007, 2010b) compared articulatory acoustics in individuals with PD (treated and untreated) and a healthy control group. In one study, Sapir et al. (2007) found that both second formant frequency of /u/ (F2u) and the ratio of F2i and F2u (F2i/F2u) variables improved (changed significantly toward normalcy) in the participants who received LSVT LOUD and were significantly correlated with perceptual improvements in vowel ratings. No such improvement was observed in the two control groups participating in the study. In another study using a complex acoustic metric of vowel articulation, the Formant Centralization Ratio (FCR, expressed as [F2u + F2a + F1i + F1u]/[F2i + F1a]), Sapir et al. (2010b) found that LSVT LOUD markedly improved vowel articulation in individuals with PD and dysarthria who received this treatment regimen, but not in individuals with PD and dysarthria who did not receive such treatment.

The impact of treatment on facial expression was compared across participants with PD who received LSVT LOUD versus an alternative treatment using the procedures of Borod et al. (2000). Following LSVT LOUD, participants were rated significantly more expressive posttreatment, compared with an alternative treatment focusing on respiration only (Spielman, Borod, & Ramig, 2003). These data underscore the relationship between face and voice that has been demonstrated in expression studies involving individuals with neurologic disorders (Borod, Koff, Lorch, & Nicholas, 1985; Borod et al., 1990; Canino, Borod, Madigan, Tabert, & Schmidt, 1999; Porges, 1995; Porges 1997; Ross & Mesulam, 1979) and suggest that these communicative behaviors may have some overlapping neural mechanisms. A pilot study involving the assessment of the impact of LSVT LOUD on swallowing used standardized radiographic studies to define any changes that may have resulted posttreatment (El-Sharkawi et al., 2002). Results indicated a 51% reduction in the number of overall swallow disorders after LSVT LOUD on several bolus types (El-Sharkawi et al., 2002). The nature of the swallow disorders that resolved with LSVT LOUD were oral tongue and tongue base disorders, indicating that the effect of treatment extended to orofacial-swallowing musculature from a focus on treatment of respiratory-laryngeal movement amplitude. These findings suggest that the impact of vocal loudness training may go beyond a simple scale up of respiratory-laryngeal movement amplitude to include the orofacial articulatory system as well as nonspeech orofacial functions (face and swallow), even though these functions were not intentionally targeted in speech therapy.

Brain imaging studies using O^{15} positron emissions tomography (PET) have also documented marked changes in brain function consistent with speech improvement following LSVT LOUD (Liotti et al., 2003; Narayana et al., 2010). Specifically, although stimulated loud phonation prior to the administration of LSVT LOUD activated cortical premotor areas, particularly the supplementary motor area (SMA), post-LSVT LOUD SMA activity was normalized and activity in the basal ganglia (right putamen) increased, suggesting a shift from abnormal cortical motor activation toward normal subcortical organization of speech-motor output. The post-LSVT LOUD changes also indicated an increase in activity in right anterior insula and right dorsolateral prefrontal cortex, suggesting that LSVT LOUD recruits a phylogenetically old, preverbal communication system that is involved in vocalization and emotive communication (consistent with multisystem effects of LSVT LOUD). Another study (Liotti et al., 2000) involving evoked response potentials (ERPs) found excessive activity in the auditory cortex prior to LSVT LOUD treatment. This activity was markedly reduced to near-normal levels following the treatment , thus providing additional evidence for improvement in neural function post-LSVT LOUD.

Neural changes induced by LSVT LOUD as measured with PET imaging (Liotti et al., 2003; Narayana et al., 2010) reflect improvements in the basal ganglia, limbic system, prefrontal cortex, and right hemisphere functions. As indicated previously, these neural systems are involved in vocalization, loudness regulation and vocal learning, which collectively may account for the significant and long-term effects of LSVT LOUD on speech in individuals with PD. These neural systems are also involved in the control of nonspeech movements, such as swallowing and facial expression of emotions (Jurgens, 2009; Larson, 1985; Miller, 2002; Sapir, Campbell, & Larson, 1981), a fact that may explain why these functions are affected by training vocal loudness. Perspectives such as these elucidate why LSVT LOUD improves voice and speech production in PD and other neural conditions. They also may explain why previous treatments that have focused on rate or articulation, which involve primarily cortical, phylogenetically newer neural centers, typically have shown only moderate or minimal success.

Unique Aspects of LSVT LOUD. LSVT LOUD is a standardized, research-based approach, delivered by an LSVT Certified speech clinician and differs from traditional speech therapy regimens in a number of key ways. First, the target of the treatment is the voice. Specifically, LSVT LOUD trains amplitude (increased healthy vocal loudness) as a single motor control parameter. Second, the mode of treatment delivery is intensive and high effort, consistent with principles that drive activity-dependent neural plasticity (Fox et al., 2006), theories of motor learning (Ofer-Noy, Dudai, & Karni, 2003), and skill acquisition (Tillerson & Miller, 2002). Third, the "calibration" aspect of the treatment directly addresses the sensory, internal cuing, and neuropsychological deficits (e.g., impaired attention to action or vocal vigilance) that can make generalization and lasting treatment effects difficult to obtain for individuals with PD.

Target: Vocal Loudness (Amplitude). We hypothesize that the LSVT LOUD training-induced increase in movement amplitude (i.e., vocal loudness) targets the proposed pathophysiologic mechanisms underlying bradykinesia/hypokinesia-inadequate muscle activation (Berardelli, Rothwell, Thompson, & Hallet, 2001). The muscle activation deficits that occur in bradykinesia are believed to result from inadequate merging of kinesthetic feedback, motor output and context feedback with the basal ganglia that is necessary to select and reinforce an appropriate gain in the motor command (Berardelli et al., 2001; Desmurget et al., 2004). The single target of training vocal loudness (increased amplitude of motor output) in LSVT LOUD is a unique approach to treatment. In addition to increasing movement amplitude, the distributed effects of vocal loudness training on articulation, facial expression, and swallowing are consistent with the concept of global parameters, whereby a single treatment target impacts common control mechanisms that, in turn, influence motor behaviors beyond the specific targeted function (Allen, 1973; Dromey & Ramig, 1998; Gandour, Dechongkit, Ponglorpisit, & Khunadorn, 1994).

The neurologic bases of such global motor parameters are not known. However, vocal loudness might be regulated, or at least influenced, by a biomechanical and neurophysiologic linkage between articulatory and phonatory systems (Cookman & Verdolini, 1999; Higgins, Netsell, & Schulte, 1998; Larson & Sapir, 1995; McClean & Tasko, 2002;

Sapir, 1989; Sapir et al., 2007). Specifically, articulatory positions or movements have been shown to be correlated with, or influence laryngeal muscle activity, vocal fold closure, laryngeal tension, transglottal air flow, maximum airflow declination rate, and air pressure with some of these adjustments also correlating strongly with vocal sound pressure level (VocSPL) or vocal loudness levels (Cookman & Verdolini, 1999; Higgins et al.,1998; Larson & Sapir 1995; McClean & Tasko 2002; Sapir, 1989). These studies suggest that a potential source of this observed neural coupling might be from efferent drive from a common brain network to motor neurons innervating orofacial, laryngeal, and respiratory muscles. Studies of brain mechanisms underlying animal vocalization suggest that this network might involve the reticular formation of the pons and medulla oblongata and the input it receives from the anterior cingulate cortex via the periaqueductal gray (PAG), the latter serving to gate corticofugal and sensorimotor inputs to and from the vocal apparatus (Jurgens, 2009). Reflexogenic mechanisms also may be part of the coupling between the respiratory, laryngeal, and articulatory systems, with the latter affecting the former (Higgins et al., 1998; Larson & Sapir 1995; Sapir, 1989). Such common neural structures and coupling may explain, in part, the potential spread of effects from stimulation of increased vocal effort and loudness (respiratory and laryngeal systems) to orofacial muscles and swallowing function.

Another explanation for the distributed and lasting impact of LSVT LOUD is that it involves and stimulates phylogenetically old neural systems, especially the emotive brain. Speech production is a learned, highly practiced motor behavior, with many of its movements regulated in a quasi-automatic fashion (Ackermann, Wildgruber, Daum, & Grodd, 1998; Hirano et al., 1996; Jurgens, Kirzinger, & von Cramon, 1982); loudness scaling is a task that both animals and humans engage in all their lives (Ho et al., 1999b; Ho et al., 2000; Jurgens et al., 1982; Kitchen, Cheney, & Seyfarth, 2005; Leinonen, Laakso, Carlson, & Linnankoski, 2003). Thus, the regulation of vocal loudness for speech may involve a phylogenetically old system that has been adapted, through learning, for speech production and comprehension purposes.

Mode: Intensive, High Effort. The mode of delivery of LSVT LOUD is intensive and high effort. It is consistent with theories of motor learning (Ofer-Noy et al., 2003) and skill acquisition (e.g., increased practice, sensory processing), as well as principles that drive activity dependent neural plasticity (e.g., intensity, complexity, saliency) (Tillerson & Miller 2002). LSVT LOUD dosage is 60-minute individual treatment sessions, 4 days per week for 4 consecutive weeks, each session lasting 50 to 60 minutes. In addition, there are daily homework and carryover assignments the entire month of therapy (i.e., all 30 days). Within each treatment session, the first half of the session is spent on three daily tasks, which are core exercises designed to rescale the amplitude of motor output. These daily tasks are completed with multiple repetitions (e.g., minimum of 15 repetitions/per task/per day), and continually increased requirements for effort, consistency, and accuracy of vocal loudness (Ramig, Pawlas, & Countryman, 1995). The second half of the session is spent on the speech hierarchy. The rescaled vocal loudness achieved in the daily tasks is now systematically trained into speech. Across the weeks of the hierarchy, the duration of time that a person needs to keep his or her voice loud and the complexity of the speech task increase from words/phrases, to sentences, continuous reading and finally conversational speech.

Within the structured setting of the LSVT LOUD treatment sessions, many elements of exercise that promote activity-dependent neural plasticity are embedded (Kleim & Jones, 2008; Kleim, Jones, & Schallert, 2003). For example, the dosage across treatment sessions (4 consecutive days per week for 4 consecutive weeks) as well as within treatment sessions (multiple repetitions, high effort, increased accuracy) is intensive. The speech materials and carryover assignments are tailored to each individual client, thus allowing for saliency of treatment tasks. The more meaningful or rewarding the task, the greater the potential impact on neural plasticity (Alexander & Crutcher, 1990; Graybiel, 1998). The positive, long-term therapeutic impact of intensive behavioral rehabilitation on disorders associated with degenerative diseases has important implications for neural plasticity. It has been shown in animal models that where dopamine cells are allowed to degenerate to levels equivalent to humans at the time of diagnosis of PD, progressive exercise promotes functional recovery (neural restorative) and increases levels of dopamine in the striatum (Fisher et al., 2004). It has also been shown in animal models of PD that increased physical activity can be neurally protective if initiated at the time of exposure to a toxin (Tillerson, Caudle, Reveron, & Miller, 2003; Tillerson et al., 2001). Key elements of exercise that promoted neural plasticity, neural protection and neural restoration in these studies included intensive training of motor tasks, increased practice of motor tasks, active engagement in tasks, complexity of tasks, saliency, and the sensory experience of the motor task Tillerson et al., 2001; Tillerson et al., 2003). These key elements of exercise also have been shown to contribute to neural plasticity and brain reorganization in human stroke-related hemiparesis (Liepert et al., 1998). The LSVT LOUD, which targets sensory-motor deficits and high level self-regulation abnormalities in people with PD, incorporates all of these elements. Importantly, the therapeutic effects of the LSVT LOUD are more dramatic if treatment is administered in the initial stages of the degenerative process. This is in line with the findings that neural plasticity in animal models of PD is more likely to occur if key exercises are delivered during the initial stages of the degenerative process. Thus, to optimize the effects of behavioral treatments such as speech therapy, physiotherapy, and occupational therapy, these treatments may need to be administered as soon as the symptoms appear, or as soon as the disease is diagnosed and not during advanced stages of disease, as some authors suggest (Rajput & Rajput, 2006). The improvement in voice, speech, swallowing, and facial expression and brain activity with LSVT LOUD in the context of degenerative disease, strongly suggest the potential roles of this behavioral treatment in neural plasticity.

Calibration: Sensory, Internal Cuing and Neuropsychological Barriers to Generalization. As discussed above, the etiology of the speech and voice disorder in individuals with PD is complex. Addressing the motor deficit in isolation is not sufficient for lasting treatment outcomes that generalize beyond the treatment room. Thus, LSVT LOUD specifically trains individuals with PD to "re-calibrate" their motor and perceptual systems so that they are less inclined to downscale (reduce amplitude) speech movement parameters. As well, it is geared toward overcoming or compensating for deficits in sensory processing and internal cuing, as well as self-regulation of vocal effort during speech production. We hypothesize that LSVT LOUD retrains amplitude planning via intensive sensorimotor training that teaches the person with PD to recognize the effort needed to use louder speech during everyday living. By directly addressing this sensory mismatch, LSVT LOUD teaches individuals with PD to recalibrate their perception of normal loudness so that by the end of 1 month of therapy, they spontaneously speak with greater vocal loudness. This improvement may be due to some restoration of the internal cuing mechanism, or improved vocal vigilance. Although the treatment delivery is complex for the clinician who is administering the therapy, the focus for the individual with PD is kept purposefully simple and redundant (think LOUD, speak LOUD) which may maximize the ability of individuals with PD to learn this one target and generalize it to spontaneous, functional speech production. If one treatment target can make an impact across multiple levels of the speech production system, this may allow us to improve efficiency and effectiveness of treatment while limiting cognitive load on the individuals with PD.

Key Features of LSVT LOUD

- Consistent with principles of motor learning, muscle training and activity-dependent neural plasticity
- Targets healthy (nonabusive, nonstrenuous) production of vocal loudness
- Delivered intensively with high effort
- Targets barriers to generalization (sensory disorders, internal cueing deficits, neuropsychological challenges) through "calibration" of the speaker to the new vocal effort and loudness

To date, LSVT LOUD is the behavioral therapy with most data to support positive outcomes addressing the type of speech impairments experienced by individuals with PD (Yorkston et al., 2003; Yorkston et al, 2007). The effectiveness of the LSVT LOUD program may be variably compromised by several factors, including severe depression or dementia, atypical parkinsonism, and neurosurgery (deep brain stimulation, DBS). Although data have been reported documenting improvements in individuals postthalamotomy (Countryman & Ramig, 1993), postfetal cell, Post-DBS (Halpern, Spielman, Ramig, Down, & Gilley, 2010; Sapir et al., 2010a; Tassoreli et al., 2009] as well as in individuals with multiple system atrophy (MSA), progressive supranuclear palsy (PSP), and Parkinson-plus syndrome (PPS) (Countryman, Ramig, & Pawlas, 1994), the most predictable outcomes are when administering LSVT LOUD to individuals with idiopathic PD.

Technology-Enhanced Accessibility. It is recognized that there are practical challenges to delivering speech treatment intensively (four individual sessions per week for 4 weeks). In fact, any treatment regime (speech, physical or occupational therapy) that is consistent with plasticity promoting principles and incorporates elements such as intensity and multiple repetitions will need to go beyond the one-to-one (patient to clinician) classic paradigm of treatment delivery. There are not enough therapists to deliver this efficacious dosage of treatment to all the people with PD; a need that will only increase dramatically in the coming years with the aging of the baby boomer population. Furthermore, some individuals with PD may not be well enough to travel to a clinic, whereas others may suffer from fatigue as a result of travel, thus rendering treatment less effective. In addition, continued exercise following the conclusion of speech treatment and "tune-up" sessions may be needed for maintenance of vocal loudness as the disease progresses. Moreover, intensive treatment can be costly, especially for the elderly, whose source of income might be limited. Thus, there is a need for expanding service delivery while containing costs and human resources.

Advances in computer and Web-based technology offer potentially powerful solutions to the problems of delivering an intensive efficacious dosage of treatment, treatment accessibility and long-term maintenance in rehabilitation. LSVT LOUD delivered by telepractice (LSVT eLOUD) has documented positive outcomes in people with PD (Theodoros et al., 2006). Recent advances in software delivery of LSVT LOUD, through the LSVT Companion (Halpern, Matos, Ramig, Petska, & Spielman, 2005) allows for independent practice by the person with PD. Outcome data following the use of the LSVT Companion for half the dose, revealed findings similar to previously published data on 16 face-to-face sessions both immediately posttreatment and at 6-month follow-up (Halpern et al., 2005).

When to Refer for Speech Treatment

It has been suggested that behavioral treatment (e.g., speech therapy, occupational therapy, physiotherapy) should be deferred until later phases of the disease (Rajput & Rajput, 2006). However, there are a number of reasons why behavioral therapy should be initiated as early as possible after the symptoms of the disease appear. Speech and voice disorders have deleterious effects on communication, health, psychological well-being, and quality of life (Dowding, Shenton, & Salek, 2006; Findley, 2007; Miller, Noble, Jones, & Burn, 2006a; Miller et al., 2006b; Miller et al., 2007; Pell, Cheang, & Leonard, 2006; Pitcairn et al., 1990). Without access to effective speech treatment, affected individuals often become disabled or retire early, are forced to give up activities they enjoy, incur substantial medical costs and have increased mortality. Treatment may be optimally efficient early in the disease when the patient has the cognitive abilities, motivation, and level of optimism necessary to learn, practice and master the therapeutic behaviors. In a degenerative disease such as PD, there often is a deterioration in cognitive and executive functions, and an increase in depression, fatigue, and pessimism as the disease progresses (Rajput & Rajput, 2006). These factors can hinder training and therapeutic outcomes.

Another reason for initiating behavioral treatment early in the course of the disease is to maximize the potential for positive neural plasticity changes and disease modification. It has been shown that neural plasticity induced by intensive training is most likely to occur during the earlier stages of PD, when the dopaminergic and nondomaminergic systems are not fully depleted or impaired and there is potential for recovery or development of a compensatory mechanism (Kleim et al., 2003; Taub, 2004; Tillerson et al., 2003). Thus, behavioral treatment of voice, speech, and swallowing disorders in PD should be administered as soon as the disease is diagnosed, and when these disorders are of mild or moderate severity, for the training to be most effective. The third reason is that many individuals with PD are aware of their speech problems early in the course of their illness, even before other people notice these problems (Miller et al., 2006b). Moreover, these problems, along with related problems such as dysphagia, affect their ability to communicate and socialize, as well as their overall psychological well-being and quality of life (Miller et al., 2006b; Miller et al., 2007; Pitcairn et al., 1990). Thus, early treatment of the speech disorder in PD is likely to prevent some of the adverse consequences of speech impairment, including social isolation and depression.

Summary

Speech, voice, and swallowing problems occur in nearly 90% of individuals with PD and are likely to impact negatively on communication, socialization, occupation, health, and overall quality of life. Although traditionally voice and speech disorders have been attributed to dopamine deficits and rigidity, more recent studies indicate other etiologic factors, such as deficits in scaling movement amplitude, sensory processing, internal cuing, and other neuropsychological challenges. Medical and surgical treatments alone have not sufficiently alleviated speech and voice disorders for people with PD, and in some cases have exacerbated or resulted in voice and speech impairment. Thus, a combination of behavioral speech therapy, specifically the LSVT LOUD approach, in medically managed people with PD appears at present to be the most effective type of speech intervention. LSVT LOUD, has been extensively documented to be a successful approach in terms of magnitude and long term effects on these disorders. Although the degenerative course of PD cannot be altered at this time, improving oral communication is key element in developing the highest levels of functioning and independence for these individuals. There are many exciting avenues of ongoing and future speech research that will clarify our understanding of the underlying mechanism of speech disorders in PD and impact development of rehabilitation strategies in the future.

Acknowledgment. Research presented in this chapter has been funded by the National Institutes of Health (NIH) grant R01 DC1150 from the National Institutes of Deafness and Other Communication Disorders (Ramig, Fox, & Sapir).

Disclosure. Dr. Ramig receives a lecturer honorarium and has ownership interest in LSVT Global, Inc. Dr. Fox receives a lecturer honorarium and has ownership interest in LSVT Global, Inc.

Statement on Disclosure and Conflict. All members of this research team have fully disclosed any conflict of interest (Ramig and Fox) and their conflict of interest management plan has been approved by the Office of Conflict of Interest and Commitment at the University of Colorado, Boulder.

References

Ackermann, H., Konczak, J., & Hertrich, I. (1997). The temporal control of repetitive articulatory movements in Parkinson's disease. *Brain and Language, 56*, 312–319.

Ackermann, H., Wildgruber, D., Daum, I., & Grodd, W. (1998). Does the cerebellum contribute to cognitive aspects of speech production? A functional magnetic resonance imaging (fMRI) study in humans. *Neuroscience Letters, 247*, 187–190..

Ackermann, H., & Ziegler, W. (1991). Articulatory deficits in parkinsonian dysarthria: An acoustic analysis. *Journal of Neurology, Neurosurgery, and Psychiatry, 54*, 1093–1098.

Adams, S. G. (1997). Hypokinetic dysarthria in Parkinson's disease. In M. R. McNeil (Ed.), *Clinical management of sensorimotor speech disorders.* (pp. 261–285). New York, NY: Thieme.

Ahlskog, J. E. (2007). Beating a dead horse: Dopamine and Parkinson disease. *Neurology, 69*, 1701–1711.

Albin, R. L., Young, A. B., & Penny, J. B. (1989). The functional anatomy of basal ganglia disorders. *Trends in Neuroscience, 12*, 366–375.

Alexander, G. E., & Crutcher, M. D. (1990). Functional architecture of basal ganglia circuits: Neural substrates of parallel processing. *Trends in Neuroscience, 13*, 266–271.

Allan, C. M. (1970). Treatment of non-fluent speech resulting from neurological disease: Treatment of dysarthria. *British Journal of Disorders Communication, 5,* 3–5.

Allen, G. (1973). Segmental timing control in speech production. *Journal of Phonetics, 1,* 219–237.

Baker K. K., Ramig L. O., Johnson A. B., & Freed C. R. (1997). Preliminary speech and voice analysis following fetal dopamine transplants in 5 individuals with Parkinson disease. *Journal of Speech and Hearing Research, 40,* 615–626.

Baker, K., Ramig, L. O., Luschei, E., & Smith, M. (1998). Thyroarytenoid muscle activity associated with hypophonia in Parkinson disease and aging. *Neurology, 51,* 1592–1598.

Bartels, A. L., & Leenders, K. L. (2009). Parkinson's disease: The syndrome, the pathogenesis and pathophysiology. *Cortex, 45,* 915–921.

Baumgartner, C. A., Sapir, S., & Ramig, L. O. (2001). Voice quality changes following phonatory-respiratory effort treatment (LSVT®) versus respiratory effort treatment for individuals with Parkinson disease. *Journal of Voice, 15,* 105–114.

Berardelli, A., Dick, J. P., Rothwell, J. C., Day, B. L., & Marsden, C. D. (1986). Scaling of the size of the first agonist EMG burst during rapid wrist movements in patients with Parkinson's disease. *Journal of Neurology, Neurosurgery, and Psychiatry, 49,*1273–1279.

Berardelli, A., Rothwell, J.C., Thompson, P. D., & Hallett, M. (2001). Pathophysiology of bradykinesia in Parkinson's disease. *Brain, 124,* 2131–2146.

Bohnen, N. I., Kaufer, D. I., Hendrickson, R., Ivanco, L., Lopresti, B., Constantine, G., . . . Dekosky, S. (2006). Cognitive correlates of cortical cholinergic denervation in Parkinson's disease and parkinsonian dementia. *Journal of Neuro*logy, *253,* 242–247.

Borod, J. C., Koff, E., Lorch, M. P., & Nicholas, M. (1985). Channels of emotional expression in patients with unilateral brain damage. *Archives of Neurology, 42,* 345–348.

Borod, J. C., Pick, L. H., Hall, S., Sliwinski, M., Madigan, N., Obler, L. K., . . . Tabert, M. (2000). Relationships among facial, prosodic, and lexical channels of emotional perceptual processing. *Cognition and Emotion, 14,* 193–211.

Borod, J. C., Welkowitz, J., Alpert, M., Brozgold, A. Z., Martin, C., Peselow, E., & Diller, L. (1990). Parameters of emotional processing in neuropsychiatric disorders: Conceptual issues and a battery of tests. *Journal of Communication Disorders, 23,* 7–71.

Brown, R. G., & Marsden, C. D. (1991). Dual task performance and processing resources in normal subjects and patients with Parkinson's disease. *Brain, 114,* 215–231.

Caligiuri, M. (1989). The influence of speaking rate on articulatory hypokinesia in parkinsonian dysarthria. *Brain and Language, 36,* 493–502.

Caligiuri, M., & Abbs, J. H. (1987). Response properties of the perioral reflex in Parkinson's disease. *Experimental Neurology, 98,* 563–572.

Canino, E., Borod, J. C., Madigan, N., Tabert, M. H., & Schmidt, J. M. (1999). Development of procedures for rating posed emotional expressions across facial, prosodic, and lexical channels. *Perceptual Motor Skills, 89*, 57–71.

Comery, T. A., Shar, R., & Greenough, W. T. (1995). Differential rearing alters spine density on medium-sized spiny neurons in the rat corpus striatum: Evidence for association of morphological plasticity with early response gene expression. *Neurobiology of Learning and Memory, 63*, 217–219

Cookman, S., & Verdolini, K. (1999). Interrelation of mandibular laryngeal functions. *Journal of Voice, 13*, 11–24.

Countryman, S., Hicks, J., & Ramig, L. (1997). Supraglottic hyperadduction in an individual with Parkinson disease: Treatment outcome. *American Journal of Speech Language Pathology, 6*, 85–94.

Countryman, S., & Ramig, L. (1993). Effects of intensive voice therapy on voice deficits associated with bilateral thalamotomy in Parkinson's disease: A case study. *Journal of Medical Speech-Language Pathology, 1*, 233–250.

Countryman, S., Ramig, L., & Pawlas, A. (1994). Speech and voice deficits in parkinsonian plus syndromes: Can they be treated? *Journal of Medical Speech-Language Pathology, 2*, 211–225.

Cramer, W. (1940). De spaak bij patienten met Parkinsonisme. *Logopaedics and Phoniatrics, 22*, 17–23.

Cunnington, R., Iansek, R., & Bradshaw, J. (1999). Movement-related potentials in Parkinson's disease: External cues and attentional strategies. *Movement Disorders, 14*, 63–68.

Cunnington R., Iansek R., Bradshaw J.L., & Phillips J.G. (1995). Movement-related potentials in Parkinson's disease. Presence and predictability of temporal and spatial cues. *Brain, 118*, 935–950.

Darley, F. L., Aronson, A. E., & Brown, J. R. (1969a). Clusters of deviant speech dimensions in the dysarthrias. *Journal of Speech and Hearing Research, 12*, 462–469.

Darley, F. L., Aronson, A. E., & Brown, J. (1969b). Differential diagnostic patterns of dysarthria. *Journal of Speech and Hearing Research, 12*, 246–269.

Demirci, M., Grill, S., McShane, L., & Hallet, M. (1995). Impairment of kinesthesia in Parkinson's disease. *Neurology, 45*, A218.

Demirci, M., Grill, S., McShane, L., & Hallett, M. (1997). A mismatch between kinesthetic and visual perception in Parkinson's disease. *Annals of Neurology, 41*, 781–788.

Desmurget, M., Grafton, S. T., Vindras, P., Gréa, H., & Turner, R. S. (2003). Basal ganglia network mediates the control of movement amplitude. *Experimental Brain Research, 153*, 197–209.

Desmurget, M., Grafton, S. T., Vindras, P., Gréa, H., & Turner, R. S. (2004). The basal ganglia network mediates the planning of movement amplitude. *European Journal of Neuroscience, 19*, 2871–2880.

Diamond, S. G., Schneider, J. S., & Markham, C. H. (1987). Oral sensorimotor defects in people with Parkinson's disease. *Advances in Neurology, 45*, 335–338.

Dowding, C. H., Shenton, C. L., & Salek, S. S. (2006). A review of the health-related quality of life and economic impact of Parkinson's disease. *Drugs and Aging, 23*, 693–721.

Downie, A. W., Low, J. M., & Lindsay, D. D. (1981). Speech disorders in parkinsonism: Usefulness of delayed auditory feedback in selected cases. *British Journal of Disorders of Communication, 16*, 135–139.

Dromey, C., & Ramig, L. (1998). Intentional changes in sound pressure level and rate: Their impact on measures of respiration, phonation, and articulation. *Journal of Speech Language and Hearing Research, 41*, 1003–1018.

Dromey, C., Ramig, L. O., & Johnson, A. (1995). Phonatory and articulatory changes associated with increased vocal intensity in Parkinson disease: A case study. *Journal of Speech Language and Hearing Research, 38*, 751–763.

El-Sharkawi, A. E., Ramig, L., Logemann, J. A., Pauloski B. R., Rademaker A. W., Smith C. H., . . . Werner C. (2002). Swallowing and voice effects of Lee Silverman Voice Treatment (LSVT®): A pilot study. *Journal of Neurology, Neurosurgery, and Psychiatry, 72*, 31–36.

Faherty, C. J., Raviie Shepherd, K., Herasimtschuk, A., & Smeyne, R. J. (2005). Environmental enrichment in adulthood eliminates neuronal death in experimental Parkinsonism. *Molecular Brain Research, 134*, 170–179.

Findley, L. J. (2007). The economic impact of Parkinson's disease. *Parkinsonism and Related Disorders, 13*(Suppl.), S8–S12.

Fisher, B. E., Petzinger, G. M., Nixon, K., Hogg, E., Bremmer, S., Meshul, C. K., & Jakowec, M. W. (2004). Exercise-induced behavioral recovery and neuroplasticity in the 1-methyl-4-phenyl-1,2,3,6-tetrahydropyridine-lesioned mouse basal ganglia. *Journal of Neuroscience Research, 77*, 378–390.

Flint, A. J., Black, S. E., Campbell-Taylor, I., Gailey, G. F., & Levinton, C. (1993). Abnormal speech articulation, psychomotor retardation, and subcortical dysfunction in major depression. *Journal of Psychiatric Research, 27*, 309–319.

Forrest, K., Weismer, G., & Turner, G. S. (1989). Kinematic, acoustic, and perceptual analyses of connected speech produced by parkinsonian and normal geriatric adults. *Journal of Acoustic Society of America, 85*, 2608–2622.

Fox, C. M., Morrison, C. E., Ramig, L. O., & Sapir, S. (2002). Current perspectives on the Lee Silverman Voice Treatment (LSVT) for people with idiopathic Parkinson's disease. *American Journal of Speech Language Pathology, 11*, 111–123.

Fox, C., & Ramig, L. (1997). Vocal sound pressure level and self-perception of speech and voice in men and women with idiopathic Parkinson disease. *American Journal of Speech Language Pathology, 2*, 29–42.

Fox C. M., Ramig L. O., Ciucci M. R., Sapir S., McFarland D. H., & Farley B. G. (2006). The science and practice of LSVT/LOUD: Neural plasticity-principled approach to treating individuals with Parkinson disease and other neurological disorders. *Seminars in Speech and Language, 27*, 283–299.

Gallena, S., Smith, P. J., Zeffiro, T., & Ludlow, C. L. (2001). Effects of levodopa on laryngeal muscle activity for voice onset and offset in Parkinson disease. *Journal of Speech Language and Hearing Research, 44*, 1284–1299.

Gandour, J., Dechongkit, S., Ponglorpisit, S., & Khunadorn, F. (1994). Speech timing at the sentence level in Thai after unilateral brain damage. *Brain and Language, 46*, 419–438.

Gentil, M., Chauvin, P., Pinto, S., Pollak, P., & Benabid, A. L. (2001). Effect of bilateral stimulation of the subthalamic nucleus on parkinsonian voice. *Brain and Language, 78*, 233–240.

Gentil, M., Garcia-Ruiz, P., Pollak, P., & Benabid, A. L. (2000). Effect of bilateral deep-brain stimulation on oral control of patients with parkinsonism. *European Neurology, 44*, 147–152.

Gentil, M., Pinto, S., Pollak, P., & Benabid, A. L. (2003). Effect of bilateral stimulation of the subthalamic nucleus on parkinsonian dysarthria. *Brain and Language, 85*, 190–196.

Goberman, A.M., & Elmer, L.W. (2005). Acoustic analysis of clear versus conversational speech in individuals with Parkinson disease. *Journal of Communication Disorders, 38*, 215–230.

Graber, S., Hertrich, I., Daum, I., Spieker, S., & Ackermann, H. (2002). Speech perception deficits in Parkinson's disease: Underestimation of time intervals compromises identification of durational phonetic contrasts. *Brain and Language, 82*, 65–74.

Graybiel, A. M. (1998). The basal ganglia and chunking of action repertoires. *Neurobiology of Learning and Memory, 70*, 119–136.

Greene, H. C. L. (1980). *The voice and its disorders*. London, UK: Pitman Medical.

Hallet, M. (1997). Sensorimotor integration and mysterious sensory phenomena in movement disorders. In M. Hallet (Ed.), *Motor control*: American Academy of Neurology.

Halpern, A., Matos, C., Ramig, L., Petska, J., & Spielman, J. (2005). *LSVTC—A PDA supported speech treatment for Parkinson's disease.* Paper presented at 9th International Congress of Parkinson's Disease and Movement Disorders. New Orleans, LA.

Halpern, A., Spielman, J., Ramig, L., Down, I., & Gilley, P. (2010). *Speech treatment for individuals with IPD post deep brain stimulation: LSVT-DBS.* Paper presented at the 15th Biennial Conference on Motor Speech, Savannah, GA.

Hammen, V. L., & Yorkston, K. M. (1996). Speech and pause characteristics following speech rate reduction in hypokinetic dysarthria. *Journal of Communication Disord*ers, *29*, 429–444.

Hammen, V. L., Yorkston, K. M., & Minifie, F. D. (1994). Effects of temporal alterations on speech intelligibility in parkinsonian dysarthria. *Journal of Speech and Hearing Research, 37*, 244–253.

Hammer, M. J, & Barlow, S. M. (2010). Laryngeal somatosensory deficits in Parkinson's disease: Implications for speech respiratory and phonatory control. *Experimental Brain Research, 201*, 401–409.

Hanson, D. G., Gerratt, B. R., & Ward, P. H. (1984). Cinegraphic observations of laryngeal function in Parkinson's disease. *Laryngoscope, 94*, 348–353.

Hartelius, L., & Svensson, P. (1994). Speech and swallowing symptoms associated with Parkinson's disease and multiple sclerosis: A survey. *Folia Phoniatrica et Logopaedica , 46*, 9–17.

Helm, N. (1979). Management of palilalia with a pacing board. *Journal of Speech and Hearing Disorders, 44*, 350–353.

Higgins, M. B., Netsell, R., & Schulte, L. (1998). Vowel-related differences in laryngeal articulatory and phonatory function. *Journal of Speech Language and Hearing Research, 41*, 712–724.

Hirano, S., Kojima, H., Naito, Y., Honjo, I., Kamoto, Y., Okazawa, H., . . . Konishi, J. (1996). Cortical speech processing mechanisms while vocalizing visually presented languages. *NeuroReport, 8*, 363–367.

Ho, A. K., Bradshaw, J. L., & Iansek, T. (2000). Volume perception in parkinsonian speech. *Movement Disorders, 15*, 1125–1131.

Ho, A. K., Bradshaw, J. L., Iansek, R., & Alfredson. R. (1999a). Speech volume regulation in Parkinson's disease: Effects of implicit cues and explicit instructions. *Neuropsychologia, 37*, 1453–1460.

Ho, A. K., Iansek, R., & Bradshaw, J. L. (1999b). Regulations of parkinsonian speech volume: The effect of interlocuter distance. *Journal of Neurology, Neurosurgery, and Psychiatry, 67*, 199–202.

Ho, A. K., Iansek, R., & Bradshaw, J. L. (2001). Motor instability in parkinsonian speech intensity. *Journal of Neuropsychiatry, Neuropsychology, and Behavioral Neurology, 14*, 109–116.

Ho A. K, Iansek, R., Bradshaw, J. L. (2002). The effect of a concurrent task on Parkinsonian speech. *Journal of Clinical Experimental Neuropsychology, 24*, 36–47.

Ho, A. K., Iansek, R., Marigliani, C., Bradshaw, J. L., & Gates, S. (1998). Speech impairment in a large sample of people with Parkinson's disease. *Behavioral Neurology, 11*, 131–137.

Huber, J., Stathopoulos, E., Ramig, L., & Lancaster, S. (2003). Respiratory function and variability in individuals with Parkinson disease: Pre and post Lee Silverman Voice Treatment (LSVT®). *Journal of Medical Speech-Language Pathology, 11*, 185–201.

Jobst, E. E., Melnick, M. E., Byl, N. N., Dowling, G. A., & Aminoff, M. J. (1997). Sensory perception in Parkinson's disease. *Archives of Neurology, 54*, 450–454.

Jones, T. A., Chu, C. J., Grande, L. A., & Gregory, A. D. (1999). Motor skills training enhances lesion-induced structural plasticity in the motor cortex of adult rats. *Journal of Neuroscience, 19*, 10153–10163.

Jürgens, U. (2009). The neural control of vocalization in mammals: A review. *Journal of Voice, 23*, 1–10.

Jurgens, U., Kirzinger, A., & von Cramon, D. (1982). The effects of deep-reaching lesions in the cortical face area on phonation. A combined case report and experimental monkey study. *Cortex, 18*, 125–130.

Kempler, D., & Van Lancker, D. (2002). Effect of speech task on intelligibility in dysarthria: A case study of Parkinson's disease. *Brain and Language, 80*, 449–464.

King, J., Ramig, L., Lemke, J. H., & Horii, Y. (1994). Parkinson disease: Longitudinal changes in acoustic parameters of phonation. *Journal of Medical Speech-Language Pathology, 2*, 29–42.

Kitchen, D. M., Cheney, D. L., & Seyfarth, R. M. (2005). Male chacma baboons (Papio hamadryas ursinus) discriminate loud call contests between rivals of different relative ranks. *Animal Cognition, 8*, 1–6.

Kleim, J. A., & Jones, T. A.(2008). Principles of experience-dependent neural plasticity: Implications for rehabilitation after brain damage. *Journal of Speech, Language, and Hearing Research, 51*, S225–S239.

Kleim, J., Jones, T., & Schallert, T. (2003). Motor enrichment and the induction of plasticity before or after brain injury, *Neurochemical Research, 11*, 1757–1769.

Kleim, J. A., Lussnig, E., Schwarz, E. R., Comery, T. A., & Greenough, W. T. (1996). Synaptogenesis and Fos expression in the motor cortex of the adult rat after motor skill learning. *Journal of Neuroscience, 16*, 4529–4535.

Kleinow, J., Smith, A., & Ramig, L. (2001). Speech stability in idiopathic Parkinson disease: Effects of rate and loudness manipulations. *Journal of Speech Language and Hearing Research, 44*, 1041–1051.

Klockgether, T., Borutta, M., Rapp, H., Spieder, S., & Dichgans, J. (1997). A defect of kinesthesia in Parkinson's disease. *Brain, 120*, 460–465.

Klosterman, F., Ehlen, F., Vesper, J., Nubel, K., Gross, M., Marzinzik, F., Curio, G., & Sappok, T. (2008). Effects of subthalamic deep brain stimulation on dysarthrophonia in Parkinson's disease. *Journal of Neurology, Neurosurgery, and Psychiatry, 79*, 522–529.

Kompoliti, K., Wang, Q. E., Goetz, C. G., Leurgans, S., & Raman, R. (2000). Effects of central dopaminergic stimulation by apomorphine on speech in Parkinson's disease. *Neurology, 54*, 458–462.

Larson, C.R. (1985). The midbrain periaqueductal gray: a brainstem structure involved in vocalization. *Journal of Speech and Hearing Research, 28*, 241–249.

Larson, K. K., & Sapir, S. (1995). Orolaryngeal reflex responses to changes in affective state. *Journal of Speech Language and Hearing Research, 38*, 990–1000.

Leinonen, L., Laakso, M. L., Carlson, S.,& Linnankoski, I. (2003). Shared means and meanings in vocal expression of man and macaque. *Logopedics, Phoniatrics, Vocology, 28*, 53–61.

Liepert, J., Miltner, W., Bauder, H, Sommer M., Dettmers C., Taub E., & Weiller C. (1998). Motor cortex plasticity during constraint-induced movement therapy in stroke patients. *Neuroscience Letters, 250*, 5–8.

Liotti, M., Ramig, L. O., Vogel, D., New P., Cook C. I., Ingham R.J., Ingham J. C., & Fox P. T. (2003). Hypophonia in Parkinson's disease: Neural correlates of voice treatment revealed by PET. *Neurology, 60*, 432–440.

Liotti, M., Vogel, D., Sapir, S., Ramig, L., New, P., & Fox, P. (2000). *Abnormal auditory gating in Parkinson's disease before & after LSVT®*. Paper presented at the annual meeting of the American Speech, Language, and Hearing Association, Washington DC.

Liss, J. M., Spitzer, S. M., Caviness, J. N., & Adler, C. (2002). The effects of familiarization on intelligibility and lexical segmentation in hypokinetic and ataxic dysarthria. *Journal of the Acoustic Society of America, 112*, 3022–3030.

Liss, J. M., White, L., Mattys, S. L., Lansford, K., Lotto, A. J., Spitzer, S. M., & Caviness, J. N. (2009). Quantifying speech rhythm abnormalities in the dysarthrias. *Journal of Speech Language and Hearing Research, 52*, 1334–1352.

Logemann, J., Boshes, B., & Fisher, H. (1973). The steps in the degeneration of speech and voice control in Parkinson's disease. In J. Siegfried (Ed.), *Parkinson's diseases: Rigidity, akinesia, behavior.* Vienna, Austria: Hans Huber.

Logemann, J., Fisher, H., Boshes, B., & Blonsky, E. (1978). Frequency and concurrence of vocal tract dysfunctions in the speech of a large sample of Parkinson patients. *Journal of Speech and Hearing Disorders, 43*, 47–57.

Ludlow, C. L., & Bassich, C. J. (1984). Relationships between perceptual ratings and acoustic measures of hypokinetic speech. In M. R. McNeil, J. C. Rosenbek, & A. E. Aronson (Eds.), *The dysarthrias: Physiology, acoustics, perception, management* (pp. 163–195). San Diego, CA: College-Hill Press.

Luschei, E. S., Ramig, L. O., Baker, K. L., Baker, K. L., & Smith, M. E. (1999). Discharge characteristics of laryngeal single motor units during phonation in young and older adults and in persons with Parkinson disease. *Journal of Neurophysiology, 81*, 2131–2139.

McClean, M. D., & Tasko, S. M. (2002). Association of orofacial with laryngeal and respiratory motor output during speech. *Experimental Brain Research, 146*, 481–489.

McNamara, P., Obler, L. K., Au, R., Durso, R., & Albert, M. L. (1992). Speech monitoring skills in Alzheimer's disease, Parkinson's disease, and normal aging. *Brain and Language, 42*, 38–51.

Miller, A. (2002). Oral and pharyngeal reflexes in the mammalian nervous system: their diverse range in complexity and the pivotal role of the tongue. *Critical Review in Oral Biology and Medicine*, 13, 409–425.

Miller, N., Allcock, L., Jones, D., Noble E., Hildreth, A. J., & Burn, D. J. (2007). Prevalence and pattern of perceived intelligibility changes in Parkinson's disease. *Journal of Neurology, Neurosurgery, and Psychiatry, 78*, 1188–1190.

Miller, N., Noble, E., Jones, D., Allcock, L., & Burn, D. J. (2008). How do I sound to me? Perceived changes in communication in Parkinson's disease. *Clinical Rehabilitation, 22*, 14–22.

Miller, N., Noble, E., Jones, D., & Burn, D. (2006a). Hard to swallow: Dysphagia in Parkinson's disease. *Age and Ageing, 35*, 614–618.

Miller, N., Noble, E., Jones, D., & Burn, D. (2006b). Life with communication changes in Parkinson's disease. *Age and Ageing, 35*, 235–239.

Möbes, J., Joppich, G., Stiebritz, F., Dengler, R., & Schröder, C. (2008). Emotional speech in Parkinson's disease. *Movement Disord*ers, *23*, 824–829.

Morris, M., Iansek, R., Matyas, T., & Summers, J. (1998). Abnormalities in the stride length-cadence relation in parkinsonian gait. *Movement Disorders, 13*, 61–69.

Mutch, R., Strucwick, A., Roy, S., & Downie, A.W. (1986). Parkinson's disease: Disability review and management. *British Medical Journal, 293*, 675–677.

Narayana, S., Fox, P. T., Zhang, W., Franklin, C., Robin, D. A., Vogel, D., & Ramig, L. O. (2010). Neural correlates of efficacy of voice therapy in Parkinson's disease identified by performance-correlation analysis. *Human Brain Mapping, 31*, 222–236.

Nijkrake, M. J., Keus, S. H., Oostendorp, R. A., Overeem, S., Mulleners, W., Bloem, B. R., & Munneke, M. (2009). Allied health care in Parkinson's disease: Referral, consultation, and professional expertise. *Movement Disorders, 24*, 282–286.

Ofer-Noy, N., Dudai, Y., & Karni, A. (2003). Skill learning in mirror reading: How repetition determines acquisition. *Cognitive Brain Research, 17*, 507–521.

Oliveira, R. M., Gurd, J. M., Nixon, P., Marshall, J. C., & Passingham, R. E. (1997). Micrographia in Parkinson's disease: The effect of providing external cues. *Journal of Neurology, Neurosurgery, and Psychiatry, 63*, 429–433.

Pell, M. D., Cheang, H. S., & Leonard, C. L. (2006). The impact of Parkinson's disease on vocal-prosodic communication from the perspective of listeners. *Brain and Language, 97*, 123–134.

Penny, J. B., & Young, A. B. (1983). Speculations on the functional anatomy of basal ganglia disorders. *Annual Review of Neuroscience, 6*, 73–94.

Perez, K., Ramig, L. O., Smith, M., & Dromey, C. (1996). The Parkinson larynx: Tremor and videostroboscopic findings. *Journal of Voice, 10*, 354–361.

Pinto, S., Gentil, M., Fraix, V., Benabid, A. L., & Pollak, P. (2003). Bilateral subthalamic stimulation effects on oral force control in Parkinson's disease. *Journal of Neurology, 250*, 179–187.

Pinto, S., Ozsancak, C., Tripoliti, E., Thobois S., Limousin-Dowsey P., & Auzou P. (2004). Treatments for dysarthria in Parkinson's disease. *Lancet Neurology, 3*, 547–556.

Pisani, A., Centonze, D., Bernardi, G., & Calabresi P. (2005). Straital synaptic plasticity: implications for motor learning and Parkinson's disease. *Movement Disorders, 20*, 395–402.

Pitcairn, T. K., Clemie, S., Gray, J. M., & Pentland, B. (1990). Non-verbal cues in the self-presentation of parkinsonian patients. *British Journal of Clinical Psychology, 29*, 177–184.

Plautz, E. J., Milliken, G. W., & Nudo, R. J. (2000). Effects of repetitive motor training on movement representations in adult squirrel monkeys: Role of use versus learning. *Neurobiology of Learning and Memory, 74*, 27–55.

Porges, S. W. (1995). Orienting in a defensive world: Mammalian modifications of our evolutionary heritage. A polyvagal theory. *Psychophysiology, 32*, 301–318.

Porges, S. W. (1997). Emotion: An evolutionary by-product of the neural regulation of the autonomic nervous system. *Annals of the New York Academy of Sciences, 807*, 62–77.

Rajput, A., & Rajput, A. H. (2006). Parkinson's disease management strategies. *Expert Review of Neurotherapeutics, 6*, 91–99.

Ramig, L. O. (1992). The role of phonation in speech intelligibility: a review and preliminary data from patients with Parkinson's disease. In R. D. Kent (Ed.), *Intelligibility in speech disorders: Theory, measurement, and management* (pp. 119–156). Amsterdam, the Netherlands: John Benjamin.

Ramig, L., O, Bonitati, C., Mead, Lemke, J. H, & Horii, Y. (1994). Voice treatment for patients with parkinson disease: Development of an approach and preliminary efficacy data. *Journal of Medical Speech-Language Pathology, 2*, 191–209.

Ramig, L. O., & Dromey, C. (1996). Aerodynamic mechanisms underlying treatment-related changes in SPL in patients with Parkinson disease. *Journal of Speech and Hearing Research, 39*, 798–807.

Ramig, L. O., Fox, C., & Sapir, S. (2008). Speech treatment for Parkinson disease. *Expert Review of Neurotherapeutics, 8*, 299–311.

Ramig, L. O., Fox, C., & Sapir, S. (In press). *Speech and voice disorders in Parkinson disease.* In W. Olanow, W. Stocchi, & A. Lang (Eds.), *The non-motor and non-dopaminergic features of Parkinson's disease.* Oxford, UK: Blackwell.

Ramig, L. O., Pawlas, A., & Countryman, S. (1995). *The Lee Silverman Voice Treatment (LSVT®): A practical guide to treating the voice and speech disorders in Parkinson disease.* Iowa City, IA: National Center for Voice and Speech and LSVT® Foundation.

Ramig, L. O., Sapir, S., Countryman, S., Pawlas A. A., O'Brien C., Hoehn M., & Thompson L. L. (2001a). Intensive voice treatment (LSVT®) for patients with Parkinson's disease: A 2-year follow-up. *Journal of Neurology, Neurosurgery, and Psychiatry, 71*, 493–498.

Ramig, L., Sapir, S., Fox, C., & Countryman, S. (2001b). Changes in vocal intensity following intensive voice treatment (LSVT") in individuals with Parkinson disease: A comparison with untreated patients and normal age-matched controls. *Movement Disorders, 16*, 79–83.

Ramig, L. O., Scherer, R., Titze, I., & Ringel, S. (1988). Acoustic characteristics of voice of patients with neurological disease: A preliminary report. *Annals of Otology, Rhinology, and Laryngology, 97*, 164–172.

Rektorova, I., Barrett, J., Mikl, M., Rektor, I., & Paus, T. (2007). Functional abnormalities in the primary orofacial sensorimotor cortex during speech in Parkinson's disease. *Movement Disord*ers, *22*, 2043–2051.

Rickards, C., & Cody, F. W. (1997). Proprioceptive control of wrist movements in Parkinson's disease. *Brain, 120*, 977–990.

Rosen, K. M., Kent, R. D., & Duffy, J. R. (2005). Task-based profile of vocal intensity decline in Parkinson's disease. *Folia Phoniatrica et Logopaedica, 57*, 28–37.

Ross, E. D., & Mesulam, M. M. (1979). Dominant language functions of the right hemisphere? Prosody and emotional gesturing. *Archives of Neurol*ogy, *36*, 144–148.

Rowe J., Stephan K. E., Friston K., Frackowiak R., Lees A., & Passingham R. (2002). Attention to action in Parkinson's disease: Impaired effective connectivity among frontal cortical regions. *Brain, 125*, 276–278.

Sanabria, J., Ruiz, P. G., Gutierrez, R., Marquez, F., Escobar, P., Gentil, M., & Cenjor, C. (2001). The effect of levodopa on vocal function in Parkinson's disease. *Clinical Neuropharmacology, 24*, 99–102.

Sapir, S. (1989). The intrinsic pitch of vowels: Theoretical, physiological, and clinical considerations. *Journal of Voice, 3*, 44–51.

Sapir, S., Campbell, C., & Larson, C. (1981). Effect of geniohyoid, cricothyroid and sternothyroid muscle stimulation on voice fundamental frequency of electrically elicited phonation in rhesus macaque. *Laryngoscope, 91*, 457–468.

Sapir, S., Halpern, A., Spielman, J., Ramig, L., & Giley, P. (2010a). *Speech treatment for individuals with idiopathic Parkinson's disease post-DBS-STN.* Paper presented at the Second International Symposium on Basal Ganglia Speech Disorders and Deep Brain Stimulation, Aix-en-Provence, France.

Sapir, S., Pawlas, A., Ramig, L., Countryman, S., O'Brien, C., Hoehn, M., & Thompson, L. (2001). Voice and speech abnormalities in Parkinson disease: Relation to severity of motor impairment, duration of disease, medication, depression, gender, and age. *Journal of Medical Speech-Language Pathology, 9*, 213–226.

Sapir, S., Ramig, L., & Fox, C. (2008a). Voice, speech and swallowing disorders. In S. Factor & W. Weiner (Eds.), *Parkinson disease: Diagnosis and clinical management* (pp. 77–97). New York, NY: Demos Medical.

Sapir, S., Ramig, L., & Fox, C. (2008b). Speech and swallowing disorders in Parkinson's disease. *Current Opinion in Otolaryngology and Head and Neck Surgery, 16,* 205–210.

Sapir, S., Ramig, L., Hoyt, P., O'Brien, C., & Hoehn, M. (2002). Speech loudness and quality 12 months after intensive voice treatment (LSVT) for Parkinson's disease: A comparison with an alternative speech treatment. *Folia Phoniatrica, 54,* 296–303.

Sapir, S., Ramig, L .O., Spielman, J. L., & Fox, C. (2010b). Formant centralization ratio (FCR): A proposal for a new acoustic measure of dysarthric speech. *Journal of Speech Language and Hearing Research, 53,* 114–125.

Sapir, S., Spielman, J., Ramig, L., Story, B., & Fox, C. (2007). Effects of intensive voice treatment (LSVT®) on vowel articulation in dysarthric individuals with idiopathic Parkinson disease: Acoustic and perceptual findings. *Journal of Speech Language and Hearing Research, 50,* 889–912.

Sarno, M. T. (1968). Speech impairment in Parkinson's disease. *Archives of Physical Medicine and Rehabilitation, 49,* 269–275.

Schneider, J. S., Diamond, S. G., & Markham, C. H. (1986). Deficits in orofacial sensorimotor function in Parkinson's disease. *Annals of Neurology, 19,* 275–282.

Schneider, J. S., & Lidsky, T. I. (1987). *Basal ganglia and behavior: Sensory aspects of motor functioning.* Toronto, Canada: Hans Huber.

Skodda, S., Rinsche, H., & Schlegel, U. (2009). Progression of dysprosody in Parkinson's disease over time—a longitudinal study. *Movement Disorders, 24,* 716–722.

Skodda, S., Visser, W., & Schlegel, U. (2010). Vowel articulation in Parkinson's disease. *Journal of Voice.* Epub ahead of print.

Smith, M., Ramig, L. O., Dromey, C., Perez, K., & Samandari, R. (1995). Intensive voice treatment in Parkinson's disease: Laryngostroboscopic findings. *Journal of Voice, 9,* 453–459.

Solomon, N. P., & Hixon, T. J. (1993). Speech breathing in Parkinson's disease. *Journal of Speech Language and Hearing Research, 36,* 294–310.

Solomon, N. P., Robin, D. A., Lorell, D. M., Rodnitzky, R. L., & Luschei, E. S. (1994). Tongue function testing in Parkinson's disease: Indicators of fatigue. In J. A. Till, K. M. Yorkston, & R. Beukelman (Eds.), *Motor speech disorders: Advances in assessment and treatment* (pp. 147–160). Baltimore, MD: Paul H. Brookes.

Spielman, J., Borod, J., & Ramig, L. (2003). The effects of intensive voice treatment on facial expressiveness in Parkinson disease: Preliminary data. *Cognitive and Behavioral Neurology, 16,* 177–188.

Stewart, C., Winfield, L., Hunt, A., Bressman S. B., Fahn S., Blitzer A.,& Brin M. F. (1995). Speech dysfunction in early Parkinson's disease. *Movement Disorders, 10,* 562–565.

Tassorelli, C., Buscone, S., Sandrini, G., Pacchetti, C., Furnari, A., Zangaglia, R., . . . Martignoni, E. (2009). The role of rehabilitation in deep brain stimulation of the subthalamic nucleus for Parkinson's disease: A pilot study. *Parkinsonism and Related Disorders, 15,* 675–681.

Taub, E. (2004). Harnessing brain plasticity through behavioral techniques to produce new treatments in neurorehabilitation. *American Psychologist, 59,* 692–704.

Theodoros, D. G., Constantinescu, G., Russell, T. G., Ward, E.C., Wilson, S. J.,& Wootton, R. (2006). Treating the speech disorder in Parkinson's disease online. *Journal of Telemedicine and Telecare, 12* (Suppl. 3), 88–91.

Tillerson, J., & Miller, G. (2002). Forced limb-use and recovery following brain injury. *Neuroscientist, 8,* 574–585.

Tillerson, J., Caudle, W. M., Reveron, M. E., & Miller, G. W. (2003). Exercise induces behavioral recovery and attenuates neurochemical deficits in rodent models of Parkinson's disease. *Neuroscience, 119,* 899–911.

Tillerson, J., Cohen, A. D., Philhower, J., Miller, G. W., Zigmond, M. J., & Schallert, T. (2001). Forced limb-use effects on the behavioral and neurochemical effects of 6-hydroxydopamine. *Journal of Neuroscience, 21,* 4427–4435.

Tjaden, K., &Wilding, G. E. (2004). Rate and loudness manipulations in dysarthria: Acoustic and perceptual findings. *Journal of Speech Language and Hearing Research, 47,* 766–783.

Trail, M., Fox, C., Ramig, L. O, Sapir S., Howard J., & Lai, E. C.(2005). Speech treatment for Parkinson's disease. *NeuroRehabilitation, 20,* 205–221.

Tripoliti, E., Zrinzo, L., Martinez-Torres, I., Tisch, S., Frost, E., Borrell, E., Hariz, M. I., & Limousin, P. (2008). Effects of contact location and voltage amplitude on speech and movement in bilateral subthalamic nucleus deep brain stimulation. *Movement Disorders, 23,* 2377–2383.

Weiner, W. J., & Lang, A. E. (1989). *Movement disorders: A comprehensive survey.* Mount Kisco, NY: Futura.

Winholtz, W., & Ramig, L. (1992). The vocal demodulator for analysis of vocal tremor. *Journal of Speech and Hearing Research, 35,* 562–573.

Yorkston, K. M. (1996). Treatment efficacy: Dysarthria. *Journal of Speech and Hearing Research, 39,* S46–S57.

Yorkston, K. M., Hakel, M., Beukelman, D. R., & Fager, S. (2007). Evidence for effectiveness of treatment of loudness, rate, or prosody in dysarthria: A systematic review. *Journal of Medical Speech-Language Pathology, 15,* 11–36.

Yorkston, K. M., Spencer, K. A., & Duffy, J. R. (2003). Behavioral management of respiratory/phonatory dysfunction from dysarthria: A systematic review of the evidence. *Journal of Medical Speech-Language Pathology, 11,* 13–38.

5

Cognitive-Linguistic Disorder in Parkinson Disease

ADRIENNE HANCOCK
LEONARD LaPOINTE
BROOKE-MAI WHELAN

Communication barriers for people with Parkinson disease (PD) are embedded in the speech production of their hypokinetic dysarthria as well as their masklike affect and facial expression. Yet, most people with PD will face cognitive-linguistic impairment as well. Less is known about the latter, but it is not unexplored. Even as recently as 20 years ago, the communication difficulty of people with PD was thought solely to be the artifact of movement-based disruption of speech and voice. Linguistic processing disorder was thought to be confined to the purview of aphasia. Expansion and evolving sophistication of our methods of assessing cognitive-linguistic processes has broadened our appreciation of what can go wrong in PD. Language function is difficult to assess and describe because it is difficult to parse from the complex motor speech and cognitive abilities (e.g., attention, memory, executive function) known to deteriorate with PD. The cognitive characteristics inherent in PD are gaining attention and clarity. Stocci and Brusa (2000) report 90% of people with PD have some cognitive impairment affecting daily life, with 25% classified as severe cognitive impairment. This supports the frequent complaints of our clients with PD who report losing their train of thought, forgetting appointments, and difficulty planning the temporal sequences of a typical day.

According to a review of 12 reports, 24 to 31% of people with PD are diagnosed with dementia, which would account for almost 4% of dementia in the population (Aarsland, Zaccai, & Brayne, 2005). The dementia of people with PD is similar to a dysexecutive syndrome, with some visuospatial and behavioral symptoms (Emre, 2003). This expresses itself in short attention span, poor working memory, reduced recent and short term memory, and trouble with planning and reasoning. A study of cognitive function through the course of the disease has demonstrated that mild cognitive dysfunction can be evident even at the time of initial PD diagnosis and may deteriorate to status of dementia or general cognitive impairment at a greater rate than for aging individuals without PD (Williams-Gray, Foltynie, Brayne, Robbins, & Barker, 2007).

A Belgian PD study reported 82% of their sample had cognitive dysfunction in one or more areas: 76% demonstrated executive/motor impairments, 34% attention/memory, and 10% visuospatial impairments (Verleden, Vingerhoets & Santens, 2006). More specifically, cognitive-linguistic deficits appear in immediate recall of verbal material, language production and comprehension, semantic fluency, set-formation, sequencing, and visuomotor construction (Dubois & Pillon, 1997; Grossman, Carvel, Stern, Goloomp, & Hurtig, 1992; Levin, Tomer, & Rey, 1992; Verleden et al., 2006). Even in people with PD but without dementia, deficits in executive functions (i.e., planning and monitoring goal-directed behavior), memory, attention, problem-solving, verbal learning, and visuospatial processing can be present (Goldman, Baty, Buckles, Sahrmann & Morris, 1998; Grossman, 1999; Kulisevesky, 2000; Owen et al., 1992; Verbaan et al., 2007).

Cognitive-linguistic and motor characteristics of PD can be heterogeneous due to many sources of variability. In most studies, cognitive-linguistic dysfunction or deterioration of function can be associated with a person's age, age at onset of PD, education level, and the stage of PD (Aarsland, Andersen, Larsen, Lolk, & Kragh-Sorensen, 2003; Jankovic & Kapadia, 2001; Mayeux et al., 1988; Verleden et al., 2006; Verbaan et al., 2007). Other studies of PD have reported no remarkable deterioration of cognitive-linguistic function (Bayles et al., 1996; Gilbert, Belleville, Bherer, & Chouinard, 2005, Verbaan et al., 2007). Mayeux et al. (1992) reported less than 1 percent prevalence for PD with dementia if under 50 years of age, with prevalence increasing each decade of life and reaching 68.7% for those 80 years and older. Overall, in this study

41% of 179 people with PD were diagnosed with dementia. One wonders if the discrepancy of reports of cognitive-linguistic impairment in PD is related to the sensitivity and specificity of the instruments used to unveil it. Several studies have indicated that PD characterized by postural/gait instability and akinesia is associated with greater risk for developing cognitive impairments than PD of a tremor-dominant type (Burn et al., 2006; Jankovic & Kapadia, 2001), although this may be confounded by Hoehn and Yahr severity score (Verbaan et al., 2007). One patient, Randy, reports difficulty remembering the lyrics of oft-sung songs in his appearances with his PD support group chorus. Martha loses her balance when she walks and tries to give directions to her sister's house. Malika cannot read or comprehend long paragraphs now, though she has a PhD in astrophysics. These reports are echoed in support groups of both young and older onset PD worldwide. It is not just the shuffling gait or the inaudible voice that plagues people with PD.

This chapter describes cognitive-linguistic interactions and explores the many elements of this nonmotoric yet potentially devastating deficit in PD. Pharmaceutical and surgical treatments for PD also provide information as to the neurologic underpinnings of motoric and cognitive-linguistic function, further guiding us toward understanding the complex neural circuitry affected by PD and developing treatments for the variety of challenges facing people with PD.

Cognitive-Linguistic Interactions

Various processes of cognition and language are entangled in an intricate relationship and may be most difficult to isolate, a concept widely supported and now referred to as *cognitive-linguistic* interaction (Body, 2004; Helm-Estabrooks, 2001; LaPointe et al., 2004a ; LaPointe, Maitland, Kemker, & Stierwalt, 2004b). Carefully controlled processes, such as attention and various forms of memory are coordinated during language comprehension. Working memory is often required for comprehension of both written and spoken language, particularly for comprehension of complex and long sentences, ambiguous words or phrases, referenced pronouns, and when information is irrelevant or interrupted (Engle & Conway, 1998; Jonides,1995). Working memory ability can be described as the ability to store some information for a short time while additional information necessary to solve a problem is computed simultaneously.

People with larger working memory spans are faster and more accurate on tasks of language comprehension, perhaps because they can simultaneously store previously read text while also using it to interpret a sentence in entirety (Jonides, 1995). The deleterious effects of a small or taxed working memory in dual-task conditions may only appear during more complex sentence comprehension, indicating working memory is utilized on a selective or as-needed basis.

Lengthy, complex sentences require more cognitive processing to interpret linguistic structure and derive accurate meanings, though the exact processes and extent of involvement are not wholly agreed on. Pronouns referencing characters first mentioned in previous sentences can only be comprehended if the referent was encoded and available for recall and comparison. Comprehension of complex sentence structure requires some clauses to be held in memory while other parts are decoded. For example, lexical cues such as *"after"* or *"but"* aid the reader to remember the previous phrase and reserve interpretations until after reading the phrase that follows, which often alters the meaning of the sentence. Sentences beginning with *"before"* require more computations than those beginning with *"after"*; the additional processing can be measured by event-related brain potentials and correlated with working-memory spans (Münte, Schilta, & Kutas, 1998). Some sentences, referred to in research as garden-path sentences and used to test language processes, are designed to initially mislead language comprehension simply by omitting a comma or rearranging clauses (Ferreira, Bailey, & Ferraro, 2002). For example, "Time flies like an arrow. Fruit flies like a banana" in Groucho's famous garden-path setup. Table 5–1 contains sentences to demonstrate how language comprehension occurs with the help of cognitive processes coordinating, retrieving, and comparing information across phrases.

Table 5–1. Sentences Requiring Cognitive Processes for Comprehension

The man who kissed the girl was holding white rabbits. (Who was holding rabbits?)
Frank drowned Dave. (Who drowned?)
The girl that the boy chased is older. (Who is older?)
While mom washed the dog slept in the sun.

Cognitive-Linguistic Dysfunction in Parkinson Disease

Semantic knowledge and complex linguistic constructions are sometimes found to be impaired in PD. Performance on the Test of Language Competence was significantly more impaired in people with PD who exhibited dementia (i.e., scores below 139.9 on the Mattis Dementia Rating Scale) (Lewis, LaPointe, Murdoch, & Chenery, 1998). Without dementia, people with PD still scored below healthy age-matched control participants for generating definitions and recreating sentences. A typical semantic assessment requiring some executive function is the verbal fluency or generative naming task. Verbal fluency tasks require people to generate words according to specific rules. On this task people with PD, more so than control participants, benefited from semantic cues (Lewis et al., 1998). Zgaljardic et al. (2006) found both category (e.g., list animals) and phonemic (e.g., list words beginning with letter "t") verbal fluency to be impaired in a group of 32 nondemented people with PD. In another study, people with PD showed no impairment on phonemic verbal fluency, but performed below normal control groups when required to generate words within a semantic category (Levin, Llabre, & Weiner, 1989). These few investigations of semantic abilities indicate impairment in PD, but this area is lacking research consensus. It is likely the inability to create categories and strategies is affecting semantic language skills of people with PD.

Syntax is another linguistic domain that has been found not to be normal in people with PD, and appears to be affected for both expression and comprehension (Grossman et al., 1991). Syntactic complexity of spontaneous speech deteriorates with progression of the disease (Illes, Metter, Hanson, & Iritani, 1988). Several studies have differentiated PD from control groups by manipulating complexity of syntax in sentence comprehension tasks. For example, when sentences contain propositions, people with PD perform more poorly than controls (Caplan & Waters, 1999). Grammatical complexity and semantic ambiguity compromised sentence comprehension in a study of nondemented people with PD, although this was inconsistent across people and across testing sessions (Grossman et al., 1992). Lee, Grossman, Morris, Stern, and Hurtig (2003) reported accurate performance, but slowed processing times for nondemented people with mild idiopathic PD when grammatical morphemes were omitted, and when center-embedded clauses were object-relative rather than subject-relative (e.g., "The boy that hugged the girl is friendly" required more time than "The boy that the girl hugged is friendly"). Noncanonical sentences, such as object-relative sentences, generally take longer to comprehend, but the significantly longer time required by people with PD may reflect slower lexical retrieval and working memory (Angwin, Chenery, Copland, Murdoch, & Silburn, 2006).

Presence of dementia concomitant with PD may be a significant influence in cognitive-linguistic performance. Lewis et al. (1998) found no language impairment in a group of idiopathic people with PD who have normal scores on the Mattis dementia rating scale (DRS). However, they did find that people with below normal DRS scores performed below normal on language tasks associated with cognitive processing, especially constructing sentences, naming, and metaphors. The higher-level language processes, such as understanding metaphors and ambiguous sentences, require inferences and are particularly challenging for people with even mild PD (Berg, Bjornram, Hartelius, Laakso, & Johnels, 2003). In another group of people without dementia, Taylor, Saint-Cyr, and Lang (1986) found no impairment in receptive or expressive aspects of language. These authors attribute intact language function to normal parietal and temporal lobe function. They suggest damage to the frontal lobes, particularly the supplementary motor area (SMA), is probably responsible for the deficit in planning actions guided by internal cues (these include language production as a goal-directed action). The functioning SMA receives input from the basal ganglia via the thalamus, which may explain why the deficit in action planning is noted in the PD population. We return to a discussion of planning and internal strategy, likely one of the deficits manifested in both cognitive-linguistic and motor dysfunction.

Involvement of the prefrontal area in cognitive-linguistic deficits associated with PD is clearly implicated by the differences reported in people with PD who have dementia and those who do not. Unlike a pure language disorder, the limited executive abilities and attention resources, particularly of working memory, appear to be the basis of cognitive-linguistic deficits in PD (Graceffa, Carlesimo, Peppe, & Caltagirone, 1999; Grossman, 1999). Working memory, information processing speed, shifting attention, and coordination of several cognitive processes are all involved in normal sentence comprehension, and deficient in some people with PD (Grossman, 1999; Lee et al,. 2003). The component systems of cognition impaired in PD that potentially provide explanations for the cognitive-linguistic deterioration noted with the progression of the disease, and the dysfunction of frontostriatal circuitry are discussed below.

Executive Functioning in Parkinson Disease

The executive function deficits in PD are very similar to those of people with dysexecutive syndrome resulting from frontal lobe damage, particularly damage in the dorsolateral prefrontal cortex (DLPFC): planning, sequencing, switching, monitoring, inhibitory control, and information processing speed (Dubois & Pillion, 1997; Kulisevsky, 2000; Verbaan et al., 2007; Zgaljardic et al., 2006). This is the very human area of the frontal cortex that plans our day, organizes our actions, and gets us there. People with DLPFC damage miss appointments, may dress peculiarly, show up late, and have difficulty with error correction, troubleshooting, and decision making.

Internal organization of guidelines and strategies is the most common component of impaired cognitive and motor execution in PD. It is suggested that people with PD struggle with or lose procedural learning skills even with intact declarative memory because of the implicit nature of procedural learning through repeated exposure and practice (Saint-Cyr, Taylor, & Lang, 1988; Vakil & Herishanu, 1998). However if rules are explicit, even when a cognitive task is challenging, speed may be slowed but accuracy is not impaired (Taylor et al., 1986; Brown & Marsden, 1990). Therefore, this deficit affects cognitive efficiency and learning, but does not always impact the final outcome. A person may learn to trace a picture backwards, but take twice as long to learn it. The Wisconsin Card Sorting Test (WCST) measures ability to learn, and occasionally change, the object of a task according to performance and examiner's limited accuracy feedback. This requires constant comparing and updating and occasional set-shifting to new rules. People with PD score poorly on the WCST because they do not adjust to a new objective (Monchi et al., 2004). This particular impairment, indicated by several perseverative errors on WCST, is present in all severities and stages of PD (Owen et al., 1992). Passive or automatic learning deficits can affect a variety of tasks and impede progress in therapy. Fortunately, the simple addition of external cues and more effortful learning processes can significantly change outcome and be valuable compensatory strategies.

Cognitive flexibility, ability to change thought and direction in response to new information, is important in rehabilitation and in daily life. Without it, people with PD have difficulty in unfamiliar routines, complex or multistep processes, and coping with unexpected changes, especially when walking or driving. Failure to organize or adopt strategies in response to a changing environment can place people at risk even in the early stages of PD (Levin et al., 1992). Many executive functions

Cognitive-Linguistic Dysfunctions in Parkinson Disease

- Attention
- Effort-demanding tasks
- Executive function and internal control tasks (e.g., set shifting)
- Learning
- Recall memory (but not recognition memory)
- Self-directed task planning/strategizing
- Syntatic complexity
- Verbal working memory
- Verbal fluency
- Visuospatial function

are impeded when people cannot self-assess or use feedback to change cognitive or motor processes. Executive functions can interact with other cognitive deficits in PD, making diagnoses and treatment plans even more heterogeneous in this clinical population.

Attention and Memory in Parkinson Disease

People with PD without dementia have intact verbal short-term storage and recognition memory (Flowers, Pearce, & Pearce, 1984; Gilbert et al., 2005) but impairments in immediate recall (Taylor et al., 1986; Verbaan et al., 2007). Breen (1993) reported this pattern of relative strengths and weaknesses in 15 people with PD and also observed that even when strategies were created they were not efficiently used. Perhaps, underlying the recall memory impairment is a deficit in working memory, which Higginson et al. (2003) proposed mediates executive and recall memory functions and, as discussed previously, is heavily involved in language processes.

In fact, working memory impairment is considered by Higginson et al. (2003) as a fundamental cognitive disturbance in PD. Components of working memory seem differentially affected by PD. Working memory impairments in individuals with PD are more related to certain executive impairments, such as manipulation, than to rehearsal or storage problems (Gilbert et al., 2005; Higginson et al., 2003; Stocchi & Brusa, 2000; Zgaljardic, Borod, Foldi, & Mattis, 2003). Normal neurologic function shows the caudate nuclei of the striatum, which may well be damaged in PD, as more active during working memory conditions requiring manipulation than during tasks of retrieval only (Lewis, Dove, Robbins, Barker, & Owen, 2004). Behaviorally, individuals with PD often struggle when manipulating information within working memory even with intact short-term memory (Bublak, Muller, Gron, Reuter, & von Cramon, 2002). When compared to a control group and a PD group with no executive dysfunction but equivalent maintenance and retrieval ability, people with PD and executive dysfunction demonstrated specific impairment in manipulating information, but not in maintaining or retrieving information, (Lewis et al., 2003). Caplan and Waters (1999) reported reduced verbal working memory spans with normal rehearsal and storage functions even in people with PD without dementia.

Working memory deficits clearly emerge in individuals with PD when task conditions become more demanding, which likely indicates a reduced ability to simultaneously process and store information (Bublak et al., 2002). Inhibitory mechanisms, disrupted in early PD, may contribute to impairments in working memory processes during distraction (Kensinger, Shearer, Locascio, Growdon, & Corkin, 2003). Sharpe (1996) found that PD people had more difficulty than controls when required to divide their attention between two competing auditory inputs. Performance is particularly impaired on tasks that require attention and fast cognitive processing or internal guiding of attention, such as language (Pahwa et al., 1998; Raskin, Borod, & Tweedy, 1990; Ridenour & Dean, 1999). In particular, sentence comprehension falters when simultaneously performing a secondary task (Grossman, 1999; Grossman, Kalmanson, Bernhardt, Stern, & Hurtig, 2000). For example, it is difficult to play Solitaire and answer survey questions on the telephone at the same time.

Sentence processing deficits in individuals with PD may be attributed to an inability to attend to sentence structure resulting from impaired working memory and slowed information processing (Grossman et al., 2002; Lee et al., 2003). When asked to process sentences with high demands of working memory, fMRI revealed that people with PD without dementia recruited fewer striatal regions than did normal controls; furthermore, the people with PD demonstrated more cortical activation to compensate for depleted working memory resources (Grossman et al., 2002).

Overall, the types of cognitive deficits caused by PD are exactly the type expected to interfere with language. People with PD are particularly susceptible when the required cognitive-linguistic processes become numerous, simultaneous, or complex (Sharpe, 1990). Further research is needed to explore the cognitive signs through the progression of the disease and the impact of deterioration on a person's daily life. Some difficulty isolating a correlation between cognitive status and disease stage may arise because the stages of the disease are often marked by physical signs only (e.g., Hoehn and Yahr score).

Relationship Between Cognitive-Linguistic and Motoric Impairment

Slow and rigid cognitive-linguistic behavior has long been compared to the slow and rigid physical signs of PD; Naville first coined the term "bradyphrenia" in 1922 to refer to slowness of thinking (Brown & Marsden, 1990). More recent understanding suggests that motor impairment is not always predictive of cognitive status or language ability. Furthermore, we know that motor, prefrontal, and limbic frontostriatal circuits sometimes function rather independently (Kulisevsky, 2000). For example, motor and cognitive impairments did not correlate in a study of 60 newly diagnosed, untreated people with PD who demonstrated deficits in attention and attention shifting and inefficient working memory (Cooper, Sagar, Jordan, Harvey, & Sullivan, 1991). There also is no well-established correlation between severity of motor performance and sentence comprehension accuracy, verbal fluency, or card sorting test scores (Grossman, 1999; Van Spaendonck, Berger, Horstink, Buytenhuijs, & Cools, 1996).

"Bradyphrenia" was introduced and used as an analogous term to "bradykinesia" when motor and cognitive deficits were thought to stem from the same dopaminergic pathology. However, studies supporting the parallel motoric-cognitive deficit theory have not all successfully separated the speed of motor responses from speed of information processing (Rafal, Posner, Walker, & Friedrich, 1984). In other words, it is difficult to know whether cognitive, motor, or both stages of a response are responsible for a slow response time. Changes in motor function, such as in "on" versus "off" states of pharmaceutical therapy, did not correspond with cognitive slowing in three within-subject experiments designed to test the "bradyphrenia" hypothesis (Rafal et al., 1984). Cooper et al. (1991) offer an explanation of two dissociable processes, at least in the earliest stages of PD: motor control (most influenced by dopamenergic pathology) and cognition (more similar to frontal system dysfunction reflecting impaired attention or vigilance). It still is unclear whether the more advanced stages of PD perhaps involve breakdowns in an integrated process regulated by frontostriatal circuitry. Motoric deficits in PD may actually reflect impaired motoric, cognitive, and integrative processes.

The conundrum of separating the influences of motor impairment in cognitive decline continues to puzzle. If movement is conceptualized as goal-directed, purposeful behavior, then cognitive processes are involved to generate and execute motor plans, monitor and regulate actions, and update information to learn new motor programs. Intact memory, attention, and feedback systems are required for motor programs to set the parameters based on past experience and current environment. The reduced initiation, speed, and overall amount of movement in PD may be attributed to a person's cognitive slowness to prepare in advance (i.e., strategize) or the inability to learn and modify movement without visual feedback (Brown & Jahanshahi, 1996).

Some studies have shown associations when measuring severity of extrapyramidal signs (EPS) and neuropsychological tests of memory, orientation, reasoning, language, construction, and psychomotor speed (Mortimer, Pirozzolo, Hansch, & Webster, 1982; Richards, Stern, Marder, Cote, & Mayeux, 1993). Vakil and Herishanu-Naaman (1998) found significantly impaired procedural learning in people with the bradykinesia subtype of PD, but not in those with tremor subtype. Thus, not only the severity of motor impairment, but the type and neuropathologic basis should be considered when investigating motor-cognitive correspondence. Cognitive deficits of the prefrontal cortex, shifting and dividing attention, may explain the additional motoric errors observed in paradigms testing speed and accuracy of simultaneous movements (Brown & Jahanshahi, 1996). Performance on activities of daily living (ADLs) is a functional and important measure when considering the interdependence of cognitive and motor function. Executive functioning, not simple motor functioning, is a significant predictor for instrumental ADL (e.g., shopping, dialing the phone, feeding the cockatoo) performance (Cahn et al., 1998). Although the comparison has limitations, bradykinesia and bradyphrenia share consequences of vocational limitation and social isolation.

Berger et al. (1999) suggested a correlation between motor and cognitive dysfunction is dependent on whether the cognitive task requires externally or internally controlled processing. As discussed previously, people with PD demonstrate reliance on explicit rules and external cues and have difficulty internally guiding behavior and movement. In a patient group with only mild/moderate physical symptoms, a positive association demonstrated that people with PD and bradykinesia are more dependent on an externally guided learning strategy although they can use an internally guided strategy (i.e., semantic organization) when the preferred external strategy is prevented (Berger et al, 1999). This explanation fits nicely with the hypothesis that people with PD have intact internal motor programs, but have deficits executing them to achieve a motor goal. External cuing greatly improves limb and speech motor performance in people with PD (Hiraoka, Matuo, Iwata, Onishi & Abe, 2006; Lewis et al., 1998; Rochester et al., 2005). Similarly, tasks with explicit instructions or which are easy to self-monitor are not affected by PD, yet performance deteriorates when tasks require generation of a plan or strategy (Taylor et al., 1986; Lee et al., 2003). Implications for behavioral treatment are tremendous: if cognitive ability and resources are available but not accessed, then treatment must target generation and implementation of plans to use what is held hostage in the prefrontal cortex.

Neurologic Bases of Cognitive-Linguistic Dysfunction in Parkinson Disease

Although a thorough discussion of the neurologic bases of PD is provided in Chapters 1 and 2, it is worth highlighting select components here as they explain, and in fact have helped predict, motoric and cognitive-linguistic signs of PD. Later in this chapter, findings about cognitive-linguistic performance after neurosurgical or pharmaceutical treatment of PD are described in terms of the contribution of each subcortical structure to language processing. However, it is important first to recognize that PD is not simply a disorder of the basal ganglia, but rather the striatal system.

Disruption in the *frontostriatal circuitry* connecting frontal cortex and the basal ganglia is clearly related to the cognitive and behavioral impairments of PD (Cummings, 1993). Specifically, dysfunction of three of the frontostriatal circuits: dorsolateral prefrontal cortex (DLPFC), anterior cingulate cortex (ACC), and orbitofrontal cortex (OFC), are responsible for the nonmotoric skills commonly impaired in PD. These frontostriatal circuits can be disrupted by striatal dysfunction resulting from neurochemical imbalance. For example, reduced dopamine outflow from the anterodorsal head of the caudate to the frontal cortex is one proposed basis for neurocognitive impairment in PD (Kulisevsky, 2000). Although the substantia nigra appears as a continuous band in brain sections, anatomic studies have found that it actually consists of two parts with very different connections and functions, the *pars compacta* and *pars reticulata*. The *pars compacta* serves mainly as an input to the basal ganglia circuit, supplying the striatum with dopamine. The *pars reticulata*, on the other hand, serves mainly as an output, conveying signals from the basal ganglia to numerous other brain structures. This circuitry is complex and allows for constant intercommunication among subcortical and cortical structures. Movement and cognition are interwoven into this circuitry and it is no wonder that parsing them is difficult when these structures and pathways are damaged. Figures 5–1, 5–2, and 5–3 depict some of the structures and circuitry that is involved in this parkinsonian puzzle of intertwined characteristics.

Zgaljardic et al. (2003) reviewed several studies and arrived at the consensus that the DLPFC is a likely suspect in PD, causing central executive deficits. The DLPFC is the primary area responsible for executive functions such as sustained attention and working memory (Cummings, 1993). The ACC, associated with conflict-monitoring, motivation, and response-inhibition functions, and OFC, more related to emotional regulation, are also likely to be affected in PD and help explain the emotional and behavioral characteristics of PD (Chow & Cummings, 1999; Zgaljardic et al., 2003). In 2006, Zgaljardic et al. administered several neuropsychological measures to people with PD without dementia and a matched-control group, categorizing the measures based on the frontostriatal circuits' known functions. Trends suggested DLPFC and ACC functions were more affected by PD than OFC's functions, and the DLPFC index was the only factor discriminating PD and control groups.

Consequently, anticipated cognitive deficits in PD encompass the following skills: complex visuospatial functions, free recall memory, working memory, effort demanding tasks (e.g., rapid processing and complex problem-solving), set-formation and set shifting entailing the internal control of attention, sequencing, temporal order and recency discrimination, as well as executive function (Saint-Cyr & Trepanier, 2000). Neuropsychological test batteries, therefore, typically include the following psy-

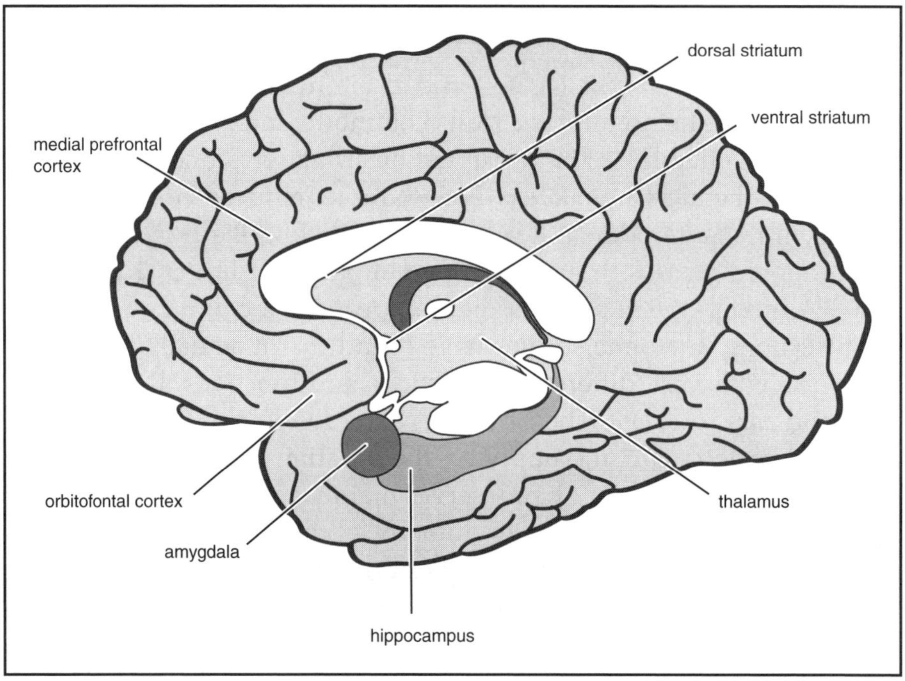

FIGURE 5–1. Simplified version of subcortical structures important in Parkinson disease for both movement and cognitive-linguistic impairment. Adapted with permission from *Acquired Language Disorders: A Case-Based Approach* (p. 13) by E. R. Klein and J. M. Mancinelli. Copyright © 2010 Plural Publishing, Inc. All rights reserved.

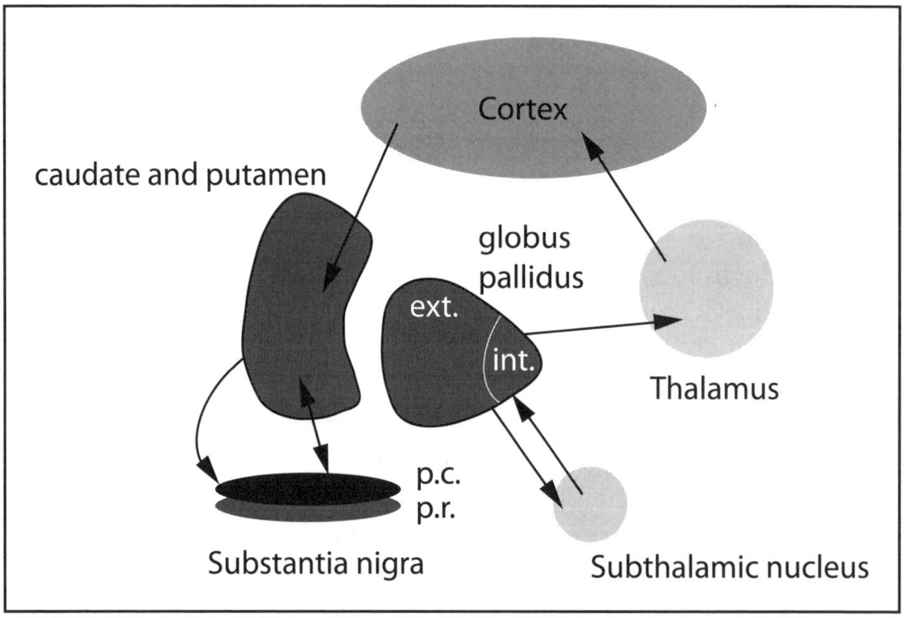

FIGURE 5–2. Schematic diagram of subcortical-frontal cortical circuitry (pc = pars compacta; pr = pars reticulate).

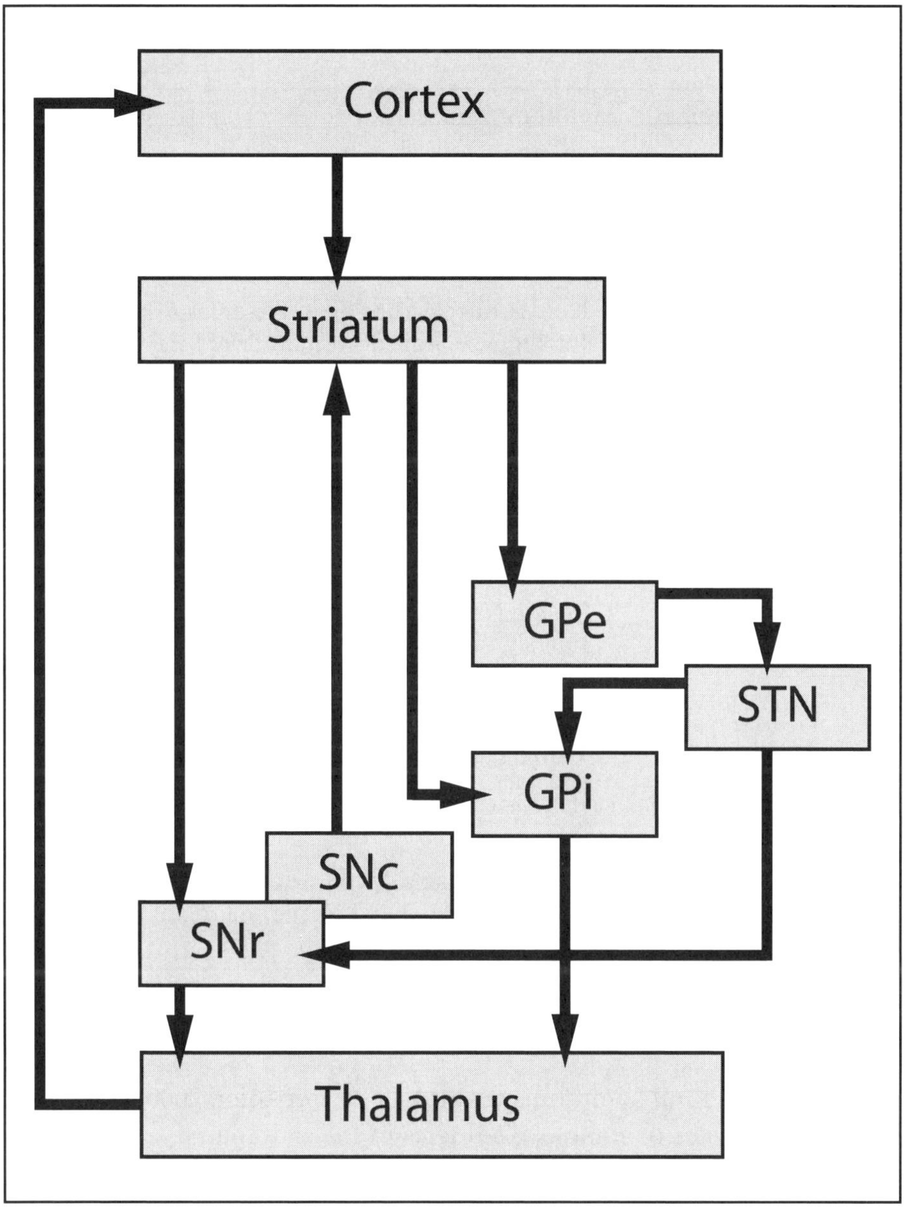

FIGURE 5–3. Schematic of thalamocorticostriatal circuitry (Key: SNc = pars comacta; SNr = pars reticulata; GPe = Globus Pallidus externus; GPi = Globus Pallidus internus; STN = Subthalamic nucleus).

chometric domains: brief cognitive screens, estimates of premorbid and current intelligence quotients, attention/working memory/psychomotor processing speed, frontal executive functioning, language, verbal learning/memory, visuospatial learning/memory, and mood and frontal per-

Table 5–2. Standard Neuropsychological Assessment Domains and Test Battery Examples

Neuropsychological Domain	*Test Battery*
Brief cognitive screenings	Mini-Mental Status Evaluation, Mattis Dementia Rating Scale, Montreal Cognitive Assessment (MoCA)
Intelligence quotients	New Adult Reading Test, Weschler Adult Intelligence Scale, Kaufman Brief Intelligence Test
Attention/working memory/psychomotor processing speed	Digit span, trail making test (A & B)
Frontal executive functioning	Odd man out, Wisconsin Card Sorting Test, Stroop test, Tower of London test, Raven's Progressive Matrices, Continuous Performance Test II
Language	Boston Naming Test, phonemic and semantic fluency, alternating fluency, Examining for Aphasia-4
Verbal learning and memory	California Verbal Learning Test, Rey Auditory Verbal Learning Test, Hopkins Verbal Learning Test
Visuospatial learning and memory	Rey-Osterrieth Complex Figure Test
Personality/behavior symptoms	Beck Depression Inventory, Geriatric Depression Scale, Beck Anxiety Inventory, Frontal Lobe Personality Scale

sonality/behavioral symptoms (Saint-Cyr & Trepanier, 2000). Table 5–2 presents examples of standardized tests in these domains.

Effects of Drug Therapy and Neurosurgical Procedures on Cognitive-Linguistic Functioning

Neurosurgical procedures are now routinely applied techniques in the management of severe or end-stage PD. These complex and precise procedures involve circumscribed lesioning or high-frequency stimulation of specific subcortical nuclei. The mid-1970s and 1980s heralded a resurgence of interest in neurosurgical interventions for the treatment of PD, largely instigated by observed long-term limitations of drug therapy; a better understanding of pathophysiologic models of PD; as well as improvements in stereotactic techniques and equipment (Gildenberg, 1984; Speelman & Bosch, 2002; Movement Disorders Society, 2002). The remainder of this chapter focuses on the effects of conventional drug therapies, as well as ablative lesions and high- frequency deep brain stimulation of specific subcortical nuclei, on cognitive-linguistic functioning in people with PD.

Effects of Drug Therapy on Cognitive-Linguistic Functioning in PD

Parkinson disease typically arises as a result of dopaminergic neuronal degeneration within the substantia nigra and ventral tegmental area (Agid, Javoy-Agid, & Ruberg, 1987). From these regions originate projection systems involved in motor and cognitive/effective functioning, namely, the nigrostriatal and mesolimbic-cortical systems, respectively (McNamara & Durso, 2006). Drug therapies in relation to the treatment of PD almost exclusively have been developed on the hallmark pathophysiologic finding of a dopamine deficiency in these patients, with levodopa and dopamine agonists subsequently representing the most widely prescribed pharmaceutical agents (Hermanowicz, 2007).

The consensus of experts appears to indicate that dopaminergic drug therapies more commonly provide relief for the associated motor symptoms of PD, yet fail to alleviate nonmotor symptoms, including cognitive deficits (Hermanowicz, 2007). Although tremor and motor impairment may be dramatically alleviated, thinking and speech may remain impervious. In fact, it has been suggested that dopaminergic therapies that achieve a person's optimal motor state may actually shift the same individual away from his or her optimum level of cognitive functioning (Cools, Barker, Sahakian, & Robbins, 2003). This profile has been hypothesized by some to be the result of a "dopamine overdose," whereby dopaminergic activation may serve to replenish depleted circuits (e.g., motor), yet overdose intact circuits (i.e., cognitive) (Swainson et al., 2000). At dose ranges adequate to eradicate motor symptoms, however, both negative and positive effects on cognition (particularly executive functioning) have been documented (McNamara & Durso, 2006). For example, verbal fluency performance has been reported to improve as a consequence of levodopa administration in people with PD (Gotham,

Brown, & Marsden, 1988), as have scores on tasks of set shifting, working memory, Tower of London test, and spatial attention (Lange, Paul, Naumann, & Gsell, 1995; Lange et al., 1992). Dopamine agonists such as bromocriptine, pergolide, and apomorphine, however, have resulted in both positive and negative effects on verbal fluency performance in people with PD (Brusa et al., 2003; Kimberg & D'Esposito, 2003; Kompoliti, Wang, Goetz, Leurgans, & Raman, 2000; McNamara & Durso, 2006); impairments on tasks of short-term verbal memory (Brusa et al., 2003); as well as short-lived improvements in verbal and visual memory, and other tasks of executive functioning (Kulisevsky et al., 2000).

In relation to language processing, dopaminergic activation has been observed to improve sentence comprehension (Grossman et al., 2001; McNamara, Krueger, O'Quin, Clark, & Durso, 1996; Morris et al., 1998), suggesting that dopamine deficiency may result in impaired sentence comprehension as a consequence of slower automatic lexical activation (Grossman et al., 2002). A number of semantic priming studies have attempted to probe the influence of dopamine on lexical activation mechanisms. The semantic priming or lexical decision task is a widely used task in cognitive psychology that was initially used to investigate the nature of semantic memory or the organization of general world knowledge. In this task, participants are asked to determine as quickly as possible whether a letter string is a word. In 1971, Meyer and Schvaneveldt used the lexical decision task to show that lexical decision responses are made more quickly when the current word is related to the previous word. People more quickly recognize DOCTOR as a word when it follows the word NURSE than if it follows the word CHAIR. The effect came to be known as "semantic priming" and is often cited as evidence for the associative strength between concepts in semantic memory.

Results of semantic priming studies indicate that in the case of healthy individuals, the administration of levodopa may speed the time course of lexical activation, as evidenced by faster onset and decay of priming effects (Angwin et al., 2004). Furthermore, enhanced direct (i.e., TIGER-STRIPES) versus indirect (i.e., LION-STRIPES) priming effects also have been observed in healthy controls as a result of levodopa ingestion, potentially indicative of increased signal to noise ratios within semantic networks as a consequence of dopaminergic activation (Kischka et al., 1996). In Parkinson disease, consistent results have been identified. Semantic priming effects have been identified in drug "on" condition as opposed to levodopa withdrawal condition, suggesting that lexical activation is delayed as consequence of dopamine depletion (Angwin, Chenery, Copland, Murdoch, & Silburn, 2007; Angwin, Copland, Chenery, Murdoch, & Silburn, 2006). In addition, reduced signal to noise ratios within parkinsonian semantic networks have been suggested, as indicated by disrupted semantic priming effects in people with PD (Angwin, Chenery, Copland, Murdoch, & Silburn, 2003).

Effects of Neurosurgical Procedures on Cognitive-Linguistic Functioning in PD

Ablative Techniques: Pallidotomy and Thalamotomy

Ablative surgical techniques constitute the procedures that were most commonly applied during the neurosurgical renaissance of the 1970s and 1980s. These techniques involve the generation of permanent lesions typically within the thalamus (i.e., thalamotomy) or globus pallidus (i.e., pallidotomy) (Kleiner-Fisman, Fisman, & Sime, 2003; Vitek, Bakay, & Freeman, 2003), by way of radiofrequency-mediated electrocoagulation that aimed to permanently ablate/disrupt or inactivate the relevant target (Benabid, Caparros-Lefebvre, & Pollak, 1998). In revisiting models of PD, a loss of dopaminergic neurons within the SNc results in hyperactivity of the *indirect pathway* and reduced activity within the *direct pathway*, causing disinhibition of GPi/SNr inhibitory outputs to the thalamus and brainstem (Lang & Lozano, 1998). This alteration in neurophysiology leads to the manifestation of cardinal parkinsonian signs and symptoms including akinesia, bradykinesia, rigidity, and tremor. Ablative lesions within motor components of this circuit aim to reduce excessive inhibitory outflow from the GPi/SNr complex (Obeso, Guridi, & DeLong, 1997) via the inactivation of target nuclei (Movement Disorders Society, 2002). In relation to target specificity, ablative neurosurgical procedures pinpoint two primary structures which may be functionally overactive as a result of the Parkinson disease process: namely, the thalamus and globus pallidus (Movement Disorders Society, 2002). The ventral intermediate (Vim) thalamus and posteroventral (PV) portion of the globus pallidus internus (GPi), constitute sensorimotor subdivisions of these structures and, hence, optimal neurosurgical targets.

Variability may exist from patient to patient in relation to primary sign and symptom presentation, perhaps as a consequence of individual pathophysiologic mechanisms or the same mechanisms influencing distinct motor subcircuits (Wichmann & DeLong, 1998). As a result, different surgical targets may be selected across candidates for surgical intervention. In more detail, lesioning Vim thalamus (i.e.,Vim thalamotomy) has been shown to be effective in relieving tremor-dominant symptoms; and lesioning of posteroventral portion of the GPi (i.e., PV pallidotomy [PVP]) has been reported to ameliorate the symptoms of akinesia, rigidity, drug-induced dyskinesias, gait, and postural disturbances (Movement Disorders Society, 2002).

Proposed Roles for the Basal Ganglia and Thalamus in Language. A number of models of subcortical participation in language postulate roles for the basal ganglia and/or thalamus in the mediation of language processes (Crosson, 1985; Nadeau & Crosson, 1997; Wallesch & Papagno, 1988). The above models collectively propose roles for the striatum, globus pallidus, thalamus (specifically VA and VL nuclei, pulvinar, CM and NR), and cerebral cortex in language processing; executed via the presence of these structures within a hypothesized basal ganglia-thalamocortical language circuit. Figure 5–4 depicts some relevant substructures of the thalamus.

Relevant to the current chapter are the potential roles of the GPi and Vim thalamus in executing language functions, which may be explored via the effects of ablative neurosurgical techniques (i.e., pallidotomy and thalamotomy), that primarily aimed to eradicate motor dysfunction. More specifically, the response-release semantic feedback model (Crosson, 1985) postulates the GPi to participate in the tonic arousal of the cerebral cortex as well as regulating the release of semantically verified language segments for verbal output, in tandem with the caudate nucleus. Lesions of the GPi are hypothesized to result in fluent language pathology, including the generation of extraneous verbal output such as semantic paraphasias (e.g., saying *truck* for *bus*; *chocolate* for *wristwatch*; *koala* for *wombat*), as a consequence of thalamic disinhibition and overexcitation of the ALC (Crosson, 1992). The lexical decision-making model (Wallesch & Papagno, 1988) incorporates the GPi within a frontal lobe system, capable of manipulating multiple degrees of freedom with respect to the temporal isochronisation of cortically generated lexical and contextual modules (Wallesch, 1990). On the basis of this model, GPi lesions are predicted to result in a range of potential language impairments including inappropriate lexical output, speech initiation difficulties, as well as an increased dependency on contextual constraints.

In relation to the thalamus, the ventral anterior (VA), ventral lateral (VL), and nonspecific thalamic nuclei (i.e., NR, CM, and PF) each have been hypothesized to play a role in linking and perhaps procuring language-dedicated cortical regions, by way of facilitating the transmission and even modulation of linguistic information, travelling via cortico-

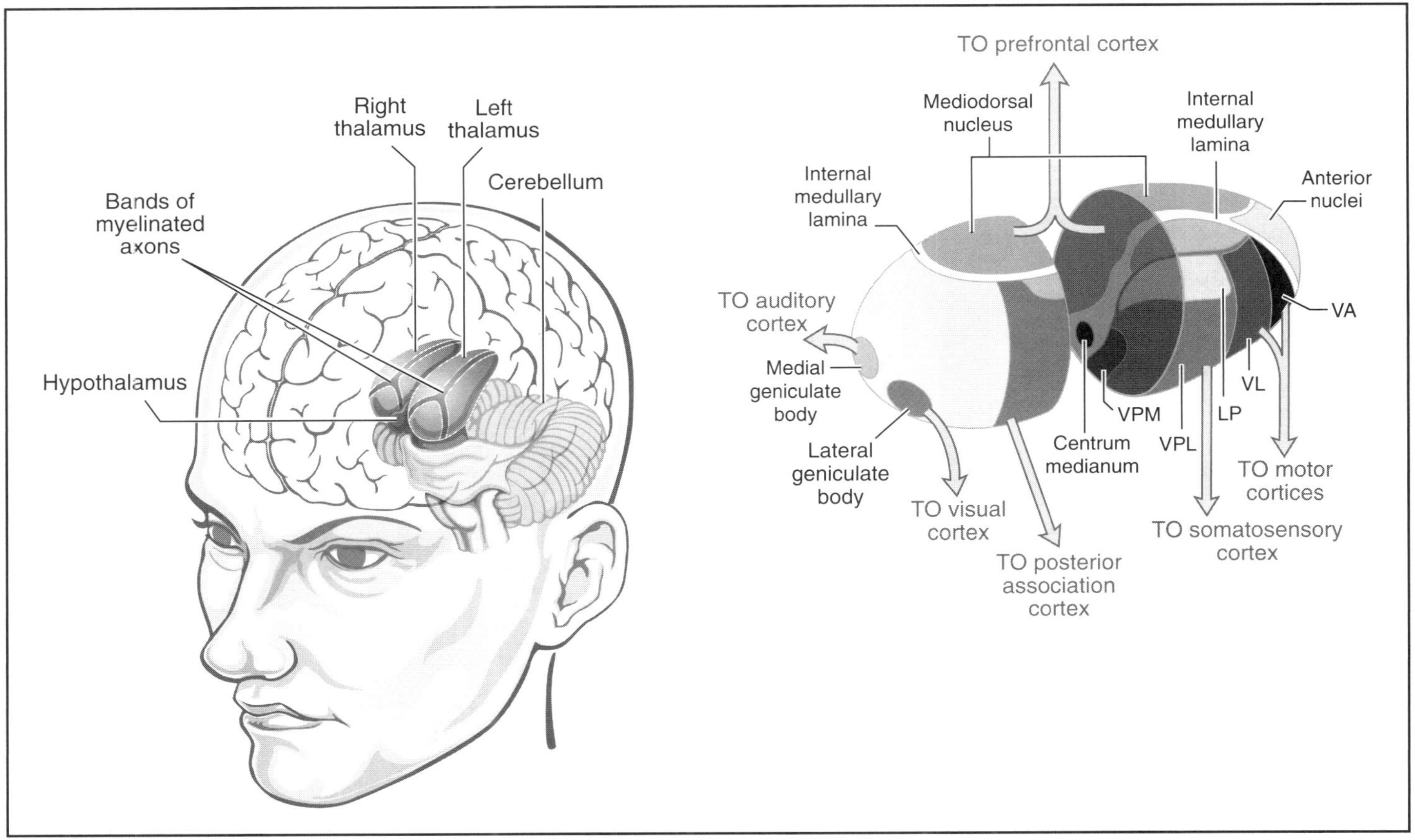

FIGURE 5–4. Thalamic nuclei.

subcortical-cortical circuits (Crosson, 1985; Nadeau & Crosson, 1997; Wallesch & Papagno, 1988). Within these circuits the thalamus has been specifically postulated to support a number of possible functions, including: (1) the facilitation of preverbal semantic monitoring and the release of semantically verified language segments for verbal production (Crosson, 1985); (2) the synchronization and gating of cortically generated lexical information (Wallesch, 1997; Wallesch & Papagno, 1988); and (3) the selective engagement of cortical nets involved in semantically driven lexical retrieval and declarative memory processes (Nadeau & Crosson, 1997). On the basis of these postulates, therefore, the thalamus has been generally perceived to represent a linguistic fulcrum relative to lexical-semantic processes.

In relation to the abovementioned theoretical frameworks of subcortical participation in language, a specific function for the Vim nucleus of the thalamus has not been proposed. Rather, only specific roles for the VA, VL and nonspecific thalamic nuclei (i.e., NR, CM, and PF) have been offered. On this basis, predictions pertaining to the impact of Vim lesions on language processes are difficult to make, yet some assumptions may be drawn, particularly in light of paradoxic clinicoanatomic findings relative to functional thalamic organization. For example, comparable aphasic profiles have been reported in cases presenting lesions both within and external to thalamic systems hypothetically implicated in the mediation of linguistic processes (Crosson, 1984). These findings suggest a potential interrelationship between anterior and posterior thalamic nuclei relative to language mechanisms (Crosson, 1999). Given the small size of the thalamus as a neural structure and the close proximity of individual nuclei to each other, circumscribed Vim lesions may influence language function in a similar manner to lesions within the general ventral region of the thalamus (e.g., VA and VL). Similarly, lesions incorporating the NR which is responsible for manipulating the firing mode of almost all thalamic output nuclei could have an impact on language function. In this case, in terms of the lexical decision-making, response-release semantic feedback, and selective engagement models, Vim lesions may result in: (1) inappropriate lexical content (e.g., semantic paraphasias, such as *plastic surgeon* for *proctologist*) as a consequence of disturbed thalamic gating mechanisms (Crosson, 1992; Wallesch & Papagno, 1988); (2) reduced spontaneous speech and paraphasic verbal output as a consequence of disturbed VA-mediated semantic release mechanisms and/or impaired cortical arousal systems mediated by intralaminar nuclei innervated by the RF (Crosson, 1985, 1992); or (3) deficits in semantically driven lexical retrieval and access to declarative memory as a consequence of disturbed thalamic engagement of language production and comprehension mechanisms (Nadeau & Crosson,

Hypothesized Roles of Globus Pallidus Internal (GPi) and Thalamus in Language

GPi	Thalamus
Tonic arousal of cerebral cortex and release of semantically verified language segments (Crosson, 1992)	Facilitates preverbal semantic monitoring and release of semantically verified language segments (Crosson, 1992)
Manipulates multiple degrees of freedom with respect to processing of cortically generated modules (Wallesch & Papagno, 1988)	Synchronization and gating of cortically generated lexical information (Wallesch & Papgno, 1988)
	Selective engagement of cortical nets involved in semantically driven lexical retrieval and declarative memory processes (Nadeau & Crosson, 1997)

1997). Directly examining the effects of pallidotomy and thalamotomy on cognitive-linguistic functioning provides an opportunity to rigorously test these postulates.

Effects of Contemporary Pallidotomy and Thalamotomy on Cognitive-Linguistic Function. The use of functional neurosurgery to treat PD has provided a novel platform from which theories of subcortical participation in language may be tested. Typically, contemporary studies pertaining to the impact of pallidotomy and thalamotomy on cognitive functions, including language, have been neuropsychologically based. The main aim of baseline neuropsychological evaluations of Parkinsonian populations has been to identify whether cognitive and behavioral profiles are consistent with the diagnosis of PD, and an absence of co-existing dementia and/ or neurological and psychiatric comorbidity (Saint-Cyr & Trepanier, 2000). Literature relating to the effects of ablative neurosurgical procedures on neuropsychological performance can be broadly divided into three groups: (1) bilateral posteroventral pallidotomy (BPVP); (2) unilateral posteroventral pallidotomy (UPVP); and (3) unilateral Vim thalamotomy.

Unilateral and Bilateral Pallidotomy: Neuropsychological Findings and Implications for Language. Conflicting results between studies have been reported on the effects of pallidotomy on cognitive functioning. The main corpus of neuropsychological literature primarily has focused on the effects of unilateral lesions (Turner, Reid, Homewood, & Cook, 2002). The comparatively smaller number of published BPVP studies may reflect the finding of a higher incidence of cognitive decline and speech dysfunction following BPVP (Lang et al., 1999). Indeed, BPVP has been described as a more psychologically toxic procedure when compared to the effects of UPVP (Trepanier, Kumar, Lozano, Lang, & Saint-Cyr, 2000), with unacceptably high rates of adverse effects limiting its general application (Alkhani & Lozano, 2001; Parkin et al., 2002). Bilateral lesions have drawn special attention, given that data report more frequent declines in cognitive performance as a consequence of left-sided lesions (Obwegeser et al., 2000). Consequently, bilateral lesions may be associated with greater risks to general levels of cognitive functioning. It is understandable that candidates for bilateral surgery may not want to risk sharp declines in thinking and talking for the promise of tremor reduction. Within the scant BPVP cognitive literature, however, the following postoperative findings have been reported across studies: reduced verbal fluency scores (Ghika et al., 1999; Scott et al., 1998); absence of decline in verbal fluency, but presence of deficits in planning (Turner et al., 2002); confrontation naming abilities, attention, verbal memory, visuospatial abilities and executive functioning (Ghika et al., 1999).

With reference to UPVP, inconsistent cognitive outcomes also have been reported across studies, with some investigations revealing declines in neuropsychological functioning as a consequence of the procedure (Alegret et al., 2003; Alegret et al., 2000; Carr, Honey, Marci Sinden, Phillips, & Martzke, 2003; de Bie et al., 2001; Masterman et al., 1998; Obwegeser et al., 2000; Trepanier et al., 2000; Trepanier, Saint-Cyr, Lozano, & Lang, 1998; Troster, Woods, & Fields, 2003; Troster, Woods, Fields, Hanisch, & Beatty, 2002), others failing to identify any postoperative changes in cognitive functioning (Fukuda, Kameyama, Yoshino, Tanaka, & Narabayashi, 2000; Gironell et al., 2003; Kuzis et al., 2001; Soukup et al., 1997), and others still, reporting improvements in a range of cognitive skills (Alegret et al., 2003; Lacritz et al., 2000; Obwegeser et al., 2000; Rettig et al., 2000; Trepanier et al., 2000). In general, declines in verbal fluency have been reported as most common following UPVP, followed by declines in working memory as well as verbal learning and memory (Carr et al., 2003). Less common changes and mixed postoperative results have been reported for executive functioning, visual memory, psychomotor speed, visuospatial abilities, and naming (Carr et al., 2003).

Despite the above inconsistencies, definitive hemispheric effects have been identified following UPVP (Rettig et al., 2000). Of specific interest to the speech-language pathologist (SLP), is the finding of significant declines in verbal fluency scores as a consequence of UPVP, in greater than 70% of studies that assess this variable (Troster et al., 2003). Furthermore, out of 20 studies that have documented declines in semantic and/or phonemic fluency following pallidotomy, left-sided lesions were responsible for 65 percent (13/20) of these decrements (Troster

Documented Neuropsychological Effects of Posteroventral Pallidotomy (PVP)

Bilateral PVP

- more psychologically toxic than UPVP
- ↓ executive functioning
- ↓ verbal fluency
- ↓ planning
- ↓ confrontation naming
- ↓ attention
- ↓ verbal memory
- ↓ visuospatial abilities

Unilateral PVP

- ↓ verbal fluency
- ↓ verbal memory
- ↓ working memory
- ↓ verbal learning

Hemispheric effects

- Left hemisphere effects
  - greater impairments in verbal fluency
- Right hemisphere effects
  - ↓ visuospatial abilities
  - ↓ visual memory

et al., 2003). In contrast, right-sided lesions more commonly have been associated with changes in visuospatial functions and visual memory (Carr et al., 2003; Olzak et al., 2006). Consequently, it has been postulated that the right and left basal ganglia, respectively, differentially mediate visuospatial and verbal abilities (Green & Barnhart, 2000), akin to the cerebral cortex. The emergence of the left to the position of relative dominance, but not complete supremacy is a traditionally familiar story.

Verbal fluency has been described as a complex task involving the engagement of numerous cognitive modules typically described as semantic or executive in nature (e.g., conceiving and applying retrieval strategy, shifting between subcategories, accessing vocabulary and semantic processing) (De Gaspari et al., 2006a). The identification, via functional neuroimaging studies, of a frontotemporal network mediating verbal fluency tasks give credence to the above explanation, in that the inferior frontal gyrus incorporating Broca's area (BA 44 and 45), the anterior cingulate cortex and superior temporal regions (Gourovitch et al., 2000; Schlosser et al., 1998) have been observed as the neural substrates underpinning semantic and executive functions (De Gaspari et al., 2006a). The reliable finding of impaired verbal fluency as a consequence of pallidotomy suggests that language systems, specifically those involving complex word retrieval mechanisms that demand frontal lobe participation, may be seriously implicated as a consequence of basal ganglia lesions. Rapid word retrieval, or generating attributes or functions of nouns, may deteriorate with basal ganglia damage.

So how does one interpret the potential language risks for candidates for subcortical invasion? Conclusions no doubt will await further refinements in both surgery and linguistic assessment. An inherent limitation of previous studies is that they have failed to routinely assess both semantic and phonemic fluency within the same test battery (Troster et al., 2003). Of 18 studies that have simultaneously assessed phonemic and semantic fluency in people post-UPVP, 33% (6/18) report an exclusive decline in phonemic fluency, and only 1 study (6%), an exclusive decline in semantic fluency (Gironell et al., 2003; Troster et al., 2003). Troster et al. (2003) extrapolated these results further by demonstrating that people with left UPVP ($n = 16$) presented greater declines in phonemic fluency performance than people with right sided UPVP ($n = 11$), with no similar observable interaction for semantic fluency. These findings suggest that phonemic fluency may be more susceptible to the effects of UPVP in the left hemisphere.

Indeed, measures of frontal lobe function have been reported as more sensitive to the effects of left UPVP lesions (Green & Barnhart, 2000). Evident verbal fluency deficits as a consequence of pallidal lesions have been attributed to disruptions in the functioning of frontal-basal ganglionic circuits involved in word search and retrieval processes, rather than as a result of more typical language disturbances associated with aphasia (Troster et al., 2003). In support of this proposal, phonemic fluency has been conceptualised to involve executive processes and therefore to be more reliant on the frontal lobes as opposed to semantic fluency, which is dependent on semantic networks within the temporal lobes (Troyer, Moscovitch, Winocur, Alexander, & Stuss, 1998).

Furthermore, qualitative analyses of verbal fluency performance post-UPVP also have revealed interesting findings that further support suggestions of frontal lobe dysfunction as a consequence of this procedure. For example, the integrity of two dissociable component processes known as clustering and switching, determine performance success relative to verbal fluency tasks (Troyer, Moscovitch, & Winocur, 1997). Clustering refers to the ability to generate words within subcategories or clusters, and switching refers to the ability to change between clusters. Relative to UPVP populations, a significantly reduced number of switches, but not clusters has been identified on both phonemic and semantic fluency tasks (Demakis et al., 2003; Troster et al., 2002; York, Levin, Grossman, & Hamilton, 1999; York, Levin, Grossman, Lai, & Krauss, 2003), and left UPVP persons have been observed to present significantly greater declines in number of switches postoperatively, when compared to right UPVP subjects (York et al., 2003). Importantly, cluster size has been reported as dependent on temporal lobe integrity and access to semantic stores (Troyer et al., 1998), and switching, upon frontal-subcortical circuit integrity mediating cognitive flexibility and mental set shifting (Troyer et al., 1997).

In summary, a functional dissociation relative to post-PVP motor and cognitive abilities represents a well-documented phenomenon common to both unilateral and bilateral cohorts (Ghika et al., 1999; Lang et al., 1999; Scott et al., 1998; Scott et al., 2002; Turner et al., 2002). Improvements in motor outcomes and declines in cognitive functioning represent a typical postoperative profile. These findings suggest not only that surgically induced lesions targeting motor portions of the GPi impact cognitive functions, but that this procedure evokes differential effects within hypothetically segregated yet parallel motor and cognitive circuits. The infiltration of proximal cognitive circuits that encompass prefrontal and inferotemporal areas of the cerebral cortex (Middleton & Strick, 2000), due to large, surgically induced lesions of motor portions of the GPi, may be the most plausible mechanism underlying the aforementioned symptom complex (Middleton & Strick, 2000). Alternatively, these results may support the notion of circuitry "convergence" (Percheron &

Filion, 1991) or "integration" (Joel & Weiner, 1994), challenging currently accepted models of functional organization of the basal ganglia.

Thalamotomy: Neuropsychological Findings and Implications for Language. In comparison to the vast body of literature detailing the affects of pallidotomy on cognitive function, the impact of thalamotomy has been modestly represented. Perhaps, this is a consequence of negative early thalamotomy reports, with estimates of over 30% of unilateral lesions and 60% of bilateral lesions associated with language and memory dysfunction (Burchiel, 1995). Analogous to pallidotomy research, however, studies investigating the effects of thalamotomy on cognitive status have been for the most part neuropsychologically based, overtly lacking in-depth language analyses (Fukuda et al., 2000; Hugdahl & Wester, 2000; Hugdahl, Wester, & Asbjornsen, 1990). Similar to pallidotomy findings, general reports of impairments in cognitive function (Almgren, Andersson, & Kullberg, 1972; Modesti & Blumetti, 1980; Van Buren, Shapiro, Henderson, & Sadowsky, 1973), no change, (Fukuda et al., 2000; Levita, Riklan, & Cooper, 1967), or improvements in cognitive status (Hugdahl & Wester, 2000; Lund-Johansen, Hugdahl, & Wester, 1996) may be found. It must be stated, however, that such inconsistencies among reports largely may be due to the fact that the majority of early thalamotomy studies targeted different thalamic nuclei (i.e., ventrolateral) to contemporary studies (i.e., ventral intermediate) (Troster, Wilkinson, Fields, Miyawaki, & Koller, 1998), making the generalization of results difficult.

Nonetheless, laterality effects also have been investigated in relation to thalamotomy and cognition, with interesting implications for language/verbal functioning. It has been reported that left thalamotomy lesions incur greater deficits in verbal fluency (Petrovici, 1980; Riklan & Levita, 1970; Riklan, Levita, Zimmerman, & Cooper, 1969; Schuurman, Bruins, Merkus, Bosch, & Speelman, 2002; Vilkki & Laitinen, 1974; 1976), executive functioning (Almgren, Andersson, & Kullberg, 1969; Almgren et al., 1972; Schuurman et al., 2002), receptive and expressive verbal "performance" (Modesti & Blumetti, 1980; Vilkki & Laitinen, 1976), attention (Modesti & Blumetti, 1980), dichotic listening (Wester & Hugdahl, 1997), and recall of word pairs (Almgren et al., 1969). In addition, a greater incidence of language deficits of a high-level nature have been reported following left-sided as well as bilateral thalamotomy lesions (Darley, Brown, & Swenson, 1975). A paucity of bilateral thalamotomy outcomes may be related to the belief that bilateral thalamic lesions present a greater risk of neurobehavioral anomalies than unilateral

Documented Neuropsychological Effects of Unilateral Thalamotomy

Compared to right thalamotomy, left thalamotomy creates greater impairments in:

- Verbal fluency
- Executive functioning
- Expressive and receptive verbal performance
- Attention
- Dichotic listening
- Verbal memory
- High-level language skills

lesions (Troster, 2000), and, as such, a lack of discussion within the current chapter.

Pallidotomy and Thalamotomy: Effects on Language Function. As demonstrated by the above summary, the majority of studies to date investigating the effects of pallidotomy and thalamotomy on cognition, and consequently language have been largely neuropsychologically based. Assessment batteries typically have included cognitive measures of intelligence, attention, memory, executive functioning, language, and visuospatial abilities. Regarding language, the effects of pallidotomy and thalamotomy on confrontation naming, verbal learning and of course verbal fluency have been given some consideration, however, the impact of these procedures on a wider range of linguistic processes that incorporate complex comprehension and sentential level production tasks, until recently, has remained unknown.

A series of recent investigations, however, have sought to provide a comprehensive assessment of language function utilizing measures of both general and high-level linguistic functioning (single word and sentential level comprehension and production tasks), not routinely included within neuropsychological test batteries, as well as measures of online semantic processing (Murdoch, Whelan, Theodoros, & Cahill, 2004; Murdoch, Whelan, Theodoros, Hall, & Silburn, 2003; Whelan, Murdoch, Theodoros, Silburn, & Hall, 2002, 2004a, 2005a). These studies aimed to evaluate the effects of bilateral pallidotomy and unilateral thalamotomy on language function, and to examine post-operative language profiles within the context of working theories of subcortical participation in language.

Pallidotomy: Language Effects. A group study of six people post-BPVP (Whelan et al., 2004a) failed to identify differences between three groups (i.e., PD post-BPVP, nonsurgical PD, and non-PD) in language performance, suggesting that BPVP produces benign effects on language processing mechanisms. Subsequent case-by-case studies (Murdoch et al., 2003; Whelan et al., 2004a; 2005a), however, have revealed significant individual variations in postpallidotomy language performance. For example, a study comparing the post-BPVP language profiles of two individuals with PD with opposing primary symptom presentations (i.e., akinetic versus dyskinetic) (Murdoch et al., 2003; Whelan et al., 2005a) revealed reliable changes in postoperative performance (including both improvements and declines) to be largely restricted to higher level language functions across participants. Higher level language functions included tasks involving lexical semantic operations relating to elaborate linguistic relationships; the repetition and manipulation of lengthy verbal material; and the production of divergent, novel language at single word and sentence level (e.g., *How many uses can you generate for a brick?*). Furthermore, dyskinetic symptoms were associated with an initial improvement in high-level language function that diminished over a 12-month period. Hypokinetic symptoms, however, were associated with a more stable longitudinal linguistic profile, albeit defined by higher proportions of reliable decline versus improvement in postoperative assessment scores over time. These findings lent support to postulates of hyper- and hypokinetic linguistic homologues akin to parkinsonian motor behavior. The potentially preferential implication of more complex language functions as a consequence of BPVP suggests the GPi may play a role in frontal lobe mediated lexical semantic manipulation and selection, as well as cognitive-linguistic resource allocation. Once again, the intertwining of cognitive and language behaviors are evident.

In relation to theories of subcortical participation in language, behaviors observed lent most support to models that included the GPi as part of a frontal lobe system mediating language functions, in particular, a role in manipulating multiple competing lexical elements in both the context of verbal expression (Wallesch & Papagno, 1988) and comprehension (Nadeau & Crosson, 1997).

Thalamotomy: Language Effects. Thalamic dominance has been investigated by comparing the language profiles of two right-handed males with tremor dominant PD and unilateral lesions of the left and right thalami, respectively (Whelan et al., 2002). Results supported an exclusive role for the dominant thalamus in language, specifically in relation to performance on tasks of higher level language processing (e.g., recreating sentences, remembering word pairs, for example, *sausage–honeymoon*) and the temporal processing of semantic information. More specifically, lesioning of the left thalamus impacted negatively on higher level language abilities involving the complex manipulation of semantic elements, and potentially, the speed of lexical retrieval. Lesioning of the right Vim thalamus, however, failed to produce any negative effects on language abilities.

The findings of this study support the hypothesis of a corticosubcortical-cortical circuit subserving language function, which incorporates the dominant thalamus (Crosson, 1985; Nadeau & Crosson, 1997; Wallesch & Papagno, 1988). Despite the fact that a specific role for the Vim nucleus of the thalamus has not been previously proposed in models of subcortical participation in language, it is postulated that postthalamotomy neurophysiologic changes in nuclei that lie in close proximity to the Vim target, including those previously implicated in language (e.g., VA, VL, pulvinar and NR) may account for the results observed.

When consulting theories of subcortical participation in language, an impaired ability to create sentences using particular words within a specified context, suggests that left Vim thalamotomy may disrupt the efficient organization, integration, and production of specified lexical content (Wallesch & Papagno, 1988) within appropriate syntactic structures. Alternatively, thalamocortical disconnection may result in concept generation deficits which include vague conceptual markers and a lack of detail in verbal expression (Nadeau & Crosson, 1997). In addition, reduced performance in the ability to recall word pairs was consistent with the findings of Almgren et al., (1972) who suggested that Vim thalamotomy may impair the processing of verbal language and the subsequent ability to retrieve words from short-term memory. This hypothesis was consistent with the models of: (1) Crosson (1985) based on the work of Ojemann (1975, 1976) that the thalamus acts to influence attentional mechanisms that gate the storage and retrieval of items held in short-term memory; and (2) Nadeau & Crosson (1997), that left thalamotomy may prohibit the selective engagement of cortical nets dedicated to the storage and generation of verbal language.

In relation to performance on the semantic processing/lexical decision-making task, the left Vim patient in the Whelan et al. (2002)

study demonstrated prolonged reaction times for all word types, with a possible reaction time advantage for few meaning words. In terms of spreading activation theory (Rubenstein, Garfield, & Millikan, 1970), it was hypothesized that left Vim thalamotomy may have served to alter word-processing mechanisms, or rather, implicate the efficiency of information transfer via nodal networks. This explanation fits well with Nadeau and Crosson's (1997) selective engagement theory, whereby thalamic lesions are postulated to interfere with thalamus-mediated engagement of lexical-semantic cortical nodes.

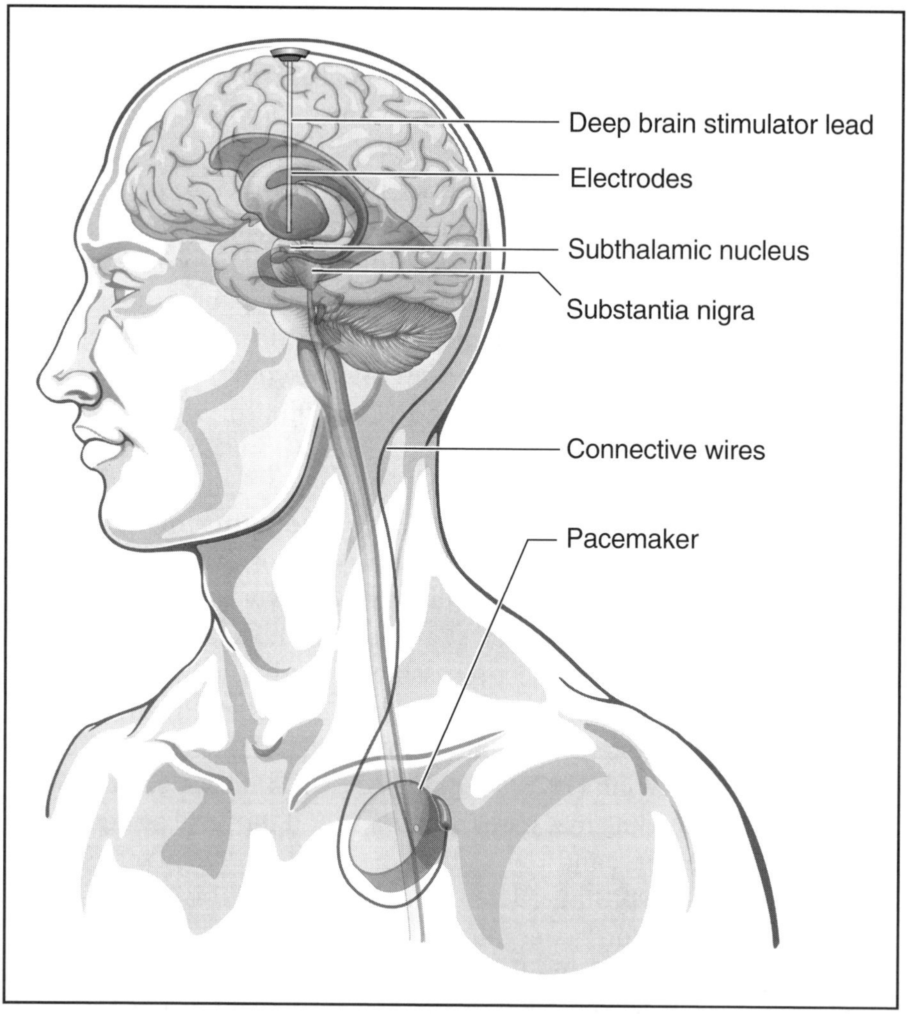

FIGURE 5–5. Deep brain stimulation.

Nonablative Techniques: Deep Brain Stimulation of the STN

In contrast to the ablative procedures described earlier, which permanently destroy neural tissue, deep brain stimulation (DBS; Figure 5–5) involves minimal destruction of brain tissue (Lozano & Mahant, 2004) via the implantation of electrodes within a range of potential subcortical targets (Wichmann & DeLong, 2006). The implanted electrodes deliver high-frequency electrical signals to the target nuclei by way of attachments to pulse generators, inserted within the chest wall. Targets utilized in the management of PD include the GPi, STN, thalamus, and pedunculopontine nucleus; however, the STN (specifically the dorsolateral motor nucleus) is currently recognized as the preferred target, given that stimulation in this region is associated with potent antiparkinsonian effects (Wichmann & DeLong, 2006) (Figure 5–6). The DBS procedure has been hailed as the gold standard in movement disorders surgery, given that its side effects are reversible (i.e., via removal or turning "off" electrodes) and parameters adjustable in maximizing clinical benefit (i.e., stimulation parameters may be programmed to different therapeutic levels) (Kopell, Rezai, Chang, & Vitek, 2006).

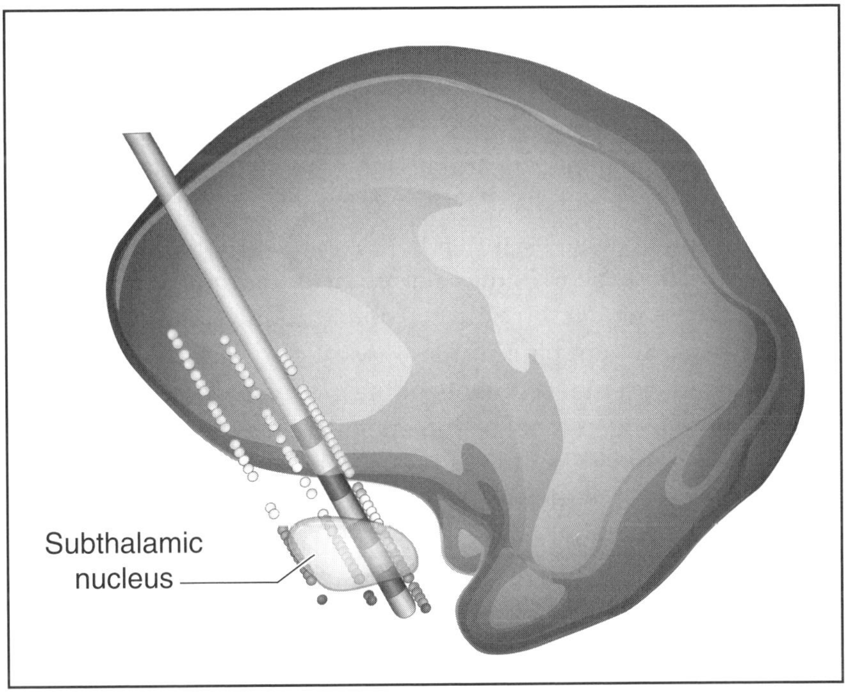

FIGURE 5–6. Subthalamic nucleus with electrode.

Proposed Roles for the Subthalamic Nucleus in Language. The original models of subcortical participation in language previously described in relation to ablative lesions of the GPi and thalamus (Crosson, 1985; Nadeau & Crosson, 1997; Wallesch & Papagno, 1988), failed to offer a role for the STN. In short, seminal models of subcortical participation in language proffered what we currently recognize as the direct (i.e., corticostriato-Gpi-thalamocortical) pathway to represent the neural turnpike underpinning linguistic processes. The subsequent expansion of functional schemas of basal ganglia organization since the inception of these language models, however, has culminated in the conceptualization of a direct-indirect basal ganglia pathway dichotomy, which proposes an indirect (i.e., corticostriatoglobus pallidus externus (Gpe)-STN-Gpi/ substantia nigra reticulata (SNr)-thalamocortical) pathway to lie in parallel with the aforementioned direct pathway (Albin, Young, & Penney, 1989; Alexander & Crutcher, 1990).

Representing a crucial component of the classical indirect pathway, the STN facilitates communication between striatal efferents (i.e., pathways travelling away from the striatum) and principle output nuclei of the basal ganglia (i.e., Gpi/ SNr) by way of an intermediary Gpe-STN projection (Parent & Hazrati, 1995). Together with the striatum, the STN has been documented to receive a diffuse array of cortical outputs (Hazrati & Parent, 1993), some reports detailing projections from the entire cortical mantle (Rouzaire-Dubois & Scarnati, 1985). This anatomical schema supports a potential role for the STN in the processing of cortical information, which may include input from language-dedicated cortical regions. The integration of corticostriatal and corticosubthalamic outputs, however, has been postulated to occur at the level of the globus pallidus, given that striatal and STN axons have been observed to terminate upon homogeneous neurons within the Gpi and Gpe (Hazrati & Parent, 1992). Thus, the STN may represent an essential component of a language processing circuit, with the ability to integrate cortical inputs and regulate basal ganglia outputs by way of direct connections with the internal and external segments of the globus pallidus.

In relation to the established Response-Release Semantic Feedback model (Crosson, 1985; Crosson & Early, 1990), the STN, in concert with the striatum, was hypothesized to potentially regulate the release of semantically verified language segments, by way of a push-pull system. Lesions of the STN resulting in direct pathway control of pallidal outputs were predicted to disrupt response-release and potentially semantic monitoring mechanisms as a consequence of thalamic disinhibition. Unimpeded thalamic excitation of the ALC was hypothesized to result in manifestations of fluent language pathology, including the production of semantically inappropriate output such as semantic paraphasias.

The lexical decision-making model proffers a frontal lobe system (i.e., the caudate nucleus, Gpi, VA and VL thalamus, and ALC) to underly the synchronization of language and non-language cortical modules processed in parallel, in addition to the regulation of cortical activity within the ALC (Wallesch, 1997; Wallesch & Papagno, 1988). Extending this frontal lobe system to include previously disregarded indirect basal ganglia pathways, proposes implications for net pallidal activity.

Given evidence of Gpe and wide-ranging cortical inputs, in addition to a proposed ability to "cross-talk" between functionally distinct regions of the basal ganglia (Feger et al., 1994) the STN was postulated to represent a subcortical component with the ability to consolidate and perhaps modulate cortical modules. STN lesions were predicted primarily to produce nonfluent language disturbances (e.g., difficulty initiating or sustaining speech) as a consequence of enforced "direct" pathway dominance. In addition, disturbed associative-limbic integration mechanisms as a result of STN lesions may be responsible for the presentation of inappropriate semantic content in verbal output (e.g., semantic paraphasias). Inappropriate striatal activation of subordinate alternatives may offer an explanation for manifestations of this behavior, in the presence of STN lesions.

Selective engagement theory proposes a frontal-ITP-NR-CM system principally to regulate cortical functions by way of the NR and its inherent ability to modulate the firing mode of thalamic output neurons, relative to cortical activation (Nadeau & Crosson, 1997). Excitatory STN influences upon pallidal outputs have the potential indirectly to regulate the thalamic engagement of language cortices. The existence of reciprocal STN-Gpe innervations and concomitant inhibitory Gpe projections to the NR, suggest that this regulatory role indeed may extend to the establishment of the firing mode of thalamic output nuclei hypothesized to underpin language processes, including the pulvinar and CMPFC.

Based on theories of motor control, however, lesions of the STN have been postulated to instigate "direct" pathway control of striato-pallidal interactions. In relation to seminal SE theory, deficits in semantically driven lexical retrieval and access to declarative memory have been indexed as the most common linguistic impairments associated with damage to frontal-ITP-NR-CM mechanisms. Lesions of the STN may contribute to manifestations of this symptom complex by disrupting basal ganglia

Hypothesized Roles for the STN in Language

1. STN (in concert with striatum) regulates release of semantically verified language segments by way of push-pull mechanism (following on from Crosson, 1985)
2. Consolidates and modulates cortical modules
3. Determines which representation most appropriate for verbal production via associative-limbic cross-talk mechanisms that overshoot activation threshold for relevant representation (following on from Wallesch & Papagno, 1988)
4. Indirectly regulates thalamic engagement of cerebral cortex via robust excitatory influences on GPi and GPe
5. May establish firing mode of thalamic nuclei subserving engagement of language dedicated cortices (following on from Nadeau & Crosson, 1997)

mechanisms that regulate the switching of thalamocortical engagement between neural nets (Malapani, Pillon, Dubois, & Agid, 1994).

Impact of Deep Brain Stimulation of the Subthalamic Nucleus on Cognitive-Linguistic Function. The impact of bilateral STN-DBS on motor systems has been well established in comparison to its effects on nonmotor functions (Voon, Kubu, Krack, Houeto, & Troster, 2006). In general, STN-DBS has been described as having relatively benign effects on cognition, yet there is documented evidence of both improvements and decrements in certain domains of cognition within some research reports (Voon et al., 2006), confusing perceptions relating to the genuine impact of this procedure.

STN-DBS: Neuropsychological Findings and Implications for Language. Postoperative STN-DBS improvements in mental flexibility (Alegret et al., 2001; Jahanshahi et al., 2000; Witt et al., 2004), working memory (Jahanshahi et al., 2000), visuomotor sequencing (Ardouin et al., 1999; Daniele et al., 2003; Jahanshahi et al., 2000; Pillon et al., 2000), conceptual reasoning (Daniele et al., 2003; Jahanshahi et al., 2000), and general cognitive functioning (Daniele et al., 2003) have been reported in a number of studies. Other reports, however have identified declines in verbal memory (Alegret et al., 2001; Daniele et al., 2003; Dujardin,

Defebvre, Krystkowiak, Blond, & Destee, 2001; Morrison et al., 2004; Saint-Cyr, Trepanier, Kumar, Lozano, & Lang, 2000; Trepanier et al., 2000; Wojtecki et al., 2006), conditional associative learning (Jahanshahi et al., 2000), visuospatial memory (Alegret et al., 2001; Saint-Cyr et al., 2000; Trepanier et al., 2000), processing speed (Saint-Cyr et al., 2000), and certain indices of executive functioning (Trepanier et al., 2000).

Similar to ablative lesions, it is apparent that studies pertaining to the impact of STN-DBS on cognition largely have been neuropsychologically based. Perhaps of most interest to the speech-language pathologist again, is the fact that reduced verbal fluency scores are the most consistently reported neuropsychological sequela of STN-DBS in people with PD (Alegret et al., 2001; Ardouin et al., 1999; Berney, Vingerhoets, & Perrin, 2002; Daniele et al., 2003; De Gaspari et al., 2006a; De Gaspari et al., 2006b; Funkiewiez et al., 2004; Gironell et al., 2003; Moretti et al., 2003; Moro et al., 1999; Morrison et al., 2004; Pillon et al., 2000; Saint-Cyr et al., 2000; Schroeder et al., 2003; Smeding et al., 2006; Wojtecki et al., 2006; Woods, Fields, & Troster, 2002).

STN-DBS: Effects on Language Function. The reliable finding of impaired verbal fluency post STN-DBS suggests that language systems, specifically those involving complex word retrieval mechanisms that demand frontal lobe participation, may be seriously implicated as a consequence of STN disruption. More recent studies have attempted to evaluate the immediate and long-term effects of bilateral and unilateral STN-DBS on language function utilizing a comprehensive test battery, and to discuss postoperative language profiles within the context of working theories of subcortical participation in language (Whelan, Murdoch, Theodoros, Hall, & Silburn, 2003, 2004b, 2005b). As for findings from pallidotomy and thalamotomy research, variable changes in language function have been identified following STN-DBS. A group study of people following STN-DBS revealed a limited number of postoperative language changes (Whelan et al., 2003). The only significant statistical results observed related to prolonged reaction times for a range of word types on an online lexical decision task. When results were examined on a case-by-case basis, however, considerable individual variation was observed. For example, participants demonstrated greater postoperative improvements on a multiple definitions subtest when compared to a nonsurgical PD group, as well as greater declines in the ability to accurately identify words with many meanings and a high degree of relatedness between meanings (i.e., MH words).

These findings suggested that STN-DBS positively as well as adversely may affect basal ganglia activity within neural circuits mediating language functions. In reference to high-level language abilities, it was apparent that STN-DBS potentially enhanced basal ganglia functioning particularly within circuits mediating linguistic flexibility in the production of definitions constrained by semantically distinct criteria.

This profile speaks to the lexical decision-making model (Wallesch & Papagno, 1988) whereby enhanced basal ganglia circuitry dynamics resulted in more flexible lexical selection mechanisms that may be active during complex or frontally taxing language tasks. Uncertainty remains, however, as to why additional high-level linguistic assessments that also required the formulation of self-generated complex language (e.g., synonym and antonym generation, semantic absurdity explanation, verbal fluency) failed to reveal a similar profile of significant postoperative improvement.

In interpreting semantic processing performance evidenced as a generalized postoperative prolongation of reaction times for all word types and reduced accuracy of decisions relating to MH words, spreading activation theory was consulted. According to this theory, word recognition is dependent upon the coherence of orthographic, phonological, and semantic features, made possible by the correlation of activation patterns between lexical (i.e., orthographic/phonological input) and semantic nodes (Van Orden & Goldinger, 1994). Rapid coherence, and consequently reaction time are contingent upon strong correlations. Deep brain stimulation has been hypothesized to disrupt neural networks through the production of artificial nerve impulses, a phenomenon defined as neural jamming (Benazzouz & Hallet, 2000). The findings of Whelan et al. (2003b) suggested that STN-DBS may indeed alter the efficiency of neural communication at the lexical-semantic interface, resulting in delayed or contaminated coherence correlations, perhaps as a consequence of neural jamming. In relation to theories of subcortical participation in language, STN-DBS may disturb GPe-NR exchanges resulting in abnormal firing nodes within thalamic nuclei subserving the efficient engagement of lexical and semantic nodes (Nadeau & Crosson, 1997). STN-DBS may result in unimpeded thalamocortical activation, and in relation to language, the engagement of multiplex versus definitive lexical-semantic representations. A postlesional inability to suppress or disengage subordinate lexical-semantic alternatives hypothetically would result in increased reaction times on the lexical decision task. Whether suppression or disengagement is the culprit, however, remains to be discovered.

Words with many meanings have been hypothesized to have a probability advantage for nodal activation, given a high concentration of interrelated nodes (Rubenstein et al., 1970). In the study by Whelan et al. (2003), reduced accuracy of lexical decisions pertaining to MH words was interpreted as a reflection of inefficient coherence mechanisms whereby intricate nodal networks underlying MH words perhaps are more susceptible to neural disturbances facilitated by DBS. In relation to selective engagement theory (Nadeau & Crosson, 1997), MH words may have failed to reach recognition thresholds with respect to the coherence of orthographic and semantic representations. STN-DBS may have disturbed the assimilation of lexical information within convoluted neural networks resulting in "incoherence" and the subsequent engagement of subordinate representations.

In a follow-up study, two of the five STN-DBS participants previously described in Whelan et al. (2003) were monitored over a 12-month postoperative period in relation to their general and high-level language abilities (Whelan et al., 2005b). STN-DBS primarily affected clinically reliable fluctuations (i.e., both improvements and declines) in performance across participants on tasks demanding cognitive-linguistic flexibility in the formulation and comprehension of complex language. Of additional interest, both participants demonstrated a cumulative increase in the proportion of reliable postoperative improvements achieved over time.

The findings of this study again provided support for the hypothesis of a STN contribution to language processes. Bilateral STN-DBS affected alterations in language performance at both three and 12 months following electrode implantation and the commencement of active stimulation. Overall, a cumulative increase in the proportion of reliable improvements in performance was demonstrated by both participants across testing phases, suggesting that bilateral STN-DBS may serve to enhance the proficiency of basal-ganglia thalamocortical linguistic circuits over time.

Notably, a greater number of high-level language, in comparison to general language, variables were subject to reliable change (including both improvements and decrements) during bilateral STN-DBS, at both 3 and 12 months following surgery, in both participants. Furthermore, general language variables demonstrating reliable postoperative changes were typically representative of more high-level linguistic measures (e.g., verbal fluency, token test, sentence construction, etc.) enmeshed within a general language battery. Bilateral STN-DBS principally affected divergent language production proficiency (e.g., verbal fluency) and lexical semantic manipulation skills (e.g., The Word Test-Revised (Huisingh et al., 1990). These findings potentially implicated the cognitive-linguistic basal ganglia thalamocortical pathways involved in the enlistment and directed interplay of frontal and temporoparietal cortical activity. Despite individual differences among participants, the current results supported an adaptation hypothesis with respect to the nature of neural network responses to continuous patterns of stimulation (Benazzouz & Hallet, 2000). A general trend towards improved linguistic performance over time implied the prospective enhancement of synaptic efficiency as a consequence of chronic bilateral STN-DBS. The findings again lent support to models of subcortical participation in language that specifically integrate the STN within a frontal lobe system of language processing.

A further study has examined the effects of left versus right functional inhibition of the STN on language function in two cases (i.e., one case with left ablative lesion of STN and one case with right STN-DBS) (Whelan et al., 2004b). Neuropsychological reports have described higher proportions of postoperative deterioration among executive function-dependent variables such as planning, spatial working memory, verbal memory, and attention in persons with left versus right ablative lesions of the STN (McCarter, Walton, Rowan, Gill, & Palomo, 2000). Given that language is considered to be entwined with executive function (Denckla, 1996), Whelan et al. (2004b) proposed that functional inhibition of the left as opposed to right STN may serve to disproportionately disturb linguistic processes.

On inspection of individual profiles, variability with respect to magnitudes and directions of reliable change was demonstrated both between participants and across assessment variables. Overall, each of the cases demonstrated a general reliable decline on tests of high-level language function, yet failed to demonstrate comparable declines on tests of general language function. The results of this study largely failed to provide support for the hypothesis of left STN dominance, relevant to the mediation of linguistic processes. Left subthalamic nucleotomy and right STN-DBS affected similar fluctuations in language performance in the two PD cases presented. Overall, surgically induced functional inhibition of the STN largely evoked declines in complex language function, suggesting that STN disruption has the potential to disturb frontally loaded cognitive-linguistic operations, regardless of hemispheric orientation. On the basis of these findings, a potential interhemispheric regulatory function for the STN was postulated, relative to higher level linguistic processing mechanisms.

In relation to models of subcortical participation in language, selective engagement theory (Nadeau & Crosson, 1997) provided the most viable interpretation of these findings. As mentioned previously, the original theory proposed a frontal-ITP-NR-CM system to regulate language functions by way of the NR and its inherent ability to modulate the firing mode of thalamic output neurons. STN-GPe disconnection as a consequence of surgically induced functional inhibition of the STN was postulated to alter the nature of GPe-NR interactions. Anomalous NR activity was predicted to result in the production of aberrant thalamic firing modes. Relevant thalamic nuclei project to language dedicated cortical regions within the left hemisphere, consequently resulting in linguistic disturbances.

Summary

Nonmotoric characteristics of PD are rampant and devastating. Although the most obvious signs and symptoms of PD are readily observable in the shuffling gait and abnormalities of movement, there is an increasing realization in clinical practice and in the research laboratories of the world that non-motor problems are at least as important to both successful management and understanding. Accurate diagnosis is made difficult by the overlap between organic signs and symptoms of PD and nonmotor symptoms, and it is becoming clear that without the use of objective and refined measures, appreciation of these aspects of this complex disorder is likely to occur. Cognition and language are two of the most enigmatic and entwined aspects of all of the non-motoric characteristics of PD. And cognition and language are largely what make us human. We can sing the praises of the opposable thumb, but the magic of thinking and language are truly what separate us from the gibbons, lizards, and fruit bats. This chapter has attempted to highlight some of these very specific cognitive and language domains that contribute so much to our quality of life and our enjoyment of our social networks. Cognitive and linguistic processing truly form the core of our enjoyment of the "Three Ls"; Living, Learning, and Loving (LaPointe, 2005). In this chapter we have emphasized the importance and the maddening complexity of understanding how language and cognition influence each other. Perhaps, something different is created when these two human domains interact. Perhaps, it is futile to attempt to isolate the dry ingredients from the wet ingredients in a cake batter. Or, perhaps, we must only await evolving sophistication of our methods of analysis and measurement. Either way, the influences of cognitive-linguistic interactions are not diminished in PD. We have carefully traced those elements of cognition and language that appear to be important in this disorder and have explicitly summarized the multifarious underpinnings and neural substrates of them. All of this has been supported with the most recent evidence that the clinical and research literature has to offer. We look forward to the inevitable continuing advances that will allow clarity and refined understanding of cognition, language, and Parkinson disease.

References

Aarsland, D., Andersen, K., Larsen, J. P., Lolk, A. & Kragh-Sorensen, P. (2003). Prevalence and characteristics of dementia in Parkinson disease. *Archives of Neurology, 60*, 387–392.

Aarsland, D., Zaccai, J., & Brayne, C. (2005). A systematic review of prevalence studies of dementia in Parkinson disease. *Movement Disorders, 20*, 1255–1263.

Agid, Y., Javoy-Agid, F., & Ruberg, M. (1987). Biochemistry of neurotransmitters in Parkinson disease. In C. D. Marsden & S. Fahn (Eds.), *Movement disorders, Vol. 2.* (pp. 166–230). London, UK: Butterworth.

Albin, R. L., Young, A. B., & Penney, J. B. (1989). The functional anatomy of basal ganglia disorders. *Trends in Neuroscience, 12*, 366–375.

Alegret, M., Junque, C., Valldeoriola, F., Vendrell, P., Pilleri, M., Rumia, J., & Toloso, E. (2001). Effects of bilateal subthalamic stimulation on cognitive function in Parkinson disease. *Archives of Neurology, 58*, 1223–1227.

Alegret, M., Valldeoriola, F., Tolosa, E., Vendrell, P., Junque, C., Martinez, J., & Rumia, J. (2003). Cognitive effects of unilateral posteroventral pallidotomy: A 4-year follow-up study. *Movement Disorders, 18*, 323–328.

Alegret, M., Vendrell, P., Junque, C., Valldeoriola, F., Nobbe, F. A., Rumia, J., Tolso, E. (2000). Effects of unilateral posteroventral pallidotomy on on-off cognitive fluctuations in Parkinson disease. *Neuropsychologia, 38*, 628–633.

Alexander, G. E., & Crutcher, M. D. (1990). Functional architecture of basal ganglia circuits: Neural substrates of parallel processing. *Trends in Neuroscience, 13*, 266–271.

Alkhani, A., & Lozano, A. M. (2001). Pallidotomy for Parkinson disease: A review of contemporary literature. *Journal of Neurosurgery, 94*(1), 43–49.

Almgren, P. E., Andersson, A. L., & Kullberg, G. (1969). Differences in verbally expressed cognition following left and right ventrolateral thalamotomy. *Scandinavian Journal of Psychology, 10*, 243–249.

Almgren, P. E., Andersson, A. L., & Kullberg, G. (1972). Long-term effects on verbally expressed cognition following left and right ventrolateral thalamotomy. *Confina Neurologica, 34*, 162–168.

Angwin, A., Chenery, H. J., Copland, D. A., Arnott, W. L., Murdoch, B., & Silburn, P. (2004). Dopamine and semantic activation: An investigation of masked direct and indirect priming. *Journal of the International Neuropsychological Society, 10*, 15–25.

Angwin, A., Chenery, H. J., Copland, D. A., Murdoch, B., & Silburn, P. (2003). Summation of semantic priming in Parkinson disease and healthy individuals. *Brain and Language, 87*, 96–97.

Angwin, A., Chenery, H. J., Copland, D. A., Murdoch, B., & Silburn, P. (2007). The speed of lexical activation is altered in Parkinson disease. *Journal of Clinical and Experimental Neuropsychology, 29*, 73–85.

Angwin, A., Copland, D. A., Chenery, H. J., Murdoch, B., & Silburn, P. (2006). The influence of dopamine on semantic activation in Parkinson disease: Evidence from a multipriming task. *Neuropsychology, 20*, 299–306.

Angwin, A. J., Chenery, H. J., Copland, D., Murdoch, B., & Silburn, P. A. (2006). Self-paced reading and sentence comprehension in Parkinson disease. *Journal of Neurolinguistics, 19*, 239–252.

Ardouin, C. M., Pillon, B., Peiffer, E., Bejjani, P., Limousin, P., Damier, P., . . . Pollak, P. (1999). Bilateral subthalamic or pallidal stimulation for Parkinson disease affects neither memory nor executive functions: A consecutive series of 62 patients. *Annals of Neurology, 46*, 217–223.

Bayles, K., Tomoeda, C., Wood, J., Montgomery, E., Cruz, R., Azuma, T., & McGeagh, A. (1996). Change in cognitive function in idiopathic Parkinson disease. *Archives of Neurology, 53*, 1140–1146.

Benabid, A. L., Caparros-Lefebvre, D., & Pollak, P. (1998). History of surgery for movement disorders. In I. Germano (Ed.), *Neurosurgical treatment of movement disorders* (pp. 19–35). Park Ridge, IL: American Association of Neurological Surgeons.

Benazzouz, A., & Hallet, M. (2000). Mechanism of action of deep brain stimulation. *Neurology, 55*, S13–S16.

Berg, E., Bjornram, C., Hartelius, L., Laakso, K., & Johnels, B. (2003). High-level language difficulties in Parkinson disease. *Clinical Linguistics and Phonetics, 17*, 63–80.

Berger, H., van Es, N., van Spaendonck, K., Teunisse, J., Horstink, M., van 't Hof, M., & Cools, A. (1999). Relationship between memory strategies and motor symptoms in Parkinson disease. *Journal of Clinical and Experimental Neuropsychology, 21*, 677–684.

Berney, A., Vingerhoets, F., & Perrin, A. (2002). Effect on mood of subthalmic DBS for Parkinson disease: A consecutive series of 24 patients. *Neurology, 59*, 1427–1429.

Body, R. (2004). *Methodological advances in the assessment of cognitive-linguistic ability after traumatic brain injury.* Paper presented at International Clinical Phonetics and Linguistic Association conference in Lafayette, LA.

Breen, E. K. (1993). Recall and recognition memory in Parkinson disease. *Cortex, 29*, 91–102.

Brown, R. G., & Jahanshahi, M. (1996). Cognitive-motor dysfunction in Parkinson disease. *European Neurology, 36*, 24–31.

Brown, R. G., & Marsden, C. D. (1990). Cognitive function in Parkinson disease. *Trends in Neuroscience, 13*, 21–29.

Brusa, L., Bassi, A., Stefania, A., Pierantozzi, M., Peppe, A., Caramia, M. D., . . . Stanzione, P. (2003). Pramipexole in comaprison to L-dopa: A neuropsychological study. *Journal of Neural Transmission, 110*, 373–380.

Bublak, P., Muller, U., Gron, G., Reuter, M., & von Cramon, D. (2002). Manipulation of working memory information is impaired in Parkinson disease and related to working memory capacity. *Neuropsychology, 16*, 577–590.

Burchiel, K. J. (1995). Thalamotomy for movement disorders. *Neurosurgery Clinics of North America, 6*, 55–71.

Burn, D. J., Rowan, E. N., Allan, L. M., Molloy, S., O'Brien, J. T., & McKeith, I. G. (2006). Motor subtype and cognitive decline in Parkinson disease, Parkinson disease with dementia, and dementia with Lewy bodies. *Journal of Neurology, Neurosurgery, and Neuropsychiatry, 77*, 585–589.

Cahn, D. A., Sullivan, E. V., Shear, P. K., Pfefferbaum, A., Heit, G., & Silverberg, G. (1998). Differential contributions of cognitive and motor component processes to physical and instrumental activities of daily living in Parkinson disease. *Archives of Neuropsychology, 13*, 575–583.

Caplan, D., & Waters, G. S. (1999). Verbal working memory and sentence comprehension. *Behavioral and Brain Sciences, 22*, 77–126.

Carr, J. A. R., Honey, C. R., Marci Sinden, P., Phillips, A. G., & Martzke, J. S. (2003). A waitlist control-group study of cognitive, mood, and quality of life outcome after posteroventral pallidotomy in Parkinson disease. *Journal of Neurosurgery, 99*, 78–88.

Chow, T., & Cummings, J. (1999). Frontal-subcortical circuits. In B. Miller and J. Cummings (Eds.). *The human frontal lobes: Functions and disorders.* New York, NY: Guilford Press.

Cools, R., Barker, R. A., Sahakian, B. J., & Robbins, T. W. (2003). L-Dopa medication remediates cognitive inflexibility, but increases impulsivity in patients with Parkinson disease. *Neuropsychologia, 41*, 1431–1441.

Cooper, J. A., Sagar, H. J., Jordan, N., Harvey, N. S., & Sullivan, E. V. (1991). Cognitive impairment in early, untreated Parkinson 's disease and its relationship to motor disability. *Brain, 114*, 2095–2122.

Crosson, B. (1984). Role of the dominant thalamus in language: A review. *Psychological Bulletin, 96*, 491–517.

Crosson, B. (1985). Subcortical functions in language: A working model. *Brain and Language, 25*, 257–292.

Crosson, B. (1992). *Subcortical functions in language and memory*. New York, NY: Guilford Press.

Crosson, B. (1999). Subcortical mechanisms in language: Lexical-semantic mechanisms and the thalamus. *Brain and Cognition, 40*, 414–439.

Crosson, B., & Early, T. A. (1990). *A theory of subcortical functions in language: Review and critique*. Unpublished manuscript.

Cummings, J. L. (1993). Frontal-subcortical circuits and human behavior. *Archives of Neurology, 50*, 873–880.

Daniele, A., Albanese, A., Contarino, M. F., Zinzi, P., Barbier, A., Gasparini, F., . . . Scerrati, M. (2003). Cognitive and behavioral effects of chronic stimulation of the subthalamic nucleus in patients with Parkinson disease. *Journal of Neurology, Neurosurgery and Psychiatry, 74*, 175–182.

Darley, F., Brown, J., & Swenson, M. (1975). Language changes after neurosurgery for parkinsonism. *Brain and Language, 2*, 65–70.

de Bie, R. M. A., Schuurman, P. R., Bosch, D. A., de Haan, R. J., Schmand, B., & Speelman, J. D. (2001). Outcome of unilateral pallidotomy in advanced Parkinson disease: Cohort study of 32 patients. *Journal of Neurology, Neurosurgery and Psychiatry, 71*, 375–382.

De Gaspari, D., Siri, C., Di Gioia, M., Antonini, A., Isella, V., Pizzolato, A., . . . Pezzoli, G. (2006a). Clinical correlates and cognitive underpinnings of verbal fluency impairment after chronic subthalamic stimulation in Parkinson disease. *Parkinsonism and Related Disorders, 12*, 289–295.

De Gaspari, D., Siri, C., Landi, A., Cilia, R., Bonetti, A., Natuzzi, F., . . . Antonini, A. (2006b). Clinical and neuropsychological follow up at 12 months in patients with complicated Parkinson's disease treated with subcutaneous apomorphine infusion or deep brain stimulation of the subthalamic nucleus. *Journal of Neurology Neurosurgery and Psychiatry, 77*, 450–453.

Demakis, G. J., Mercury, M. G., Sweet, J. J., Rezak, M., Eller, T., & Vergenz, S. (2003). Qualitative analysis of verbal fluency before and after unilateral pallidotomy. *Clinical Neuropsychologist, 17*(3), 322–330.

Denckla, M. B. (1996). A theory and model of executive function: A neuropsychological perspective. In G. R. Lyon & N. A. Krasnegor (Eds.), *Attention, Memory and Executive Function.* Baltimore, MD: Paul Brookes.

Dubois, B., & Pillon, B. (1997). Cognitive deficits in Parkinson disease. *Journal of Neurology, 244*, 2–8.

Dujardin, K., Defebvre, L., Krystkowiak, P., Blond, S., & Destee, A. (2001). Influence of chronic bilateral stimulation of the subthalamic nucleus on cognitive function in Parkinson Disease. *Journal of Neurology, 248*, 603–611.

Emre, M. (2003). Dementia associated with Parkinson disease. *Lancet Neurology, 2*, 229–237.

Engle, R. W., & Conway, A. R. A. (1998). Working memory and comprehension. In R. H. Logie & K. J. Gilhooly (Eds.), *Working memory and thinking.* London, UK: Psychology Press.

Feger, J., Mouroux, M., Benazzouz, A., Boraud, T., Gross, C., & Crossman, A. R. (1994). The subthalamic nucleus: A more complex structure than expected. In G. Percheron, J. S. McKenzie, & J. Feger (Eds.), *The basal ganglia IV: New ideas and data on structure and function* (pp. 371–382). New York, NY: Plenum Press.

Ferreira, F., Bailey, K. G. D., & Ferraro, V. (2002). Good-enough representation in language comprehension. *Current Directions in Psychological Science, 11*, 11–15.

Flowers, K. A., Pearce, I., & Pearce, J. M. S. (1984). Recognition memory in Parkinson disease. *Journal of Neurology, Neurosurgery, and Psychiatry, 47*, 1174–1181.

Fukuda, M., Kameyama, S., Yoshino, M., Tanaka, R., & Narabayashi, H. (2000). Neuropsychological outcome following pallidotomy and thalamotomy for Parkinson disease. *Stereotactic and Functional Neurosurgery, 74*, 11–20.

Funkiewiez, A., Ardouin, C. M., Caputo, E., Krack, P., Fraix, V., Klinger, H., . . . Pollak, P. (2004). Long-term effects of bilateral subthalamic nucleus stimulation on cognitive function, mood, and behavior in Parkinson disease. *Journal of Neurology Neurosurgery and Psychiatry, 75*, 834–839.

Ghika, J., Ghika-Schmid, F., Fankhauser, H., Assal, G., Vingerhoets, F., Albanese, A., . . . Favre, J. (1999). Bilateral contemporaneous posteroventral pallidotomy for the treatment of Parkinson disease: Neuropsychological and neurological side effects. *Journal of Neurosurgery, 91*, 313–321.

Gilbert, B., Belleville, S., Bherer, L., & Chouinard, S. (2005). Study of verbal working memory in patients with Parkinson disease. *Neuropsychology, 19*, 106–114.

Gildenberg, P. L. (1984). The present role of stereotactic surgery in the management of Parkinson's disease. In R. G. Hassler & J. F. Christ (Eds.), *Advances in neurology* (Vol. 40, pp. 447–452). New York, NY: Raven Press.

Gironell, A., Kulisevsky, J., Rami, L., Fortuny, N., Garcia-Sanchez, C., & Pascual-Sedano, B. (2003). Effects of pallidotomy and bilateral subthalamic stimulation on cognitive function in Parkinson disease: A controlled comparative study. *Journal of Neurology, 250*, 917–923.

Goldman, W., Baty, J., Buckles, V., Sahrmann, S., & Morris, J. (1998). Cognitive and motor functioning in Parkinson disease. *Archives of Neurology, 55*, 674–680.

Gotham, A. M., Brown, R. G., & Marsden, C. D. (1988). "Frontal" cognitive function in patients with Parkinson disease "on" and "off" levodopa. *Brain, 111*, 299–311.

Gourovitch, M. L., Kirkby, B. S., Goldberg, T. E., Weinberger, D. R., Gold, J. M., Esposito, G., . . . Berman, K. F. (2000). A comparison of rCBF patterns during letter and semantic fluency. *Neuropsychology, 14*, 353–360.

Graceffa, A. M. S., Carlesimo, G. A., Peppe, A., & Caltagirone, C. (1999). Verbal working memory deficit in Parkinson disease subjects. *European Neurology, 42*, 90–94.

Green, J., & Barnhart, H. (2000). The impact of lesion laterality on neuropsychological change following posterior pallidotomy: A review of current findings. *Brain and Cognition, 42*, 379–398.

Grossman, M. (1999). Sentence processing in Parkinson disease. *Brain and Cognition, 40*, 387–413.

Grossman, M., Carvel, S., Goloomp, S., Stern, M. B., Vernon, G., & Hurtig, H. I. (1991). Sentence comprehension and praxis impairment in Parkinson disease. *Neurology, 41*, 1620.

Grossman, M., Carvel, S., Stern, M. B., Gollomp, S., & Hurtig, H. (1992). Sentence comprehension in Parkinson disease: The role of attention and memory. *Brain and Language, 42*, 347–384.

Grossman, M., Glosser, G., Kalmanson, J., Morris, J., Stern, M. B., & Hurtig, H. I. (2001). Dopamine supports sentence comprehension in Parkinson disease. *Journal of Neurological Science, 184*, 123–130.

Grossman, M., Kalmanson, J., Bernhardt, N., Stern, M. B., & Hurtig, H. I. (2000). Cognitive resource limitations during sentence processing in Parkinson disease. *Brain and Language, 73*, 1–16.

Grossman, M., Zurif, E., Lee, C., Prather, P., Kalmanson, J., Stern, M. B., & Hurtig, H. I. (2002). Information processing speed and sentence comprehension in Parkinson disease. *Neuropsychology, 16*, 174–181.

Hazrati, L.-N., & Parent, A. (1992). Differential patterns of arborisation of striatal and subthalamic fibres in the two pallidal segments in primates. *Brain Research, 598*, 311–315.

Hazrati, L.-N., & Parent, A. (1993). Striatal and subthalamic afferents to the primate pallidum: Interactions between two opposite chemospecific neuronal systems. *Progress in Brain Research, 99*, 89–104.

Helm-Estabrooks, N. (2001). *Cognitive Linguistic Quick Test.* San Antonio, TX: PsychCorp.

Hermanowicz, N. (2007). Drug therapy for Parkinson disease. *Seminars in Neurology, 27*, 97–105.

Higginson, C. I, King, D. S., Levine, D., Wheelcok, V. L., Khamphay, N. O., & Sigvardt, K. A. (2003). The relationship between executive function and verbal memory in Parkinson disease. *Brain and Cognition, 52*, 343–352.

Hiraoka, K., Matuo, Y., Iwata, A., Onishi, T., & Abe., K. (2006). The effects of external cues on ankle control during gait initiation in Parkinson disease. *Parkinsonism and Related Disorders, 12*, 97–102.

Hugdahl, K., & Wester, K. (2000). Neurocognitive correlates of stereotactic thalamotomy and thalamic stimulation in Parkinson patients. *Brain and Cognition, 42*, 231–252.

Hugdahl, K., Wester, K., & Asbjornsen, A. (1990). The role of the left and right thalamus in language asymmetry: Dichotic listening in Parkinson patients undergoing stereotactic thalamotomy. *Brain and Language, 39*, 1–13.

Huisingh, R., Barrett, M., Zachman, L., Blagden, C., & Orman, J. (1990). *The word test-revised: A test of expressive vocabulary and semantics*. East Moline, IL: Linguisystems.

Illes, J., Metter, E. J., Hanson, W. R., & Iritani, S. (1988). Language production in Parkinson disease: Acoustic and linguistic considerations. *Brain and Language, 33*, 146–160.

Jahanshahi, M., Ardouin, C. M., Brown, R. G., Rothwell, J. C., Obeso, J. A., Albanese, A., . . . Limousin-Dowsey, P. (2000). The impact of deep brain stimulation on executive function in Parkinson disease. *Brain, 123*, 1142–1154.

Jankovic, J., & Kapadia, A. S. (2001). Functional decline in Parkinson disease. *Archives of Neurology, 58*, 1611–1615.

Joel, D., & Weiner, I. (1994). The organization of the basal ganglia-thalamocortical circuits: Open interconnected rather than closed segregated. *Neuroscience, 63*, 363–379.

Jonides, J. (1995). Working memory and thinking. In E. E. Smith & D. N. Osherson (Eds.), *Thinking: An initiation to cognitive science, Vol. 3* (2nd ed., pp. 215–265). Cambridge, MA: MIT Press.

Kensinger, E. A., Shearer, D. K., Locascio, J. J., Growdon, J. H., & Corkin, S. (2003). Working memory in mild Alzheimer's disease and early Parkinson disease. *Neuropsychology, 17*, 230–239.

Kimberg, D. Y., & D' Esposito, M. (2003). Cognitive effects of the dopamine receptor agonist pergolide. *Neuropsychologia, 41*, 1020–1027.

Kischka, U., Kammer, T., Maier, S., Weisbrod, M., Thimm, M., & Spitzer, M. (1996). Dopaminergic modulation of semantic network activation. *Neuropsychologia, 37*, 1107–1113.

Kleiner-Fisman, G., Fisman, D. N., & Sime, E. (2003). Long-term follow up of bilateral deep brain stimulation of the subthalamic nucleus in patients with advanced Parkinson disease. *Journal of Neurosurgery, 99*, 489–495.

Kompoliti, K., Wang, Q. E., Goetz, C. G., Leurgans, S., & Raman, R. (2000). Effects of central dopaminergic stimulation by apomorphine on speech in Parkinson disease. *Neurology, 54*, 458–462.

Kopell, B. H., Rezai, A., Chang, J.-W., & Vitek, J. L. (2006). Anatomy and physiology of the basal ganglia: Implications for deep brain stimulation for Parkinson disease. *Movement Disorders, 21*(Suppl. 14), 238–246.

Kulisevsky, J. (2000). Role of dopamine in learning and memory. *Drugs and Aging, 16*, 365–379.

Kulisevsky, J., Garcia-Sanchez, C., Berthier, M. L., Barbanoj, M., Pascual-Sedano, B., Gironell, A., & Estevez-Gonzalez, A. (2000). Chronic effects of dopaminergic replacement on cognitive function in Parkinson disease: A two-year follow-up study of previously untreated patients. *Movement Disorders, 15*, 613–626.

Kuzis, G., Sabe, L., Tiberti, C., Dorrego, F., Starkstein, S., & Merello, M. (2001). Neuropsychological effects of pallidotomy in patients with Parkinson disease. *Journal of Neurology, Neurosurgery and Psychiatry, 71*, 563–564.

Lacritz, L. H., Munro Cullum, C., Frol, A. B., Dewey, R. B., & Giller, C. A. (2000). Neuropsychological outcome following unilateral stereotactic pallidotomy in intractable Parkinson disease. *Brain and Cognition, 42*, 364–378.

Lang, A. E., Duff, J., Saint-Cyr, J. A., Trepanier, L. L., Gross, R. E., Lombardi, W. J., . . . Lozano, A. M. (1999). Posteroventral medial pallidotomy in Parkinson disease. *Journal of Neurology, 246*, 28–41.

Lang, A. E., & Lozano, A. M. (1998). Medical progress: Parkinson disease (second of two parts). *New England Journal of Medicine, 339*, 1130–1143.

Lange, K. W., Paul, G. M., Naumann, M., & Gsell, W. (1995). Dopaminergic effects on cognitive performance in patients with Parkinson disease. *Journal of Neural Transmission, 46*, 423–432.

Lange, K. W., Robbins, T. W., Marsden, C. D., James, M., Owen, A. M., & Paul, G. M. (1992). L-dopa withdrawal in Parkinson disease selectively impairs cognitive performance in tests sensitive to frontal lobe dysfunction. *Psychopharmacology, 107*, 394–404.

LaPointe, L. L., Maitland, C. G., Blanchard, A. A., Kemker, B. K., Stierwalt, J. A. G., & Heald, G. R. (2004a). *Distraction effects in cognitive-linguistic processing: Neurogenic clinical populations.* Paper presented at American Speech-Language Hearing Convention, Philadelphia, PA, November, 2004.

LaPointe, L. L., Maitland, C. G., Kemker, B. K., & Stierwalt, J. A. G. (2004b). *Cognitive-linguistic interactions: Strategies for assessment of cognitive status in*

neurogenic disorders. Workshop presented at International Association of Logopedics and Phoniatrics in Brisbane, Australia, September, 2004.
Lee, C., Grossman, M., Morris, J., Stern, M. B., & Hurtig, H. (2003). Attentional resource and processing speed limitations during sentence processing in Parkinson disease. *Brain and Language, 85*, 347–356.
Levin, B. E., Llabre, M. M., & Weiner, W. J. (1989). Cognitive impairments associated with early Parkinson disease. *Neurology, 39*, 557–561.
Levin, B. E., Tomer, R., & Rey, G. J. (1992). Cognitive impairments in Parkinson disease. *Neurologic Clinics, 10I*, 471–485.
Levita, E., Riklan, M., & Cooper, D. B. (1967). Psychological comparison of unilateral and bilateral thalamic surgery. *Journal of Abnormal Psychology, 72*, 251–254.
Lewis, F. M., LaPointe, L. L., Murdoch, B. E., & Chenery, H. J. (1998). Language impairment in Parkinson disease. *Aphasiology, 12*, 193–206.
Lewis, S., Cools, R., Robbins, T., Dove, A., Barker, R., & Owen, A. (2003). Using executive heterogeneity to explore the nature of working memory deficits in Parkinson disease. *Neuropsychologia, 41*, 645–654.
Lewis, S., Dove, A., Robbins, T. W., Barker, R., & Owen, A. M. (2004). Striatal contributions to working memory: A functional magnetic resonance imaging study in humans. *European Journal of Neuroscience, 19*, 755–760.
Lozano, A. M., & Mahant, N. (2004). Deep brain stimulation surgery for Parkinson disease: Mechanisms and consequences. *Parkinsonism and Related Disorders, 10*, 49–57.
Lund-Johansen, M., Hugdahl, K., & Wester, K. (1996). Cognitive function in patients with Parkinson disease undergoing stereotaxic thalamotomy. *Journal of Neurology Neurosurgery and Psychiatry, 60*, 564–571.
Malapani, C., Pillon, B., Dubois, B., & Agid, Y. (1994). Impaired simultaneous cognitive task performance in Parkinson disease: A dopamine-related dysfunction. *Neurology, 44*, 319–326.
Masterman, D., DeSalles, A., Baloh, R. W., Frysinger, R., Foti, D., Behnke, E., . . . Bronstein, J. (1998). Motor, cognitive and behavioral performance following unilateral ventroposterior pallidotomy for Parkinson disease. *Archives of Neurology, 55*, 1201–1208.
Mayeux, R., Denaro, J., Hemenegildo, N., Marder, K., Tang, M., Cote, L., & Stern, Y. (1992). A population-based investigation of Parkinson disease with and without dementia: Relationship to age and gender. *Archives of Neurology, 49*, 492–497.
Mayeux, R., Stern, Y., Rosenstein, R., Marder, K., Hauser, A. Cote, L., & Fahn, S. (1988). An estimate of the prevalence of dementia in idiopathic Parkinson disease. *Archives of Neurology, 45*, 260–262.
McCarter, R. J., Walton, N. H., Rowan, A. F., Gill, S. S., & Palomo, M. (2000). Cognitive Funtioning after subthalamic nucleotomy for refractory Parkinson disease. *Journal of Neurology Neurosurgery and Psychiatry, 69*, 60–66.
McNamara, P., & Durso, R. (2006). Neuropharmacological treatment of mental dysfunction in Parkinson disease. *Behavioral Neurology, 17*, 43–51.

McNamara, P., Krueger, M., O'Quin, K., Clark, J., & Durso, R. (1996). Grammaticality judgements and sentence comprehension in Parkinson disease: A comparison with Broca's aphasia. *International Journal of Neuroscience, 86*, 151–166.

Meyer, D. E., & Schvaneveldt, R. W. (1971). Facilitation in recognizing pairs of words: Evidence of a dependence upon retrieval operations. *Journal of Experimental Psychology, 90*, 227–234.

Middleton, F. A., & Strick, P. L. (2000). Basal ganglia output and cognition: Evidence from anatomical, behavioral, and clinical studies. *Brain and Cognition, 42*, 183–200.

Modesti, L. M., & Blumetti, A. E. (1980). Long term effects of stereotaxic thalamotomy on parameters of cognitive functioning. *Acta Neurochirurgica: Supplementum, 30*, 401–403.

Monchi, O., Petrides, M., Doyon, J., Postuma, R. B., Worsley, K., & Dagher, A. (2004). Neural bases of set-shiftng deficits in Parkinson disease. *Journal of Neuroscience, 24*, 702–710.

Moretti, R., Torre, E., Antonello, R. M., Capus, L., Zambito Marsala, S., Cattaruzza, T., Cazzato, G., & Bava, A. (2003). Neuropsychological changes after subthalamic nucleus stimulation: A 12-month follow-up in nine patients with Parkinson disease. *Parkinsonism and Related Disorders, 10*, 73–79.

Moro, E., Scerrati, M., Romito, L. M. A., Roselli, R., Tonali, P., & Albanese, A. (1999). Chronic subthalamic nucleus stimulation reduces medication requirements in Parkinson disease. *Neurology, 53*, 85–90.

Morris, J., Glosser, G., Kalmanson, J., Hurtig, H., Stern, M., & Grossman, M. (1998). Dopamine supports sentence comprehension in Parkinson disease. *Brain and Language, 65*, 16–19.

Morrison, C. E., Borod, J. C., Perrine, K., Beric, A., Brin, M. F., Rezai, A., . . . Olanow, C. W. (2004). Neuropsychological functioning following bilateral subthalamic nucleus stimulation in Parkinson disease. *Archives of Clinical Neurophysiology, 19*, 165–181.

Mortimer, J. A., Pirozzolo, F. J., Hansch, E. C., & Webster, D. D. (1982). Relationship of motor symptoms to intellectual deficits in Parkinson disease. *Neurology, 32*, 133–137.

Movement Disorders Society. (2002). Surgical treatment for Parkinson disease: Deep brain surgery. *Movement Disorders, 17*, S128–S147.

Münte, T. F., Schilz, K., & Kutas, M. (1998). When temporal terms belie conceptual order. *Nature, 395*, 71–73.

Murdoch, B. E., Whelan, B.-M., Theodoros, D. G., & Cahill, L. (2004). A subcortical chain of command involved in the regulation of linguistic processes? *Brain and Language, 91*, 175–176.

Murdoch, B. E., Whelan, B.-M., Theodoros, D. G., Hall, B., & Silburn, P. (2003). Correlating motor and cognitive behavior: Exploring the notion of akinetic and dyskinetic linguistic homologues. *Brain and Language, 87*, 192.

Nadeau, S. E., & Crosson, B. (1997). Subcortical aphasia. *Brain and Language, 58*, 355–402.

Obeso, J. A., Guridi, J., & DeLong, M. R. (1997). Surgery for Parkinson disease. *Journal of Neurology Neurosurgery and Psychiatry, 62*, 2–8.

Obwegeser, A. A., Uitti, R., Lucas, J. A., Witte, R. J., Turk, M. F., & Wharen, R. (2000). Predictors of neuropsychological outcome in patients following microelectrode-guided pallidotomy for Parkinson disease. *Journal of Neurosurgery, 93*, 410–420.

Ojemann, G. (1975). Improved performance in some dysnomic states after human ventrolateral thalamic stimulation. *Journal of Neurology, Neurosurgery and Psychiatry, 38*, 408.

Ojemann, G. (1976). Subcortical language mechanisms. In H. A. Whitaker & H. Whitaker (Eds.), *Studies in Neurolinguistics* (pp. 103–138). New York, NY: Academic Press.

Olzak, M., Laskowska, I., Jelonek, J., Michalak, M., Szolna, A., Gryz, J., . . . Gorzelanczyk, E. J. (2006). Psychomotor and executive functioning after unilateral posteroventral pallidotomy in patients with Parkinson disease. *Journal of the Neurological Sciences, 248*, 97–103.

Owen, A. M., James, M., Leigh, P. N., Summers, B. A., Marsden, C. D., Quinn, N. P., . . . Robbins, T. W. (1992). Fronto-striatal cognitive deficits at different staged of Parkinson disease. *Brain, 115*, 1727–1751.

Pahwa, R. Paolo, A., Troster, A., & Koller, W. (1998). Cognitive impairment in Parkinson disease. *European Journal of Neurology, 5*, 431–441.

Parent, A., & Hazrati, L.-N. (1993). Anatomical aspects of information processing in primate basal ganglia. *Trends in Neuroscience, 16*, 111–116.

Parkin, S. G., Gregory, R. P., Scott, R., Bain, P., Silburn, P., Hall, B., . . . Aziz, T. (2002). Unilateral and bilateral pallidotomy for idiopathic Parkinson disease: A case series of 115 patients. *Movement Disorders, 17*, 682–692.

Percheron, G., & Filion, M. (1991). Parallel processing in the basal ganglia: Up to a point. *Trends in Neuroscience, 14*, 55–59.

Petrovici, J. N. (1980). Speech disturbances following stereotaxic surgery in ventrolateral thalamus. *Neurosurgical Review, 3*(3), 189–195.

Pillon, B., Ardouin, C. M., Damier, P., Krack, P., Houeto, J. L., Klinger, H., . . . Agid, Y. (2000). Neuropsychological changes between "off" and "on" STN or GPi stimulation in Parkinson disease. *Neurology, 55*, 411–418.

Rafal, R. D., Posner, M. I., Walker, J. A., & Friedrich, F. J. (1984). Cognition and the basal ganglia: Separating mental and motor performance in Parkinson disease. *Brain, 107*, 1083–1094.

Raskin, S. A., Borod, J. C., & Tweedy, J. (1990). Neurological aspects of Parkinson disease. *Neuropsychology Review, 1*, 185–221.

Rettig, G. M., York, M. K., Lai, E. C., Jankovic, J., Krauss, J. K., Grossman, R. G., & Levin, H.S. (2000). Neuropsychological outcome after unilateral pallidotomy for the treatment of Parkinson disease. *Journal of Neurology, Neurosurgery and Psychiatry, 69*, 326–336.

Richards, M., Stern, Y., Marder, K., Cote, L., & Mayeux, R. (1993). Relationships between extrapyramidal signs and cognitive function in a community-dwelling cohort of patients with Parkinson disease and normal elderly individuals. *Annals of Neurology, 33*, 267–274.

Ridenour, T. A., & Dean, R. S. (1999). Parkinson disease and neurological assessment. *International Journal of Neuroscience, 99,* 1–18.

Riklan, M., & Levita, E. (1970). Psychological studies of thalamic lesions in humans. *Journal of Nervous and Mental Disease, 150,* 251–265.

Riklan, M., Levita, E., Zimmerman, J., & Cooper, I. S. (1969). Thalamic correlates of language and speech. *Journal of the Neurological Sciences, 8,* 307–328.

Rochester, L., Hetherington, V., Jones, D., Nieuwboer, A., Willems, A., Kwakkel, G., & Van Wegen, E. (2005). The effect of external rhythmic cues (auditory and visual) on walking during a functional task in homes of people with Parkinson's disease. *Archives of Physical Medicine and Rehabilitation, 86,* 999–1006.

Rouzaire-Dubois, B., & Scarnati, E. (1985). Bilateral corticosubthalamic nucleus projections: An electrophysiological study in rats with chronic cerebral lesions. *Neuroscience, 15,* 69–75.

Rubenstein, H., Garfield, L., & Millikan, J. (1970). Homographic enteries in the internal lexicon. *Verbal Learning and Verbal Behavior, 9,* 484–494.

Saint-Cyr, J. A., Taylor, A. E., & Lang, A. E. (1988). Procedural learning and neostriatal dysfunction in man. *Brain, 111,* 941–959.

Saint-Cyr, J. A., & Trepanier, L. L. (2000). Neuropsychologic assessment of patients for movement disorder surgery. *Movement Disorders, 15,* 771–783.

Saint-Cyr, J. A., Trepanier, L. L., Kumar, R., Lozano, A. M., & Lang, A. E. (2000). Neuropsychological consequences of chronic bilateral stimulation of the subthalamic nucleus in Parkinson disease. *Brain, 123,* 2091–2108.

Schlosser, R., Hutchinson, M., Joseffer, S., Rusinek, H., Saarimaki, A., Stevenson, J., . . . Brodie, J. (1998). Functional magnetic resonance imaging of human brain activity in a verbal fluency task. *Journal of Neurology Neurosurgery and Psychiatry, 64,* 492–498.

Schroeder, U., Kuehler, A., Lange, K. W., Haslinger, B., Tronnier, V. M., Krause, M., . . . Baumann, A. O. (2003). Subthalamic nucleus stimulus affects frontotemporal network: A PET study. *Annals of Neurology, 54,* 445–450.

Schuurman, P. R., Bruins, J., Merkus, M. P., Bosch, D. A., & Speelman, J. D. (2002). A comparison of neuropsychological effects of thalamotomy and thalamic stimulation. *Neurology, 59,* 1232–1239.

Scott, R. B., Gregory, R., Hines, N., Carroll, C., Hyman, N., & Papanasstiou, V. (1998). Neuropsychological, neurological and functional outcome following pallidotomy for Parkinson disease: A consecutive series of eight simultaneous bilateral and twelve unilateral procedures. *Brain, 121,* 659–675.

Scott, R. B., Harrison, J., Boulton, C., Wilson, J., Gregory, R., Parkin, S., . . . Aziz, T. Z. (2002). Global attentional-executive sequelae following surgical lesions to globus pallidus interna. *Brain, 125,* 562–574.

Sharpe, M. H. (1990). Distractibility in early Parkinson disease. *Cortex, 26,* 239–246.

Sharpe, M. H. (1996). Is there a divided attention deficit in patients with early Parkinson disease? *Cortex, 32,* 747–753.

Smeding, H. M. M., Speelman, J. D., Koning-Haanstra, M., Schuurman, P. R., Nijssen, P., van Laar, T., & Schmand, B. (2006). Neuropsychological effects of bilateral STN stimulation in Parkinson disease: A controlled study. *Neurology, 66*, 1830–1836.

Soukup, V. M., Ingram, F., Schiess, M. C., Bonnen, J. G., Nauta, H. J. W., & Calverly, J. R. (1997). Cognitive sequelae of unilateral posteroventral pallidotomy. *Archives of Neurology, 54*, 947–950.

Speelman, J. D., & Bosch, D. A. (2002). Neurosurgical treatment modalities in Parkinson disease. *Movement Disorders, 17*, S83–S85.

Stocchi, F., & Brusa, L. (2000). Cognition and emotion in different stages and subtypes of Parkinson disease. *Journal of Neurology, 247*, 114–121.

Swainson, R., Rogers, R. D., Sahakian, B. J., Summers, B. A., Polkey, C. E., & Robbins, T. W. (2000). Probabilistic learning and reversal deficits in patients with Parkinson disease or frontal or temporal lobe lesions: Possible adverse effects of dopaminergic medication. *Neuropsychologia, 38*, 596–612.

Taylor, A. E., Saint-Cyr, J. A., & Lang, A. E. (1986). Frontal lobe dysfunction in Parkinson disease: The cortical focus of neostriatal outflow. *Brain, 109*, 845–883.

Trepanier, L. L., Kumar, R., Lozano, A. M., Lang, A. E., & Saint-Cyr, J. A. (2000). Neuropsychological outcome of GPi pallidotomy and GPi or STN deep brain stimulation in Parkinson disease. *Brain and Cognition, 42*, 324–347.

Trepanier, L. L., Saint-Cyr, J. A., Lozano, A. M., & Lang, A. E. (1998). Neuropsychological consequences of posteroventral pallidotomy for the treatment of Parkinson disease. *Neurology, 51*, 207–215.

Troster, A. (2000). Introduction to neurobehavioral issues in the neurosurgical treatment of movement disorders: Basic issues, thalamotomy, and nonablative treatments. *Brain and Cognition, 42*, 173–182.

Troster, A., Wilkinson, S. B., Fields, J., Miyawaki, K., & Koller, W. C. (1998). Chronic electrical stimulation of the left ventrointermediate thalamic nucleus for the treatment of pharmacotherapy-resistant Parkinson disease: A differential impact on access to semantic and episodic memory? *Brain and Cognition, 38*, 125–149.

Troster, A., Woods, S. P., & Fields, J. (2003). Verbal fluency declines after pallidotomy: An interaction between task and lesion laterality. *Applied Neuropsychology, 10*, 69–75.

Troster, A., Woods, S. P., Fields, J., Hanisch, C., & Beatty, W. W. (2002). Declines in switching underlie verbal fluency changes after unilateral pallidal surgery in Parkinson disease. *Brain and Cognition, 50*, 207–217.

Troyer, A. K., Moscovitch, M., & Winocur, G. (1997). Clustering and switching as two components of phonemic fluency: Evidence from younger and older healthy controls. *Neuropsychology, 11*, 138–146.

Troyer, A. K., Moscovitch, M., Winocur, G., Alexander, M. P., & Stuss, D. (1998). Clustering and switching on verbal fluency: The effects of focal frontal and temporal-lobe lesions. *Neuropsychologia, 36*, 499–504.

Turner, K. R., Reid, W. G., Homewood, J., & Cook, R. J. (2002). Neuropsyhcological sequelae of bilateral posteroventral pallidotomy. *Journal of Neurology, Neurosurgery and Psychiatry, 73*, 444–446.

Vakil, E., & Herishanu-Naaman, S. (1998). Declarative and procedural learning in Parkinson disease patients having tremor or bradykinesia as the predominant symptom. *Cortex, 34*, 611–620.

Van Buren, J. M., Shapiro, D. Y., Henderson, W. G., & Sadowsky, D. A. (1973). A qualitative and quantitative evalutaion of parkinsonians three to six years following thalamotomy. *Confina Neurologica, 35*(4), 202–235.

Van Orden, G. C., & Goldinger, S. D. (1994). Interdependence of form and function in cognitive systems explains perception of printed words. *Journal of Experimental Psychology: Human Perception and Performance, 20*, 1269–1291.

Van Spaendonck, K., Berger, H., Horstink, M., Buytenhuijs, E., & Cools, A. (1996). Executive functions and disease characteristics in Parkinson disease, *Neuropsychologia, 34*, 617–626.

Verbaan, D., Marinus, J., Visser, M., van Rooden, S. M., Stiggelbout, A. M., Middelkoop, H. A. M., & van Hilten, J. (2007). Cognitive impairment in Parkinson disease. *Journal of Neurology, Neurosurgery, and Psychiatry, 78*, 1182–1187.

Verleden, S. Vingerhoets, G. & Santens, P. (2006). Heterogeneity of cognitive dysfunction in Parkinson disease. *European Neurology, 58*, 34–40.

Vilkki, J., & Laitinen, L. V. (1974). Differential effects of left and right ventrolateral thalamotomy on receptive and expressive verbal performances and face matching. *Neuropsychologia, 12*, 11–19.

Vilkki, J., & Laitinen, L. V. (1976). Effects of pulvinotomy and ventrolateral thalamotomy on some cognitive functions. *Neuropsychologia, 14*, 67–78.

Vitek, J. L., Bakay, R. A. E., & Freeman, A. (2003). Randomised trial of pallidotomy versus medical therapy for Parkinson disease. *Annals of Neurology, 53*, 558–569.

Voon, V., Kubu, C. S., Krack, P., Houeto, J. L., & Troster, A. (2006). Deep brain stimulation: Neuropsychological and neuropsychiatric issues. *Movement Disorders, 21*, 305–326.

Wallesch, C.-W. (1990). Repetitive verbal behavior: Functional and neurological considerations. *Aphasiology, 4*, 133–154.

Wallesch, C.-W. (1997). Symptomatology of subcortical aphasia. *Journal of Neurolinguistics, 10*(4), 267–275.

Wallesch, C.-W., & Papagno, C. (1988). Subcortical aphasia. In F. C. Rose, R. Whurr, & M. A. Wyke (Eds.), *Aphasia* (pp. 256–287). London, UK: Whurr.

Whelan, B.-M., Murdoch, B., Theodoros, D. G., Hall, B., & Silburn, P. (2003). Defining a role for the subthalamic nucleus (STN) within operative theoretical models of subcortical participation in language. *Journal of Neurology, Neurosurgery and Psychiatry, 74*, 1543–1550.

Whelan, B.-M., Murdoch, B., Theodoros, D. G., Hall, B., & Silburn, P. (2004a). Redefining functional models of basal ganglia organisation: A role for the posteroventral pallidum in linguistic processing. *Movement Disorders, 19*, 1267–1278.

Whelan, B.-M., Murdoch, B., Theodoros, D. G., Hall, B., & Silburn, P. (2004b). Re-appraising contemporary theories of subcortical participation in language: Proposing an interhemispheric regulatory function for the subthalamic nucleus (STN) in the mediation of high-level linguistic processes. *Neurocase, 10,* 345–352.

Whelan, B.-M., Murdoch, B., Theodoros, D. G., Hall, B., & Silburn, P. (2005b). Beyond verbal fluency: Investigating the long-term effects of bilateral subthalamic (STN) deep brain stimulation (DBS) on language function in 2 cases. *Neurocase, 11*, 93–102.

Whelan, B.-M., Murdoch, B. E., Theodoros, D. G., Silburn, P., & Hall, B. (2002). A role for the dominant thalamus in language?: A linguistic comparision of two cases subsequent to unilateral thalamotomy procedures in the dominant and non-dominant hemispheres. *Aphasiology, 16,* 1213–1226.

Whelan, B.-M., Murdoch, B. E., Theodoros, D. G., Silburn, P., & Hall, B. (2005a). Borrowing from models of motor control to translate cognitive processes: Evidence for hypokinetic-hyperkinetic linguistic homologues? *Journal of Neurolinguistics, 18*, 361–381.

Wester, K., & Hugdahl, K. (1997). Thalamotomy and thalamic stimulation: Effects on cognition. *Stereotactic and Functional Neurosurgery, 69*, 80–85.

Wichmann, T., & DeLong, M. R. (1998). Models of basal ganglia function and pathophysiology of movement disorders. *Neurosurgery Clinics of North America, 9*, 223–236.

Williams-Gray, C. H., Foltynie, T., Brayne, C., Robbins, T. W., & Barker, R. A. (2007). Evolution of cognitive dysfunction in an incident Parkinson disease cohort. *Brain, 130,* 1787–1798.

Witt, K., Pulkowski, U., Herzog, J., Lorenz, D., Hamel, W., Deuschl, G., & Krack, P. (2004). Deep brain stimulation of the subthalamic nucleus improves cognitive flexibility but impairs response inhibition in Parkinson disease. *Archives of Neurology, 61*, 697–700.

Wojtecki, L., Timmerman, L., Jorgens, S., Sudmeyer, M., Maarouf, M., Treuer, H., . . . Schnitzler, A. (2006). Frequency-dependent reciprocal modulation of verbal fluency and motor functions in subthalamic deep brain stimulation. *Archives of Neurology*, *63*, 1273–1276.

Woods, S. P., Fields, J., & Troster, A. (2002). Neuropsychological sequelae of subthalamic nucleus deep brain stimualtion in Parkinson disease: A critical review. *Neuropsychology Review, 12*, 111–126.

York, M., Levin, H. S., Grossman, R. G., & Hamilton, W. J. (1999). Neuropsychological outcome following unilateral pallidotomy. *Brain, 122*, 2209–2220.

York, M., Levin, H. S., Grossman, R. G., Lai, E. C., & Krauss, J. K. (2003). Clustering and switching in phonemic fluency following pallidotomy for the treatment of Parkinson disease. *Journal of Clinical and Experimental Neuropsychology, 25*(1), 110–121.

Zgaljardic, D. J., Borod, J. C., Foldi, N. S., & Mattis, P. (2003). A review of the cognitive and behavioral sequelae of Parkinson disease: Relationship to frontostriatal circuitry. *Cognitive and Behavioral Neurology, 16*, 193–210.

List of Abbreviations

PD	Parkinson disease
SNc	Substantia nigra compacta
GPi	Globus pallidus internus
SNr	Substantia nigra reticulata
Vim	Ventral intermediate nucleus of thalamus
PV	Posteroventral
AC	Anterior commissure
PC	Posterior commissure
MRI	Magnetic resonance image
CT	Computed tomography
VA	Ventral anterior thalamic nucleus
VL	Ventral lateral thalamic nucleus
CM	Centrum medianum
NR	Nucleus reticularis
ALC	Anterior language centre
PLC	Posterior language centre
PF	Parafascicular nucleus
BPVP	Bilateral posteroventral pallidotomy
UPVP	Unilateral posteroventral pallidotomy
BA	Brodmann's area
DBS	Deep brain stimulation
STN	Subthalamic nucleus
GPe	Globus pallidus externus
ITP	Inferior thalamic peduncle
CMPFC	Centrum medianum parafascicular complex
TWT-R	The Word Test-Revised
MH	Words with many meanings and a high degree of relatedness between meanings

6

Assessment and Treatment of Cognitive-Linguistic Disorder in Parkinson Disease

BROOKE-MAI WHELAN

As outlined in Chapter 5, cognitive deficits associated with Parkinson Disease (PD) largely have been attributed to dysfunctional striatofrontal circuitry (Dubois & Pillon, 1991), and include impairments of visuospatial functioning; free recall memory; working memory; effort demanding tasks (e.g., rapid processing and complex problem solving); set formation and set shifting entailing the internal control of attention, sequencing, temporal order, and recency discrimination; as well as executive functioning (Saint-Cyr & Trepanier, 2000). The assessment and treatment of these cognitive sequelae are routinely undertaken by the neuropsychologist, with little attention being paid to the comprehensive investigation of potential language breakdown in PD. In general, confrontation naming and verbal fluency tasks represent the mainstay of neuropsychological tools dedicated to the assessment of language functioning in PD patients, with indexes of more complex comprehension and sentential level production skills infrequently applied. Nevertheless, current evidence suggests that language deficits in PD typically extend beyond the level of single word production.

Detailed investigations into the potential language deficits associated with PD represent a very narrow scope of research; however, studies to date have revealed an interesting profile of impairment. Specific deficits have been identified on certain targeted aspects of language processing in people with PD, including syntax comprehension, and confrontation and generative naming (i.e., verbal fluency) (Auriacombe et al., 1993; Bayles & Boone, 1982; Bayles & Tomoeda, 1983; Beatty & Monson, 1989; Caltagirone, Carlesimo, Nocentini, & Vicari, 1989; Grossman et al., 1991; Grossman et al., 2002; Gurd, Master, & Oliveria, 2001; Lieberman, Friedman, & Feldman, 1990; Lieberman, Kako, Tajchman, Feldman, & Jiminez, 1992; Matison, Mayeaux, Rosen, & Fahn, 1982; Natsopoulos et al., 1991; Raskin, Sliwinski, & Borod, 1992; Tweedy, Langer, & McDowell, 1982). It also has been established from a more general viewpoint that PD patients characteristically present with difficulty on cognitively demanding language tasks, whereas more operative language functions remain intact (Lewis, LaPointe, Murdoch, & Chenery, 1998).

Essentially, basic linguistic process within the PD population remain undisturbed, yet as adjunct nonlinguistic cognitive domains (e.g., memory, attention, executive function) are affected by the disease, more complex language processes supported by the frontal lobes become impaired (Bayles, 1990; Lewis et al., 1998). Lewis et al. (1998) elegantly demonstrated this phenomenon with evidence of a broader range of complex divergent language deficits (i.e., naming, definition and multiple definition formulation, ambiguity detection, figurative language interpretation, sentence construction, and semantic fluency) in PD patients with below normal cognitive status, when compared to PD patients with normal cognitive status. On the basis of this profile it is apparent that the language deficits seen in the PD population do not conform to the traditional definition of aphasia, and therefore require specially tailored speech pathology assessment and treatment approaches.

Assessment of Cognitive-Linguistic Disorder in Parkinson Disease

Patients with PD typically present normal profiles on tests of primary language function, yet demonstrate difficulty on tasks that assess metacognitive and metalinguistic processes. When intact, these processes permit the conscious and effective manipulation of the semantic system via the interaction of primary language, cognitive, and executive processes (Hinchliffe, Murdoch, & Theodoros, 2001a). Failure to adequately evaluate these skills within this population, by way of the exclusive application of traditional aphasia assessments, may serve to mask more complex language deficits that exist as a result of subcortical pathology.

Previous studies examining the effects of TBI on language function have employed language assessment batteries that evaluate function across a range of modalities as well as a hierarchy of structure, complexity, and predictability (Hinchliffe, Murdoch, & Chenery, 1998). This selection of tests was based on a conceptual model which defined communicative competence as the endpoint of the efficient interaction of language with other cognitive processes. Assessments included clinically available tests of primary language function as well as linguistically complex/higher level language abilities. A number of these assessments have been applied subsequently to the study of subcortical language disorders associated with PD.

In previous comprehensive PD language studies (Whelan & Murdoch, 2005; Whelan, Murdoch, Theodoros, Hall, & Silburn, 2003, 2004, 2005; Whelan, Murdoch, Theodoros, Silburn, & Hall, 2002, 2004, 2005; Whelan, Murdoch, Theodoros, Silburn, & Hall, 2002, 2005; Whelan, Murdoch, Theodoros, Silburn, & Harding-Clark, 2000), language tests have been divided into two principle batteries: (1) a general language battery, consisting of assessments of primary language functions, and (2) a high-level language battery, consisting of assessments of more complex language functions. The general language battery included: the Neurosensory Centre Comprehensive Examination for Aphasia (NCCEA) (Spreen & Benton, 1977) and the Boston Naming Test (BNT) (Kaplan, Goodglass, & Weintraub, 1983), including an analysis of error types (Chenery, Murdoch, & Ingram, 1996). The high-level linguistic assessment battery included: The Test of Language Competence-Expanded Edition (TLC-E) (Wiig & Secord, 1989), The Word Test-Revised (TWT-R) (Huisingh, Barrett, Zachman, Blagden, & Orman, 1990), Test of Word Knowledge (TOWK) (Wiig & Secord, 1992), Wiig-Semel Test of Linguistic Concepts (WSTLC) (Wiig & Semel, 1974), and semantic fluency tasks (Table 6–1).

General Language Battery

Neurosensory Centre Comprehensive Examination for Aphasia (NCCEA)

The NCCEA constitutes a detailed assessment of language functions (Spreen & Benton, 1977), incorporating subtests that evaluate primary as well as high-level linguistic abilities (Murdoch & Leathlean, 1996).

Table 6–1. Language Assessment Battery

Battery 1: General Language
• Neurosensory Centre Comprehensive Examination of Aphasia (NCCEA) (Spreen & Benton, 1977) • Boston Naming Test (BNT) (Kaplan, Goodglass, & Weintraub, 1983)
Battery 2: High-Level Language Battery
• Test of Language Competence-Expanded (TLC-E) (Wiig & Secord, 1989) a. Ambiguous Sentences: providing 2 essential meanings for ambiguous sentences (e.g., *Right then and there the man drew a gun*) b. Making Inferences: utilizing causal relationships or chains in short paragraphs to make logical inferences c. Recreating Sentences: formulating grammatically complete sentences utilizing key semantic elements within defined contexts (e.g., Defined context = *At the ice cream store*; key semantic elements = *some, and, get*) d. Figurative Language: interpreting metaphorical expressions (e.g., *There is rough sailing ahead for us*) and correlating structurally related metaphors (e.g., *We will be facing a hard road*) according to shared meanings e. Remembering Word Pairs: recalling paired word associates • The Word Test-Revised (TWT-R) (Huisingh, Barrett, Zachman, Blagden, & Orman, 1990) a. Associations: identifying semantically unrelated words within a group of 4 spoken words (e.g., knee, shoulder, *bracelet*, ankle) and providing an explanation for the selected word in relation to the category of semantically related words (e.g., *The rest are parts of the body*) b. Synonym Generation: generation of synonyms for verbally presented stimuli (e.g., *afraid = scared*) c. Semantic Absurdities: identifying and repairing semantic incongruities (e.g., *My grandfather is the youngest person in my family = My grandfather is the oldest person in my family*) d. Antonym Generation: generating antonyms for verbally presented stimuli (e.g., *alive = dead*) e. Formulating Definitions: identify and describe critical semantic features of specified words (e.g., *house = person + lives*) f. Multiple Definitions: provision of 2 distinct meanings for series of spoken homophonic words (e.g., *down = position/feathers/feeling*) • Test of Word Knowledge (TOWK) (Wiig & Secord, 1992) a. Conjunctions and Transitions (e.g., evaluation of logical relationships between clauses and sentences (e.g., *It is too cold to play outside now. We will play outside (until/when/where/while) it gets warmer*) • Wiig-Semel Test of Linguistic Concepts (WSTLC) (Wiig & Semel, 1974) a. Comprehension of complex linuistic structures (e.g., *John was hit by Eric. Was John hit?*) b. Animal and tool verbal fluency • Semantic Fluency Tasks

Principally designed for the assessment of aphasic individuals, the NCCEA is composed of 20 language tasks that specifically evaluate the status of immediate verbal memory, verbal production and fluency, receptive language, reading, writing, and basic articulatory proficiency (Spreen & Benton, 1977). Overall, the assessment provides a descriptive versus taxonomic classification of linguistic abilities (Spreen & Benton, 1977).

Boston Naming Test (BNT)

The BNT is a reliable measure of confrontation naming abilities (Guilford & Nawojczk, 1988) and provides information about the effectiveness of semantic and phonemic cues in facilitating word retrieval (Kaplan et al., 1983). The person is instructed to name 60 constituent black and white line drawings of various objects ranging in frequency from *bed* to *abacus* and are permitted up to 20 seconds to respond to each item. A semantic cue is given if the person provides a response that represents a misinterpretation of the target or a lack of recognition. A phonemic cue is provided subsequent to any failure to respond or incorrect response to a semantic cue, or in the event of recognition of the item but an inability to produce its name.

Error responses also may be transcribed online and later coded for analysis. Errors may be classified according to a system devised by Chenery et al., 1996, based on the naming error taxonomies of Kushner et al. (1987), LaBarge, Balota, Stordandt, and Smith (1992), LeDorze and Nespoulous (1989), and Smith, Murdoch, and Chenery (1989). A summary of error types and examples is shown in Table 6–2.

High-Level Language Battery

The Test of Language Competence-Expanded Edition (TLC-E)

The TLC-E is an assessment of language proficiency and metalinguistic ability, consisting of a range of subtests that probe the semantic system, semantic-syntactic interfaces, and pragmatics (Wiig & Secord, 1989). Designed and standardized on 2 levels (i.e., Level 1: children 5 to 9 years and Level 2: preadolescents and adolescents aged 9 to 18+ years), the TLC-E assesses language competence by way of complex tasks that demand divergent language production, cognitive-linguistic flexibility and planning for production. The TLC-E Level 2 has been utilized in the

Table 6–2. Classification System for Errors Produced on the Boston Naming Test (BNT)

Error Type	*Description*	*Example*
1. SEMANTIC		
• Semantic paraphasia	Single word with a semantic relationship to the target	*Leash* for muzzle
• Definitional circumlocution	Informative multiword response with a semantic relationship to the target	*Remembrance flowers to go to a memorial* for wreath
• Vague circumlocution	Multiword response lacking specific definitional information but with a tangential relationship to the target	*The person who is going to be murdered* for noose
• Semantic negation	Response indicating what the target is not	*Not an otter* for beaver
• Semantically related whole/part-part/whole	Response named a part of target that formed part of its semantic specification	*Bedstead* for bed
2. NO RELATIONSHIP		
• Wild paraphasia	Single word response with no relationship to target	*Cup* for scroll
• Neutral		
a. deixis	Target labeled by non-specific pronoun	*The thing* for dart
b. empty syntax	Noninformative utterance used to describe target	*It's a funny thing too* for mask
• Deviant circumlocution	Inappropriate multiword response referring to attributes not typically associated with target	*Nice piece of elephant* for cactus
• Don't know	Statement of inability to label target	*I don't know the name of it* for palette
• No response		
• Question to examiner	Acknowledgment of examiner with inquiry as to whether response was correct or incorrect	*Is that right?* for octopus

Table 6–2. *continued*

Error Type	*Description*	*Example*
• Self-centered	Relation of target to self/ possessions or a phase or sentence relating personal experience to word meaning	*I bought that with the* . . . for mushroom
• Incomplete	Response composed of incomplete carrier phrase or sentence	*Thing around making the* . . . for compass
• Meta-task	A comment about the task or target	*I should know that one* for wreath
3. PERCEPTUAL		
• Perceptually related	Response involved label that visually was similar to target	*Snake* for pretzel
• Perceptually related: part/ whole or whole/ part	Response labeled part of the target that was perceprtually misinterpreted	*It's a bicycle* for wheelchair
4. PHONOLOGICAL		
• Phonemic paraphasia	Real word that shares some phonological elements of the target	*Corn* for accordian
• Literal paraphasia	Nonword that shares more than half the phonemes of the target word	*Mush* for mushroom
• Neologistic	Jargon nonword	*Squizzle* for octopus
• Phonemic letter cue	Response specified target letter beginning name	*It starts with "c"* for camel
5. UNRECOGNIZED CORRECT		*It's not a beaver* for beaver

Source: Adapted from Chenery, Murdoch, and Ingram (1996).

assessment of people with PD, and includes the following subtests: Ambiguous Sentences, Listening Comprehension: Making Inferences, Oral Expression: Recreating Sentences, Figurative Language, and Remembering Word Pairs. Table 6–1 presents subtest details.

The Word Test-Revised (TWT-R)

The Word Test-Revised (TWT-R) represents an assessment of expressive vocabulary and semantics (Huisingh et al., 1990), originally designed for use with the school-age child. The TWT-R specifically probes the ability to identify and express critical semantic features of the lexicon by way of tasks that involve categorization, definition, verbal reasoning, and lexical selection. This test includes the following subtests: Associations, Synonyms, Semantic Absurdities, Antonyms, Definitions, and Multiple Definitions. Table 6–1 presents specific subtest details.

Test of Word Knowledge (TOWK)

The Conjunctions and Transitions subtest of the TOWK has been employed as an additional probe of semantic integrity in people with PD. This subtest involves the evaluation of logical relationships between clauses and sentences (i.e., coherence) (Wiig & Secord, 1992). This task consists of a series of written paragraphs, each two sentences in length. The first sentence defines the relevant context and is syntactically complete (e.g., *It is too cold to play outside now*). The second sentence is incomplete, missing a conjunction or transition (e.g., *We will play outside (____) it gets warmer*). The absent word defines a logical semantic relationship between the sentences and is provided in multiple choice format as one of four possible choices (e.g., (a) *until*, (b) *when*, (c) *where*, (d) *while*). A respondent is instructed to select the linguistic marker that most adequately defines the underlying semantic relationship.

Wiig-Semel Test of Linguistic Concepts (WSTLC)

The WSTLC assesses the auditory comprehension of complex linguistic structures (Wiig & Semel, 1974). Consisting of 50 yes/no questions, correct responses are contingent on the undertaking of logical semantic operations in the manipulation of a range of complex linguistic relationships, including passive, comparative, temporal, spatial, and familial structures.

Semantic Fluency

Semantic fluency tasks entail the generation of as many item names as possible within specified semantic categories, in 60-second time intervals. An animate/ inanimate fluency dichotomy (e.g., animals/tools) often is chosen to assess the status of knowledge processing relevant to frequently dissociated semantic categories following brain injury (Ilmberger, Rau, Noachtar, Arnold, & Winkler, 2002; Tranel, Logan, Frank, & Damasio, 1997).

Strengths and Weaknesses of Recommended Assessments

The application of tests of metalinguistic competence, language integration and lexical-semantic system manipulation to populations with subcortical pathology such as PD has provided unprecedented insight into the nature of the ensuing language deficits. It is now known that tests that exclusively focus on the status of primary language functions such as traditional aphasia assessments, fail to adequately capture the true nature of subcortical language disorders that exist at the interface of language and cognition. More complex language measures, such as those listed within the high-level language battery above, provide more sensitive indices of language dysfunction within populations such as PD and, therefore, should be administered accordingly.

An inherent limitation of these assessments, however, is that they originally were designed for use with pediatric populations. Consequently, they have no accompanying standardized data relevant to normal adult or brain-impaired populations. Despite this weakness, however, these measures have been identified as sensitive to language disorders in PD within a research context (i.e., when research subjects were paired with age and education matched controls). Future research lies with the compilation of adult norms for the relevant tests summarized within this chapter, or the development of similar assessments that have been normed on nonneurologically impaired adults as well as adult brain injured populations. Current clinical recommendations for the application of these tests to adult populations, however, would be the adoption of maximal or ceiling score criteria as a bench mark for normal performance.

Assessment of Functional Communication in Parkinson Disease

The assessments outlined above primarily focus on the evaluation of language abilities from an impairment perspective, but fail to ascertain the impact of these deficits on functional communication skills (Hinchliffe, Murdoch, & Theodoros, 2001b). Additional to the assessments outlined above are those that evaluate communication activity limitation and participation restriction. As defined by Hinchliffe et al. (2001b), assessments of communication activity limitation encompass measures of functional and pragmatic communication abilities, which enable the evaluation of a person's ability to plan, deliver, and understand communication content within a range of interactive contexts. Pragmatic assessments typically appraise the ability to use language within natural contexts, including knowledge of language structure, knowledge of the environment and social rules, as well as the ability to adapt to changing environmental demands (Penn, 1999). In contrast, functional communication assessments largely aim to evaluate the quality of communication attempts (Manochiopining, Sheard, & Reed, 1992), or the impact of communication disorders on social and vocational roles, otherwise referred to as participation restrictions (Hinchliffe et al., 2001b). The incorporation of such measures is considered critical to any thorough clinical evaluation of language dysfunction resulting from PD, as opposed to an exclusive impairment-driven approach. Table 6–3 gives some suggested functional and pragmatic assessments that may be applied in the management of language disorders associated with PD.

Table 6–3. Suggested Functional and Pragmatic Communication Assessments for People with Parkinson Disease

Functional Assessments	*Author(s)*
• Functional Communication Profile	Sarno (1975)
• Everyday Communication Needs Assessment (ECNA)	Worrall (1999)
• Functional Assessment of Communication Skills for Adults (ASHA FACS)	Frattali, Thompson, Holland, Wohl, & Ferketic (1995)
• Communicative Effectiveness Index (CETI)	Lomas et al. (1989)
• Communicative Adequacy in Daily Situations	Clark & White (1995)
• The Communication Profile	Payne (1994)
Pragmatic Assessments	***Author(s)***
• The Profile of Communicative Appropriateness	Penn (1985)
• The Edinburgh Communication Functional Profile (Revised)	Wirz, Skinner, & Dean (1990)
• Communicative Abilities in Daily Living (CADL-Revised)	Holland, Frattali, & Fromm (1998)

Treatment of Cognitive-Linguistic Disorder in Parkinson Disease

Communication has been described as essential to all activities of daily living, and critical to maintaining psychosocial well-being and positive quality of life (Hinchliffe et al., 2001b). Akin to any communication deficit, the efficacious treatment of language disorders resulting from PD relies on comprehensive assessment at impairment, activity, and participation levels (Hinchliffe et al., 2001b). On the basis of these findings, appropriate therapeutic goals and treatment programs may then be developed. A range of treatment approaches, largely adopted from the school of cognitive neuropsychology (Gordon, 1990; Gross & Schultz, 1986; Mazaux & Richer, 1998) may be applied to the rehabilitation of PD. Although previously discussed within the context of language deficits resulting from TBI (Hinchliffe et al., 2001b), restorative, compensatory and behavioral treatment principles are considered translatable to all language disordered populations, including patients with PD.

Restorative Treatment Approaches

Restorative approaches operate on the premise that the repetitive undertaking of specific exercises, which train particular neuronal circuits, will improve functional abilities as a consequence of neuronal growth. In this manner, cognitive skills are re-established within the context of their premorbid status (Hinchliffe et al., 2001b). In applying this approach, specific linguistic deficits are determined by psychometric/impairment-based assessment and rehabilitation programs implemented involving the repeated execution of structured tasks (Mateer, Sohlberg, & Youngman, 1990) that target areas of deficit. In relation to language rehabilitation, such tasks may involve: lexical-semantic processing exercises (e.g., identifying synonyms and antonyms, defining words according to semantic criteria, categorization tasks); complex comprehension exercises (e.g., following instructions of increasing complexity, story retelling, defining multiple meaning words), or word retrieval exercises (e.g., word association tasks, synonym and antonym generation) (Hinchliffe et al., 2001b).

Limitations of this approach, however, exist and include a potential difficulty for some patients to generalize skills taught during structured clinical tasks to real-world situations, and may be related to an incomplete understanding of the relationship between the targeted deficit and the training task utilized (Snow & Ponsford, 1995). It has been suggested that the modification of such tasks to include functionally relevant stimuli on an individual basis, may alleviate this downfall to some extent, as would combining this approach with the development of compensatory strategies (Hinchliffe et al., 2001b).

Compensatory and Behavioral Treatment Approaches

Compensatory approaches operate on the premise that function cannot be restored once lost. Alternatively, skills and strategies are developed to establish functional competence (Mazaux & Richer, 1998). Behavioral treatment approaches adopt behavior modification techniques that aim to reinforce desired behaviors and to extinguish undesirable behaviors, or to positively reinforce the learning of new skills (Gross & Schultz, 1986). In applying compensatory approaches, patients are taught self-initiated methods by which to overcome language deficits such as the use of aids (e.g., notebooks containing word cues in the case of word-finding difficulties) and external cues (e.g., requests for repetition of information in the case of comprehension deficits), with a view to automatization over time (Hinchliffe et al., 2001b). Functional skills training may entail activity-based tasks within relevant communicative environments (e.g., telephone-answering routines, role-playing, direct instructions and scripting, fading of cues) (Hinchliffe et al., 2001b). Functional skills training also may extend to environmental manipulation techniques, whereby the person's communicative environment is modified to maximize communicative success (e.g., providing communication strategies for potential communication partners such allowing increased time for a response, or reducing environmental distractions to enhance comprehension) (Hinchliffe et al., 2001b).

Communication Strategies to Enhance Language Function

Changes in the ability to communicate have been described as unavoidable for people with PD (Miller, Noble, Jones, & Burn, 2006). Of particular relevance to the present chapter are reports by people with PD that a demise in the ability to communicate a view of oneself, as well as the need for increased effort in overcoming mental and physical limitations, present more of a concern than that of the voice difficulties frequently experienced in PD (Miller et al., 2006). In particular, people with PD have highlighted conversational difficulties such as: reduced attention

Treatment Strategies for Cognitive-Linguistic Disorders in Parkinson Disease

Treatment Approach	Treatment Strategies
■ Restorative: training of neuronal circuits thereby improves functional abilities over time	Repetitive structured tasks: ■ lexical-semantic processing (synonym judgement, word definition according to semantic criteria, categorization tasks) ■ complex comprehension (defining words with multiple meaning, following instructions of increasing complexity, story retelling) ■ word retrieval (word association, synonym/antonym generation)
■ Compensatory: function cannot be restored once lost; skills and strategies developed to establish functional competence	Self-initiated strategies: ■ use of aids (notebooks containing word cues for word finding difficulty) ■ use of external cues (requesting repetition of information not understood)
■ Functional skills training	Activity-based tasks in relevant communicative environments ■ direct instructions/scripts/routines (e.g., answering the telephone) ■ role-playing

span; distractibility; reduced ability to formulate ideas; as well as word-finding problems. Speakers specifically reported impediments to initiating and maintaining conversations, an inability to express personal needs, and perceptions of neglect by others. Furthermore, people with PD stated that listeners often "talk over" and "speak for" them, fail to give adequate time for them to respond, ignore them in conversation, and lack a general understanding of the difficulties they confront in trying to communicate (Miller et al., 2006).

The outcomes of the above research provide valuable insight into the language difficulties and associated communication barriers that carry anecdotal weight for people with PD. Central to these difficulties are maladaptive responses and strategies adopted by communication partners. Indeed, it previously has been emphasized that the role and abilities of the listener within a conversation are as pivotal to communicative success as the status of the speaker (Cruice, Worrall, Hickson, & Murison, 2003). The implementation of effective strategies for the communication partners of people with PD via timely referral to a speech-language pathologist will serve to prevent the development of maladaptive coping strategies, as well as to spare the speaker from the social isolation and withdrawal that may result from frustration associated with communication failure (Miller et al., 2006).

Focusing on improving the skills and confidence of communication partners (Simmons-Mackie, 2008), therefore, may constitute an integral part of therapy for the PD patient. Communication partner training typically involves: (1) the provision of strategies to the partner with which to assist the speaker when language breakdowns occur; and (2) encouragement by the partner of the speaker to utilize augmentative communication tools (e.g., writing) (Simmons-Mackie, 2008). Specific examples of strategies for communication partners of patients with PD adapted from Simmons-Mackie (2008) and Ylvisaker, Szekeres, and Fenney (2008) have been listed in Table 6–4.

Summary

The present chapter provides a summary of linguistic assessments identified as sensitive in detecting language deficits that may arise as a consequence of PD. In particular, it was emphasized that traditional aphasia tests fail to adequately profile the nature of language disturbances associated with PD. Attention was specifically directed to tests of complex, or higher level language function, of which component tasks demand frontal lobe participation in their execution. Limitations of these assessments include a foundation in pediatrics and a subsequent lack of normative data relevant to adults, as well as a deficiency in functional outcome measures needed to assess the impact of communication deficits on quality of life. Potential treatment approaches include restorative and compensatory/behavioral methods, functional skills training, and strategies for communication partners to enhance communicative success.

Table 6–4. Strategies for Communication Partners of People with Parkinson Disease

General Strategies	
• Slow rate of conversational speech	• Use redundancy (e.g., "Where's Jane your daughter?" instead of "Where's Jane?"
• Use pauses between topics	• Use alerting gestures or phrases (e.g., touch to gain attention)
• Use simple sentences/simplify information	• Emphasise key conversational points with stress and intonation
• Present one idea at a time	• Be tolerant of silences
• Position key information at the end of a sentence	• Use gesture and mime to supplement spoken information
• Repeat key words	• Paraphrase, summarize, clarify, elaborate, and sustain conversational topics
• Write key words to refer back to	• Use written support (e.g., drawing or written word) and/ or props (e.g., photos, magazines, etc.)
• Rephrase when there is a breakdown in understanding	• Encourage use of augmentative communication strategies prescribed for person with PD (e.g., picture book prompts)
• Use direct terms (e.g., Sue instead of "she")	• Use shared experiences to form conversational topics (e.g., shopping, gardening)
• Use nonverbal cues to initiate topic changes (e.g., gesture and gaze)	• Acknowledge feelings that are communicated nonverbally (e.g., "I can tell that you are frustrated")
• Use verbal introductions (e.g., "Let's talk about . . . ") to introduce topics	• Establish equality in your relationship by following lead of person with PD, acknowledge their opinions, etc.
• Promote environmental adaptations to encourage successful communication (e.g., reduce background noise; ensure face to face interactions with person with PD, etc.)	• Prepare for management of emergency situations (e.g., written message for taxi driver stating address, contact details in case of health problems, etc.)

continues

Table 6–4. *continued*

Specific Compensatory Strategies for Comprehension Difficulties	*Specific Compensatory Strategies for Word Retrieval Difficulties*
• Give feedback to person with PD (e.g., "Slow down," "Repeat that")	• Organized circumlocution (e.g., "What kind of thing is it?," "What does it do?," "What is it used for?," "What color is it?," "Where would I find it?")
• Request repetition in an alternative form (e.g., "Could you write that down?")	• Use gesture/signs
• Create visual props (e.g., pictures or drawings) to enhance comprehension of complex information	• Start sentences with carrier phrases (e.g., "You eat with a . . . ")
• Use large print	• Ask person with PD to try to write the word
• Use audio books	
• Eliminate visual distractions	

Source: Adapted from Simmons-Mackie et al. (2008) and Ylvisaker et al. (2008).

References

Auriacombe, S., Grossman, M., Carvell, S., Gollomp, S., Stern, M. B., & Hurtig, H. I. (1993). Verbal fluency deficits in Parkinson's disease. *Neuropsychology, 7*, 182–192.

Azuma, T., & Van Orden, G. C. (1997). Why SAFE is better than FAST: The relatedness of a word's meaning affects lexical decision times. *Journal of Memory and Language, 36*, 484–504.

Bayles, K. (1990). Language and Parkinson's disease. *Alzheimer Disease and Associated Disorders, 4*, 171–180.

Bayles, K., & Boone, D. R. (1982). The potential of language tasks for identifying senile dementia. *Journal of Speech and Hearing Disorders, 47*, 210–217.

Bayles, K., & Tomoeda, C. K. (1983). Confrontation naming in dementia. *Brain and Language, 19*, 98–114.

Beatty, W. W., & Monson, N. (1989). Lexical processing in Parkinson's disease and multiple sclerosis. *Journal of Geriatric Psychiatry and Neurology, 2*, 145–152.

Caltagirone, C., Carlesimo, A., Nocentini, U., & Vicari, S. (1989). Defective concept formation in parkinsonians is independent from mental deterioration. *Journal of Neurology, Neurosurgery and Psychiatry, 52*, 334–337.

Chenery, H. J., Murdoch, B. E., & Ingram, J. C. L. (1996). An investigation of confrontation naming performance in Alzheimer's disease as a function of disease severity. *Aphasiology, 10*, 423–441.

Clark, L. W., & White, K. (1995). Nature and efficiency of communication management in Alzheimer's disease. In R. Lubinski (Ed.), *Dementia and communication* (pp. 238–256). San Diego, CA: Singular.

Cruice, M., Worrall, L., Hickson, L. M. H., & Murison, R. (2003). Finding a focus for quality life with aphasia: Social and emotional health and psychological well-being. *Aphasiology, 17*, 333–353.

Dubois, B., & Pillon, B. (1991). Cognitive deficits in Parkinson's disease. *Journal of Neurology, 244*, 2–8.

Frattali, C. M., Thompson, D., Holland, A., Wohl, C., & Ferketic, M. (1995). *American Speech Language and Hearing Association Functional Assessment of Communication Skills for Adults*. Rockville, MD: ASHA.

Gordon, W. A. (1990). Approaches to cognitive rehabilitation. In R. L. I. Wood (Ed.), *Management of behavioral sequelae of traumatic brain injury*. Baltimore, MD: Brookes.

Gross, Y., & Schultz, L. E. (1986). Intervention models in neuropsychology. In B. Uzzell & Y. Gross (Eds.), *Clinical neuropsychology of intervention*. New York, NY: Guilford.

Grossman, M., Carvell, S., Gollomp, S., Stern, M. B., Vernon, G., & Hurtig, H. I. (1991). Sentence comprehension and praxis deficits in Parkinson's disease. *Neurology, 41*, 1620–1626.

Grossman, M., Zurif, E., Lee, C., Prather, P., Kalmanson, J., & Stern, M. (2002). Information processing speed and comprehension in Parkinson's disease. *Neuropsychology, 16*, 174–181.

Guilford, A. M., & Nawojczk, D. C. (1988). Standardisation of the Boston Naming Test at the kindergarten and elementary school levels. *Language, Speech and Hearing Services in Schools, 19*, 395–400.

Gurd, J. M., Master, N., & Oliveria, R. M. (2001). A method of investigating the relation between cognitive and motor functions in Parkinson's disease. *Journal of Neurolinguistics, 14*, 45–57.

Hinchliffe, F. J., Murdoch, B. E., & Chenery, H. J. (1998). Towards a conceptualisation of language and cognitive impairment in closed head injury: Use of clincical measures. *Brain Injury, 12*, 109–132.

Hinchliffe, F.J., Murdoch, B.E., & Theodoros, D.G. (2001a). Linguistic deficits in adults subsequent to traumatic brain injury. In B. E. Murdoch & D. G. Theodoros (Eds.), *Traumatic brain injury: Associated speech, language and swallowing disorders* (pp. 199–222). San Diego, CA: Singular.

Hinchliffe, F. J., Murdoch, B. E., & Theodoros, D. G. (2001b). Treatment of cognitive-linguistic communication disorders following traumatic brain injury. In B. E. Murdoch & D. G. Theodoros (Eds.), *Traumatic brain injury: Associated speech, language and swallowing disorders* (pp. 273–309). San Diego, CA: Singular.

Holland, A., Frattali, C. M., & Fromm, B. (1998). *Communication Activities of Daily Living (CADL-2)*. Austin, TX: Pro-Ed.

Huisingh, R., Barrett, M., Zachman, L., Blagden, C., & Orman, J. (1990). *The Word Test-Revised: A Test of Expressive Vocabulary and Semantics*. East Moline, IL: Linguisystems.

Ilmberger, J., Rau, S., Noachtar, S., Arnold, S., & Winkler, P. (2002). Naming tools and animals: Asymmetries observed during direct electrical cortical stimulation. *Neuropsychologia, 40*, 695–700.

Kaplan, E., Goodglass, H., & Weintraub, S. (1983). *Boston Naming Test*. Philadelphia, PA: Lippincott Williams & Wilkins.

Kushner, M., Reivich, M., Fieschi, C., Silver, F., Chawluk, J., Rosen, M., . . . Alavi, A. (1987). Metabolic and clinical correlations of acute ischaemic infarction. *Neurology, 37*, 1103–1110.

LaBarge, E., Balota, D. A., Stordandt, M., & Smith, D. S. (1992). An analysis of confrontation naming errors in senile dementia of the Alzheimer's type. *Neuropsychology, 6*, 77–95.

LeDorze, G., & Nespoulous, J. L. (1989). Anomia in moderate aphasia: Problems in accessing the lexical representation. *Brain and Language, 37*, 381–400.

Lewis, F. M., LaPointe, L. L., Murdoch, B., & Chenery, H. J. (1998). Language impairment in Parkinson's disease. *Aphasiology, 12*, 193–206.

Lieberman, P., Friedman, J., & Feldman, L. S. (1990). Syntax comprehension deficits in Parkinson's disease. *Journal of Nervous and Mental Disease, 178*, 360–365.

Lieberman, P., Kako, E. J. F., Tajchman, G., Feldman, L. S., & Jiminez, E. B. (1992). Speech production, syntax comprehension and cognitive deficits in Parkinson's disease. *Brain and Language, 43*, 169–189.

Lomas, J., Pickard, L., Betser, S., Elbard, H., Finlayson, A., & Zoghaib, C. (1989). The communicative effectiveness index: Development and psychometric evaluation of a functional communication measure for adult aphasia. *Journal of Speech and Hearing Disorders, 54*, 113–224.

Manochiopining, S., Sheard, C., & Reed, V. A. (1992). Pragmatic assessment in adult aphasia: A clinical review. *Aphasiology, 6*, 519–534.

Mateer, C. A., Sohlberg, M. M., & Youngman, P. K. (1990). The management of acquired attention and memory deficits. In R. L. I. Wood & I. Fussey (Eds.), *Cognitive rehabilitation in perspective* (pp. 68–95). London, UK: Taylor & Francis.

Matison, R., Mayeaux, R., Rosen, J., & Fahn, S. (1982). Tip-of-the-tongue phenomenon in Parkinson's disease. *Neurology, 19*, 124–141.

Mazaux, C. A., & Richer, E. (1998). Rehabilitation after traumatic brain injury in adults. *Disability and Rehabilitation, 20*, 435–447.

Miller, N., Noble, E., Jones, D., & Burn, D. (2006). Life with communication changes in Parkinson's disease. *Age and Aging, 35*, 235–239.

Murdoch, B., & Leathlean, J. B. (1996). Language dysfunction in subcortical arteriosclerotic encephalopathy. *Journal of Medical Speech Language Pathology, 4*, 275-288.

Natsopoulos, D., Katsarou, Z., Bostantzopoulou, S., Grouios, G., Mentenopoulos, G., & Logothetis, J. (1991). Strategies in comprehension of relative clauses by Parkinsonian patients. *Cortex, 27*, 255–268.

Payne, J. C. (1994). *Communication profile: A functional skills survey.* Tucson, AZ: Communication Skill Builders.

Penn, C. (1985). The profile of communicative appropriateness: A clinical tool for the assessment of pragmatics. *South African Journal Communication Disorders, 32,* 18-23.

Penn, C. (1999). Pragmatic assessment and therapy for persons with brain damage: What have clinicians gleaned in two decades? *Brain and Language, 68,* 535–552.

Raskin, S. A., Sliwinski, M., & Borod, J. C. (1992). Clustering strategies on tasks of verbal fluency in Parkinson's disease. *Neuropsychologia, 30,* 95–99.

Saint-Cyr, J. A., & Trepanier, L. L. (2000). Neuropsychologic assessment of patients for movement disorder surgery. *Movement Disorders, 15,* 771–783.

Sarno, M. T. (1975). *The Functional Communication Profile.* New York, NY: NYU Medical Center, Institute of Rehabilitation Medicine.

Simmons-Mackie, N. (2008). Social approaches to aphasia intervention. In R. Chapey (Ed.), *Language intervention strategies in aphasia and related neurogenic communication disorders* (5th ed., pp. 290–318). Philadelphia, PA: Lippincott Williams & Wilkins.

Smith, S. R., Murdoch, B. E., & Chenery, H. J. (1989). Semantic abilities in dementia of the Alzheimer's type. *Brain and Language, 36,* 314–324.

Snow, P., & Ponsford, J. (1995). Assessing and managing changes in communication and interpersonal skills following TBI. In J. Ponsford, S. Sloan, & P. Snow (Eds.), *Traumatic brain injury rehabilitation for everyday adaptive living* (pp. 137–164). Hillsdale, NJ: Lawrence Erlbaum Associates.

Spreen, O., & Benton, A. L. (1977). *Neurosensory Centre Comprehensive Examination for Aphasia.* Victoria, Canada: University of Victoria.

Tranel, D., Logan, C. G., Frank, R., & Damasio, A. R. (1997). Explaining category-related effects in the retrieval of conceptual and lexical knowledge for concrete entities: Operationalisation and analysis of factors. *Neuropsychologia, 35,* 1329–1339.

Tweedy, J. P., Langer, K. G., & McDowell, F. A. (1982). The effect of semantic relations on the memory deficit associated with Parkinson's disease. *Journal of Clinical Neuropsychology, 4,* 235–247.

Whelan, B. M., & Murdoch, B. E. (2005). Unravelling subcortical linguistic substrates: Comparison of thalamic versus cerebellar cognitive-linguistic regulation mechanisms. *Aphasiology, 19,* 1097–1106.

Whelan, B.-M., Murdoch, B., Theodoros, D. G., Hall, B., & Silburn, P. (2003). Defining a role for the subthalamic nucleus (STN) within operative theoretical models of subcortical participation in language. *Journal of Neurology Neurosurgery and Psychiatry, 74,* 1543–1550.

Whelan, B. M., Murdoch, B., Theodoros, D. G., Hall, B., & Silburn, P. (2004). Re-appraising contemporary theories of subcortical participation in language: Proposing an interhemispheric regulatory function for the subthalamic nucleus (STN) in the mediation of high-level linguistic processes. *Neurocase, 10,* 345–352.

Whelan, B. M., Murdoch, B., Theodoros, D. G., Hall, B., & Silburn, P. (2005). Beyond verbal fluency: Investigating the long-term effects of bilateral subthalamic (STN) deep brain stimulation (DBS) on language function in two cases. *Neurocase, 11*, 93–102.

Whelan, B. M., Murdoch, B. E., Theodoros, D. G., Silburn, P., & Hall, B. (2002). A role for the dominant thalamus in language? A linguistic comparision of two cases subsequent to unilateral thalamotomy procedures in the dominant and non-dominant hemispheres. *Aphasiology, 16*, 1213–1226.

Whelan, B. M., Murdoch, B., Theodoros, D. G., Silburn, P., & Hall, B. (2004). Redefining functional models of basal ganglia oragnisation: A role for the posteroventral pallidum in linguistic processing. *Movement Disorders, 19*, 1267–1278.

Whelan, B.M., Murdoch, B. E., Theodoros, D. G., Silburn, P., & Hall, B. (2005). Borrowing from models of motor control to translate cognitive processes: Evidence for hypokinetic-hyperkinetic linguistic homologues? *Journal of Neurolinguistics, 18*, 361–381.

Whelan, B. M., Murdoch, B. E., Theodoros, D. G., Silburn, P., & Harding-Clark, J. A. (2000). Towards a better understanding of the role of subcortical nuclei participation in language: The study of a case following bilateral pallidotomy. *Asia Pacific Journal of Speech, Language and Hearing, 5*, 93–112.

Wiig, E. H., & Secord, W. (1989). *Test of Language Competence-Expanded Edition*. New York, NY: Psychological Corporation.

Wiig, E. H., & Secord, W. (1992). *Test of Word Knowledge*. New York. NY: Psychological Corporation.

Wiig, E. H., & Semel, E. (1974). Development of comprehension of logical grammatical sentences by grade school children. *Perceptual and Motor Skills, 38*, 171–176.

Wirz, S. L., Skinner, C., & Dean, E. (1990). *Revised Edinburgh Functional Communication Profile*. Tucson, AZ: Communication Skill Builders.

Worrall, L. (1999). *The Everyday Communication Needs Assessment (ECNA)*. London, UK: Winslow Press.

Ylvisaker, M., Szekeres, S. F., & Fenney, T. (2008). Communication disorders associated with traumatic brain injury. In R. Chapey (Ed.), *Language intervention strategies in aphasia and related neurogenic communication disorders* (5th ed., pp. 879–962). Philadelphia, PA: Lippincott Williams & Wilkins.

7

Swallowing Disorders in Parkinson Disease

MICHELLE CIUCCI
LESLIE MAHLER
DAVID H. McFARLAND[1]

Swallowing is a complex sensorimotor process requiring coordinated activity in many muscles distributed across several subsystems, including respiratory, laryngeal, oral-facial, and gastrointestinal. The neural control of swallowing involves a widespread network including brainstem, basal ganglia and other subcortical structures as well as the cortex. Parkinson Disease (PD) involves the degeneration of dopaminergic neurons in the nigrostriatal (basal ganglia) pathways, other brainstem regions, and primary and association cortical areas. As these same regions are key to normal swallowing dynamics, PD can severely impact normal swallowing function. Furthermore, these control systems are involved in speech and voice production, and speech/language and swallowing disorders often co-occur in PD and other neurologic conditions (Martin & Corlew, 1990; McFarland & Tremblay, 2006; Robbins, Logemann, & Kirshner, 1986; Sapir, Ramig, & Fox, 2008). Changes in speech or swallowing often can be some of the first signs of PD (Harel, Cannizaro, & Snyder, 2004; Robbins et al., 1986; Sung et al., 2010). As outlined below, swallowing disorders may often have devastating effects on medical health and quality of life. Despite this, they often are underrepresented in both patient reporting and physician treatment.

---

[1] Please contact David H. McFarland for questions regarding this chapter.

Onset and Prevalence

The literature on incidence and prevalence of dysphagia associated with PD is conflicting with estimates ranging from 18% to 100% (Bird, Woodward, Gibson, Phyland & Fonda, 1994; Clarke, Gullaksen, Macdonald, & Lowe, 1998; Miller et al., 2009; Potulska, Friedman, Krolicki, & Spychala, 2003). Although a clear relationship has not been established between PD severity and severity of dysphagia symptoms (Monte, daSilva-Junio, Braga-Neto, Nobre e Souza, & deBruin, 2005; Hunter, Crameri, Austin, Woodward, & Hughes, 1997), it generally is accepted that swallowing disorders increase with disease severity and dysphagia is nearly ubiquitous in the late-stages of PD (Ali et al.,1996; Fuh et al., 1997; Monte et al., 2005; Robbins et al., 1986). However, it is important to note that early stage PD can also be associated with severe dysphagia. Part of the issue is that PD severity is based primarily on limb symptoms that do not necessarily correlate with problems in speech or other oral-facial movements, hence the apparent "mismatch" in the correlation between disease progression and dysphagia severity. Additionally, because swallowing impairments occur in the aerodigestive pathway, they are not as "visible" as impairments of whole body movements. Swallowing impairments may be present without the awareness of the individual with PD due to sensory impairments, and they can occur at any time during the disease process (Bushman, Dobmeyer, Leeker, & Perlmutter, 1989; Logemann, Blonsky, & Boshes, 1975; Potulska et al., 2003; Robbins et al., 1986).

Swallowing disorders have a large impact on quality of life. Social activities such as dining with friends, family, and work colleagues can be negatively impacted. People with PD may be reluctant to eat in public due to embarrassment about drooling, slowness of eating, or fear of choking (Rosenbek & Jones, 2009). Patients also may have difficulty with reach-to-eat movements that can negatively impact feeding (Doan, Melvin, Whishaw, & Suchowersky, 2008). Patient and caregiver interviews have revealed that patients are highly concerned with these consequences of swallowing disorders (Miller, Noble, Jones, & Burn, 2006). Swallowing and other gastrointestinal disorders, obviously, can also negatively impact the nutritional status of persons with PD (Barichella, Cereda, & Pezzoli, 2009). Unfortunately, due to the progressive nature of PD, swallowing abilities decline to the point that patients often require severe dietary restrictions and, depending on ethical decisions made by the patient and their family, tube feeding. Swallowing disorders, like speech impairments, therefore, may go well beyond specific physiologic impairment to negatively impact social interaction and quality of life.

Parkinson Disease and Swallowing

Swallowing is involved in airway protection, including clearing saliva during sleep and wakefulness in infants and adults (Nixon, Charbonneau, Kermack, Brouillette, & McFarland, 2008). Distributed cross-system neural control elements ensure the rapid sequential activation of a large number of cranial nerves and muscles to execute a safe swallow (Hartelius & Svensson, 1994; Jean, 1990; McFarland & Tremblay, 2006; Miller, 2002). Sensory feedback, combined with cortical and subcortical regulatory systems, are critical for swallowing. Dysphagia may result whenever there is a disruption in any of the anatomic structures or neural control mechanisms involved in swallowing.

Furthermore, there are motivational and cognitive processes involved in recognizing, obtaining, and attending to a food bolus during a meal (Leonard & Kendall, 2008; Logemann, 1998; Miller, 1999; Rosenbek & Jones, 2009). This chapter aims to familiarize the clinician, researcher, and patient with the effects of PD on swallowing and how the disease may lead to a swallowing disorder, or dysphagia. It provides a critical appraisal of the relevant literature, presents the signs/symptoms that lead to a diagnosis of dysphagia, and discusses intervention approaches based on an understanding of how PD impacts the nervous system and influences swallowing function. The chapter concludes with general recommendations for clinicians and patients regarding managing dysphagia associated with PD.

Although swallowing historically has been described as occurring in discrete stages (e.g., oral, pharyngeal, and esophageal), it is more accurately represented as a continuum of coordinated and interdependent movements resulting in the transport of the bolus from the oral cavity to the esophagus (Martin-Harris, Brodsky, Michel, Lee, & Walters, 2007; Martin-Harris, Michel, & Castell, 2005). Oral preparation involves formation of the bolus into a cohesive mass for oral transport. Depending on the size and consistency of the bolus (e.g., solid vs. liquid), this may involve more extensive preparation, including chewing, and, consequently, the duration of oral preparation of the bolus is variable. Once the bolus is formed, it is held between the hard palate and tongue for transport, which involves a quick stripping motion of the tongue transporting the bolus into the pharynx. Sequential contraction of the pharyngeal muscles creates a pharyngeal stripping wave that propels the bolus to the opening of the esophagus. The upper esophageal sphincter opens due to the propulsive forces acting on the bolus, the superior-anterior movements of the hyoid-larynx, and the relaxation of the cricopharyngeal muscle, and the bolus enters the esophagus. Peristaltic esophageal contractions then move the bolus toward the lower esophageal sphincter and the stomach. Airway protective mechanisms during swallowing include velopharyngeal closure, hyolaryngeal elevation, respiratory inhibition, and vocal fold closure.

The basal ganglia are thought to be involved in swallowing initiation and regulation and in modifying the basic swallowing pattern (in combination with other neural elements including the cortex) to accommodate bolus characteristics, such as changes in bolus volume and consistency (Wintzen, Badrising, Roos, Vielvoye, & Liauw, 1994). It is not surprising, therefore, that patients with PD often have impairments in swallowing. Decreased proprioception, hypokinesia, bradykinesia, and a progressive decline in motor function on tasks such as chewing may lead to abnormalities in producing timely and efficient bolus transfer and clearance during a meal. Additionally, PD is associated with a sensorimotor/perceptual deficit (see Chapters 3 and 4), which is clearly seen in both the speech and whole body movement domains (Fox et al, 2006; Farley, Fox, Ramig, & McFarland, 2008). For example, patients with significantly reduced vocal loudness often report that they are speaking with normal loudness (Ho, Bradshaw, Iansek, & Alfredson, 1999; Ho, Iansek, & Bradshaw, 1999). Given that sensory processing is key to many aspects of swallowing function, it is likely that deficits in sensation/perception underlie many aspects of disordered swallowing function associated with PD, and this concept should be considered when designing interventions.

Although the specific signs/symptoms of dysphagia are heterogeneous in PD, typical patient complaints and clinical signs of dysphagia can be summarized as in Table 7–1. Generally, abnormalities include decreased tongue control that can lead to difficulty in forming and transporting a bolus (including difficulty with mastication), premature loss of the bolus into the pharynx, and residue in the oral cavity after the swallow (Miller et al., 2006; Potulska et al., 2003). Difficulty in oral control of the bolus and/or delayed initiation of the pharyngeal aspect of the swallow that moves the bolus from the posterior portion of the oral cavity to the esophagus can lead to penetration into the laryngeal vestibule or aspiration into the trachea (Ali et al., 1996; Bird et al., 1994; Troche, Sapienza, & Rosenbek, 2008). Piecemeal deglutition (swallowing the bolus in small segments) and festinated tongue movement (tongue pumping) are hallmarks of dysphagia associated with PD (El Sharkawi et al., 2002). Additionally, drooling occurs in up to 75% of patients and is likely related to less frequent and efficient swallowing rather than excess saliva production (Ertekin, 2002; Mancini et al., 2003) as saliva production is reduced in PD (Proulx., de Courval, Wiseman, &

Table 7–1. Common Patient Complaints and Clinical Signs of Dysphagia

Patient Complaints/Symptoms	*Clinical Signs of Dysphagia*
• Increased coughing or choking at mealtimes	• Weight loss
• Frequently wet or gurgly voice quality	• Pneumonia
• More difficulty than usual swallowing pills	• Tremor, rigidity, hypokinesia, bradykinesia of orofacial, laryngeal, pharyngeal, esophageal, and respiratory musculature
• New difficulty eating foods that weren't difficult before	• Increased drooling/salivation
• Eating a meal takes an unusually long time	• Coughing
• Sensation that food gets stuck in the throat	• Throat clearing
• Excessive drooling	• Choking
• Weight loss	• Abnormal mastication
	• Festinated tongue movement
	• Piecemeal deglutition
	• Oral residue (Stasis)
	• Delayed onset of swallow
	• Delayed/reduced hyolaryngeal excursion
	• Pharyngeal stasis (valleculae, piriform sinuses)
	• Penetration
	• Aspiration

Panisset, 2005). Dry mouth is also a potential side effect of drug therapy for PD (Proulx et al., 2005). Saliva is especially important for the mastication and swallowing of solid food, and a dry mouth may negatively influence bolus preparation and bolus transport from the oral cavity through the pharynx and into the esophagus. This in turn may lead to increased oral and pharyngeal residue post swallow.

Reduced and delayed excursion of the base of the tongue, hyolaryngeal complex, and pharyngeal walls (Ali et al., 1996; Bird et al., 1994;

Fuh et al., 1997; Leopold & Kagel, 1997; Nagaya, Kachi, Yamada, & Igata, 1998; Potulska et al., 2003; Robbins et al., 1986; Wintzen et al., 1994) may result in deficient laryngeal closure during the swallow, leading to increased risk of bolus penetration/aspiration. Residue in the valleculae after the swallow may be present due to decreased base of tongue, hyolaryngeal, and/or posterior pharyngeal wall movement. Further, insufficient opening of the upper esophageal sphincter may result in residue in the piriform (or pyriform) sinuses. This residue subsequently may be aspirated into the trachea in disordered conditions.

Pneumonia resulting from the entry of saliva, liquid, or solid food particles into the lungs is a serious complication of PD and is the leading cause of death (Beyer, Herlofson, Arsland, & Larsen, 2001; Clarke, 2000; D'Amelio et al., 2006). The actual probability of developing pneumonia subsequent to aspiration of liquids or solids (aspiration pneumonia) is influenced by a variety of factors including oral hygiene, overall health, the amount and physical characteristics of the aspirated food or

Common Findings from Videofluoroscopy or Videoendoscopy

- Impaired mastication and lingual movements
- Increased number of swallows per bolus
- Tongue pumping (festinated tongue movement)
- Premature or uncontrolled loss of bolus from the oral cavity
- Increased oral transit duration
- Decreased suction pressure
- Residue on the tongue and anterior and lateral sulci after the swallow
- Delayed pharyngeal swallow
- Prolonged laryngeal movement
- Decreased pharyngeal contraction pressure
- Vallecular and piriform sinus residue
- Inability to adapt hyoid bone movement to changes in bolus characteristics
- Penetration/Aspiration

liquid, and the frequency of aspiration (Langmore et al., 1998). Muscle rigidity, tremor, and hypokinesia all can negatively impact the ability of PD patients to perform adequate oral care and hygiene, and PD patients have increased incidence of periodontal disease (Friedlander, Mahler, Norman, & Ettinger, 2009; Kieser, Jones, Borlase, & MacFadyen, 1999; Schwarz, Heimhilger, & Storch, 2006). As poor oral hygiene is a contributing factor to aspiration pneumonia (Langmore et al., 1998), careful attention should be given to the adequacy of oral care and regular dental examinations are recommended.

Cough often is impaired in patients with PD and this may be related to hypophonia as both voice production and cough rely on appropriate respiratory support for the generation of sufficient expiratory drive. Cough is extremely important for airway protection and expectorant clearance, and is potentially impaired in PD patients in two related ways. First, chest wall rigidity and other muscle functions limit expiratory support for adequate cough (Fontana, Pantaleo, Lavorini, Benvenuti, & Gangemi, 1998; Pitts, Bolser, Rosenbek, Troche, & Sapienza, 2008). Second, sensory mechanisms, involved in "triggering" cough may be impaired (Davenport, 2008; Pitts et al., 2008). PD patients, therefore, are often "silent aspirators" (Robbins et al., 1986) with liquids or solids entering the airway in the absence of airway protective reflexes such as cough.

In summary, oropharyngeal impairments may include difficulty initiating key oropharyngeal events (such as bolus transport and the pharyngeal transport), lingual hypokinesia and bradykinesia, and diminished airway protection. These in turn may lead to decreased bolus formation and control. Airway compromise can occur before, during, or after a swallow. The bolus may enter the airway before swallow initiation due to loss of bolus control. Delayed pharyngeal responses and/or decreased laryngeal movement/closure can lead to air penetration or aspiration. After the swallow, residue due to decreased pharyngeal contraction, tongue base movement, or sphincter opening may enter the airway.

Esophageal stage disorders associated with PD may include weak esophageal peristalsis with food remaining in the esophagus, esophageal spasm, hiatal hernia, and a higher incidence of gastroesophageal reflux (Eadie & Tyrer, 1965; Leopold & Kagel, 1997). Extended meal duration may contribute to malnutrition and weight loss making the patient more vulnerable to infection (i.e. pulmonary in the case of aspiration).

As highlighted above, impairments in any or all of these bolus flow or physiologic events can have important health consequences that include dehydration, malnutrition, infection/pneumonia, reduced quality of life, and death. Identifying the impaired physiologic processes is paramount to the appropriate diagnosis and treatment of swallowing disorders.

Impact of Medical and Surgical Management for PD on Swallowing

Historically, the treatment of PD has focused on pharmacologic management and more recently on neurosurgical procedures such as deep brain stimulation (DBS) (see Chapter 1). Although limb function is often improved with these medical interventions, voice, speech, and swallowing are more resistant and DBS actually may have negative consequences to these behaviors (Benabid, Chabardes, Mitrofanis, & Pollak, 2009). A recent systematic review of the influence of levodopa (a dopamine precursor) and apomorphine (a dopamine agonist) in improving swallowing in patients with PD highlights the conflicting literature (Baijens & Speyer, 2008). As described in this review, there are a limited number of clinical trials, and those that exist have several methodological shortcomings (Baijens & Speyer, 2008). The overall consensus in the field is that medical management for PD more positively impacts limb in contrast to oral motor function (Dromey, Kumar, Lang, & Lozano, 2000; Kompoliti, Wang, Goetz, Leurgans, & Raman, 2000; Rosenbek & Jones, 2009; Trail et al., 2005).

Information is even more limited regarding the effects of DBS on swallowing function (Bejjani, et al., 1998; Ciucci, Barkmeier-Kraemer, & Sherman, 2008; D'Alatri et al., 2008; Dromey, et al., 2000; Pinto et al., 2004; Solomon et al., 2000). DBS has been shown to negatively impact the ability to finely grade and sustain nonspeech/nonswallow oral forces whereas maximal force is not impacted (Gentil, Garcia-Ruiz, Pollak & Benabid, 1999). Ciucci et al. (2008) examined the impact of DBS of the subthalamic nucleus (STN) on swallowing function in PD patients. Although no improvement was observed in the oral stage of swallowing, results revealed that STN DBS reduced (improved) pharyngeal transit time in the stimulated versus nonstimulated condition and reduced pharyngeal residue and aspiration. Data were interpreted to suggest that movements that require more precise/fine motor control (such as tongue movements during oral stage) may not be improved but the overall transfer of the bolus through the pharynx and airway protection may be improved with STN DBS. The impact of DBS on speech and swallowing likely depends on the location of the implanted electrodes (subthalamic nucleus, pedunculopontine nucleus) and stimulation parameters (high vs. low frequency stimulation, pulse width, amplitude), as other movements, such as gait and posture, are differentially affected by these variables (Pereira, Muthusamy, De Pennington, Joint, & Aziz, 2008; Stefani et al., 2007). These findings support the need to consider the potential impact of DBS parameters on swallowing (and speech) during surgical implantation and implementation. Currently, the recommendation is to follow the standard of care prescribed by the movement disorders specialist and a team approach to adjust medical therapies according to their risks/benefits to the patient considering all of the systems affected (including speech and swallowing).

Although studies are limited, it is clear that current DBS or pharmacologic interventions are not sufficient to improve swallowing (or speech) function in PD patients. It is important, therefore, to directly target the physiologic impairments underlying the swallowing disorder to improve swallow safety and efficiency in patients with PD. A key aspect of treating any swallowing disorder is a thorough understanding of the nature of the impairments as gained through detailed swallowing assessment.

Evaluating Swallowing Function in PD

A swallowing assessment is used to elucidate the underlying anatomic and physiologic components of the swallow and to determine if there is adequate airway protection during swallowing. The assessment is also used to establish the most appropriate and least restrictive hydration and nutrition regimen for each patient, and to estimate the effects of intervention strategies in improving airway protection and efficient bolus transfer. Swallowing evaluations involve a detailed assessment of the patient's medical history, a thorough understanding of the nature of the neurologic impairments underlying PD, and clinical or bedside evaluations. Swallowing evaluations may also include instrumental assessments (e.g., videofluoroscopic or endoscopic) as needed. Although speech language pathologists (SLPs) often take the lead in the identification and treatment of swallowing disorders, dysphagia management, especially with PD, is a multidisciplinary process involving various medical and paramedical disciplines.

As with any swallowing evaluation, the medical history, chart review, and patient interview are vital in understanding the impact of the disease process and the associated functional disability. However, people with PD often are unaware of their own dysphagia and may initially deny symptoms. It is interesting to note that patients who are specifically probed with targeted questions may show additional awareness of their swallowing difficulty (Mahler, Ramig & Logemann, 2008). Increasing awareness of the difficulty potentially is very important for treatment efficacy and compliance (Mahler et al., 2008). As aspiration is the leading cause of death in PD and is often silent (without any obvious clinical signs such as coughing), the assessment of penetration or aspiration of the bolus into the airway is of vital importance. We also stress the importance of linking the nature of the disorder (i.e. the specific sensorimotor deficits that are well-known to accompany PD) to the underlying cause of the dysphagia.

Clinical Examination

When reviewing the medical chart and during the patient interview, importance should be given to weight loss and history of pneumonia. Inadequate nutrition and aspiration pneumonia are pervasive and life-threatening problems in PD, and inadequate nutrition can actually increase the risk of aspiration-related pneumonia. Understanding the time of disease onset and the current stage of the disease is important when planning any intervention and potential follow-up. Variability throughout the day with medications, energy level, and other factors strongly impact the quality of movements, including speech and swallowing, in patients with PD. Patients often will report few dysphagia symptoms during meals when they feel rested but may express some difficulties associated with fatigue or during "off" periods of the medication cycle. Thus, assessing swallowing abilities throughout the day is necessary. Most PD patients receive some ongoing medical intervention and these may lead to a range of symptoms, such as dry mouth or GI upset with anti-Parkinson medications to severe impairment of cognition with DBS (Alberts et al., 2008). As mentioned above, traditional

Components of Clinical Assessment

- Chart Review
- Medical History
- Cranial Nerve/Oral Mechanism Examination
- Bedside/Clinical Evaluation
- Modified Barium Swallow Study
- Fiberoptic Endoscopic Examination of Swallowing (FEES) Study

medical and surgical management may or may not improve dysphagia. Other medical comorbidities may also negatively impact swallowing, such as previous stroke or head/neck cancer. Finally, interviewing the patient and perhaps a caregiver about the perceived areas of difficulty (foods/liquids that patient may be self-omitting due to difficulty, drooling, and saliva management) and impact on quality of life are a key part of this assessment as they will influence the therapy approach. For further reading on the salient aspects of a chart review and medical history, please see Rosenbek and Jones (2009).

The clinical evaluation assesses general mental status (orientation, alertness, attention), general physical abilities, respiration, cranial nerve/ oromotor function (including cough, voice and speech function), and trials with food or liquid if it is deemed safe at that time. There are some special considerations for patients with PD. Cognitive deficits and dementia can emerge in PD and these may influence the patient's ability to carry out the proposed swallowing therapy. Because of this, clinical assessment should include testing of cognitive abilities. Orofacial, laryngeal, pharyngeal, and respiratory sensorimotor deficits likely will be apparent in the form of rigidity, tremor, bradykinesia, and hypokinesia. Thus, the cranial nerve examination will elucidate the degree of impairment of these systems. It also will be important to note if these abilities observed are typical of the patient at mealtimes, the variability throughout the day, and the influence of medications and other medical management. Information from this assessment is used to determine working hypotheses regarding the underlying causes of dysphagia, recommendations for diet and treatment, and if further instrument based evaluation is necessary.

Additional evaluation of swallowing typically involves videofluoroscopy (modified barium swallow study) or videoendoscopy (fiberoptic endoscopic evaluation of swallowing [FEES]). These techniques are often referred to as "instrumental" swallowing assessments. Videofluoroscopy, or modified barium swallow studies allow for both lateral and anterior/posterior views of the oral, pharyngeal and esophageal structures involved in swallowing (Figure 7–1A). A barium-coated bolus of various characteristics (e.g., solid, liquid) is used to determine the physiologic cause of the dysphagia and aspiration/penetration (if present). Standardized analysis protocols exist for the assessment of videofluoroscopic data and the identification of underlying physiologic impairments (Martin-Harris, Michel, & Castell, 2005). Videoendoscopy offers a direct view of the nasopharynx and laryngopharynx by a transnasal endoscope and can be used in sensory testing (Figure 7–1B). Furthermore, this instrument allows "online" testing of treatment

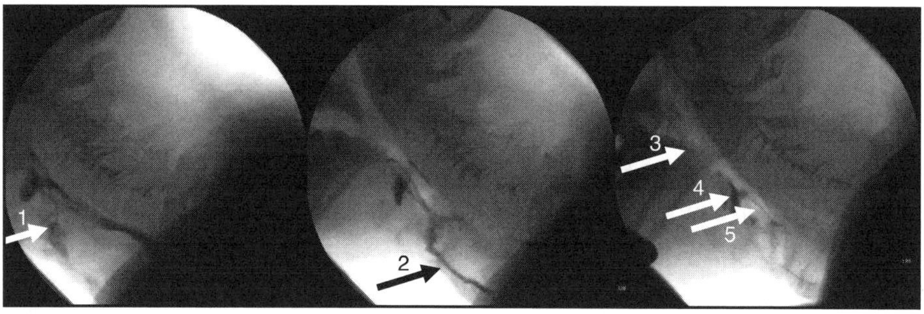

A

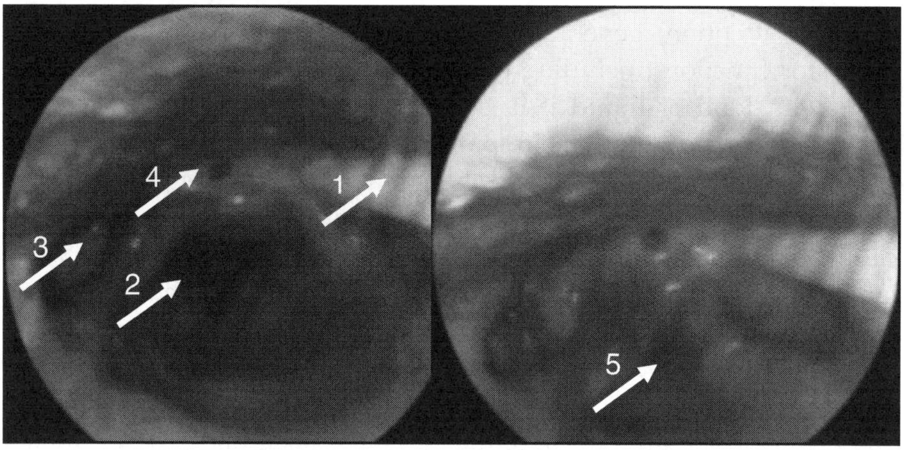

B

FIGURE 7–1. A. Lateral view of the pharynx from a videofluoroscopic swallow study of a patient with PD. Arrows indicate misdirection of the bolus: penetration into the laryngeal vestibule (1) during the pharyngeal swallow with subsequent silent aspiration into the trachea (2) and residue coating the base of tongue (3) and in the valleculae (4) and piriform sinuses (5) after swallow completion. **B.** Superior view of the larynx from a FEES study of a patient with PD. Note the presence of a feeding tube (1). Image on the left is during inspiration after a dry swallow. Vocal folds are in the abducted position; right vocal fold is on the left side (2). Secretions are present in the piriform sinuses (3, and 4). Image on the left is during a voluntary breath hold. Note the incomplete vocal fold closure (5).

strategies and can be used as a biofeedback tool without concern for radiation exposure. There is a period of "white out" during the pharyngeal swallow that obscures the view of the larynx and pharynx. Residue and potential airway entry of the bolus can be assessed before and after the swallow, but aspiration in the lungs can be missed by this examination. The specific assessment tool or tools that the clinician chooses is based on several factors, including strengths and weaknesses of the

Additional Considerations During Assessment

- Cognitive deficits
- Multiple medical comorbidities
- Negative effects from medical/surgical interventions
- Motor fluctuations
- Fatigue
- Progressive nature of PD
- Underreporting by patient
- Oral hygiene
- Nutritional status
- Quality of life

instrument, the specific swallowing events that need to be assessed, clinician's skill/level of familiarity with the instrument, and the mobility of the patient.

Treatment of Swallowing Disorders in PD

Although PD patients may share a common pathophysiology, the expression of the disorder is heterogeneous and cannot be anticipated based on the neurologic diagnosis alone. As such, the results of the swallowing evaluation are key to determine the nature of the disorder and what potential treatment strategies are most effective for that particular patient. Unfortunately, many of the treatment strategies to improve swallowing impairments that are used routinely with PD (and other neurological conditions) have not been assessed by rigorous clinical research protocols (Ashford et al., 2009).

Management strategies fall into two main categories: compensatory and intervention. Compensatory strategies include compensatory postures, swallowing maneuvers, and bolus modification. However, these strategies are not designed to address the underlying impairments and some patients find them difficult to remember and employ consistently. There is obvious interest, therefore, in treatments that target the underlying deficit. Intervention strategies typically employed in swallowing rehabilitation include strengthening exercises, sensory stimulation, and biofeedback. However, given the underlying nature of the disorder, it seems reasonable to propose that treatments involve intensive, task-specific exercises and sensory recalibration (discussed below). For further information on special considerations in the evaluation and management of dysphagia in movement disorders, including PD, the reader is referred to Rosenbek and Jones (2009).

Compensatory Strategies

Traditionally, behavioral treatment techniques for swallowing disorders associated with PD have been chosen for their perceived effectiveness in increasing swallowing safety and efficiency. Compensatory strategies are used to modify bolus flow and to accommodate any structural abnormality, weakness, or slowness of movement. There are several compensatory methods commonly employed in dysphagia treatment, and the selection of these is based on the deficit noted in the evaluation.

One strategy, termed *chin-tuck* or *chin-down* posture has been shown to reduce aspiration in 41% of patients with PD (Logemann et al., 2008), although the same study showed that thickening liquids to honey or nectar consistencies was more effective. Patients preferred the *chin-tuck* strategy to these diet modifications, even though it was somewhat less effective. A recent systematic review suggests that using the *chin-tuck* has the potential to increase swallow safety in some patients with neurogenic dysphagia, including that associated with PD (Ashford et al., 2009). Another compensatory strategy, the *supraglottic swallow,* which involves a laryngeal valsalva or breath hold before initiating the swallow, has been reported to be difficult for patients to learn and minimally effective in patients with PD to improve swallowing efficiency and airway protection (Nagaya et al., 1998). Other compensatory techniques commonly used are the *effortful swallow* and the *Mendelssohn maneuver* (prolonging laryngeal elevation with the goal of facilitating upper esophageal sphincter opening), but there has been no specific evaluation of these procedures with PD. As mentioned above, any of these strategies can be employed if they consistently improve swallow safety and efficacy and, thus, they are potentially important tools in the clinical management of swallowing disorders consequent to PD. Furthermore, it is possible that techniques typically viewed as compensatory, such as the *effortful swallow,* may be used as a swallow-specific exercise in a more direct treatment protocol.

If bolus flow modification does not improve swallow outcome through the use of compensatory postures and swallowing maneuvers, it may be necessary to modify the bolus characteristics including changing the size (small bites, single sips), consistency, or the method of delivery (no straws for liquids, alternate liquids and solids). However, there is a dearth of research on the efficacy of these approaches in improving functional outcomes. A common assumption is that a smaller bolus is more "safe" as there is less material to be aspirated. However, given that swallowing is modulated by sensory feedback, a larger bolus may provide more sensory "stimulation" which, in turn, may augment swallowing performance. Therefore, decisions to change the size of the bolus in either a larger or smaller quantity should be based on clinical observations of the safety and efficacy of this manipulation. Modifying liquids to a honey thick or nectar consistency has been shown to eliminate aspiration in 41% of PD patients and lead to a safer swallow (Logemann, et al., 2008; Troche et al., 2008). However, aspiration of thickened liquids may also be associated with increased pulmonary complications (Logemann et al., 2008). Swallowing thickened liquids may also be problematic if pharyngeal weakness is present and this in turn could lead to increased residue and risk of postswallow aspiration. As such, decisions to thicken liquids must consider therapeutic benefit and pulmonary risk.

If liquids, solids, or both are determined to be unsafe, alternatives to oral nutrition and hydration must be considered. As PD is a progressive disease and dysphagia likely will worsen over time, ethical issues must be revisited in light of current medical status, prognosis, and quality of life.

Intervention Strategies

As mentioned above, there are a limited number of well-studied interventions to specifically improve swallowing in PD. However, a few studies have shown that intensive, target specific practice of one or more of the subsystems involved in the alimentary/respiratory system leads to improved swallowing outcomes (El Sharkawi et al., 2002; Pitts et al., 2009; Robbins et al., 2005). Intensive lingual resistance exercise (i.e., pressing tongue against a bulb) improved swallow safety and efficiency in older adults and may be promising for PD (Robbins et al., 2005). Expiratory muscle strength training was shown to improve cough function and scores on the penetration/aspiration scale in patients with PD (Pitts et al., 2009). In a preliminary investigation, LSVT LOUD voice treatment led to improvement in oral tongue and tongue base movement during the oral and pharyngeal stages of swallowing and improvements in oral pharyngeal swallow efficiency (El Sharkawi et al., 2002; Jobges, Spittler-Schneiders, Renner, & Hummelsheim, 2007). All of these treatments share a common aspect of frequent, intensive and task-specific practice/exercise.

A critical component of lasting therapeutic benefit for patients with PD is training the appropriate scaling (magnitude) of movements through sensorimotor recalibration even though the new movements may "feel" much more exaggerated to the patients. The amount of effort perceived to make an accurate movement is conditioned to become the effort for a habitual movement (Farley & Koshland, 2005; Fox et al., 2006). Thus, with swallowing, the patient may need to be trained to scale and habitually perform swallow movements with this new, more appropriate dynamic range. Such sensorimotor calibration has been shown to be vital in the rehabilitation of speech and whole body movements through target specific functional exercise such as provided by LSVT LOUD (Farley et al., 2008; Fox et al., 2006).

There are numerous studies using human and nonhuman animal models of PD that demonstrate that intensive and target-specific practice leads to behavioral improvements of PD symptoms (Anstrom, Schallert, Woodlee, Shattuk, & Roberts, 2007; Ramig et al., 2001a; Ramig, Sapir, Fox, & Countryman, 2001b; Tillerson, Caudle, Reveron, & Miller, 2003) as well as lasting brain changes (Cohen, Tillerson, Smith, Schallert, & Zigmond, 2003; Faherty, Raviee Shepherd, Herasimtschuk, & Smeyne, 2005; Swain et al., 2003; van Praag, Shubert, Zhao, & Gage, 2005), especially if initiated early in the disease process either by sparing neurons or encouraging neuronal regeneration (Tillerson et al., 2001) Strikingly, discontinuation of exercise in the rat results in a reversal of treatment effects bringing them below pretreatment values (Tillerson et al., 2002). Thus, it seems reasonable that swallowing interventions involving intensive target-specific practice aimed at recalibrating functional movement amplitude should be initiated early in the disease process and continued for the duration (Hirsch & Farley, 2009).

Over the last several decades, emphasis has been placed on studying the brain's ability to slow disease progress and improve function with behavioral intervention (for a review, see Kleim and Jones, 2008). Based on our current knowledge of the neuroplasticity of the nervous system and the impact of PD on basal ganglia function, the principles of intervention for swallowing with persons with PD are proposed and presented in Table 7–2.

Obtaining a baseline of swallow function is important to monitor the progression of dysphagia as well as gauge the efficacy of treatment interventions. Monitoring should include nutrition/hydration status and weight, pulmonary status, and quality of life. The dysphagia team should consider advising assistance or supervision with eating to ensure that recommendations are followed. Supervision can range from occasional cueing to total assistance for all oral intakes. The level of supervision is

Table 7–2. Intervention Guidelines

• Encourage oral hygiene and dental care
• Monitor nutritional status
• Monitor respiratory status
• Monitor swallowing function closely
• Begin intervention early
• Continue intervention throughout the disease process
• Design the intervention to be task-specific and functionally relevant
• Minimize cognitive load when instructing therapeutic or compensatory strategies
• Make the task highly salient and rewarding
• Perform therapeutic exercises with high intensity and multiple repetitions
• Train the sensorimotor recalibration of appropriate swallowing behaviors

usually determined based on the patient's cognitive abilities to independently carry out recommendations on a consistent basis. As PD progresses, increased levels of supervision and monitoring are usually indicated.

Parkinson-Plus Syndromes and Swallowing

People who are diagnosed with Parkinson-plus syndromes typically have a more accelerated progression of swallowing disorders. Progressive supranuclear palsy, multiple system atrophy (MSA), and corticobasal-ganglionic degeneration are examples of Parkinson-plus syndromes. People with Parkinson plus syndromes have symptoms typical of Parkinson disease but are less responsive to dopaminergic treatment and typically the disease has a faster progression. Oropharyngeal dysphagia is often more prominent in progressive supranuclear palsy than idiopathic PD with potentially serious health consequences. The dysphagia associated with MSA presents like idiopathic PD, placing them at an increased risk of aspiration especially as the disease progresses (Buchholz & Robbins, 1997; Higo, Tayama, Watanabe, Nitou, & Ugawa, 2003). However, due to the more rapid progression of MSA, swallowing may deteriorate more quickly requiring more aggressive intervention (Rosenbek & Jones, 2009). Accordingly, people who are diagnosed with a Parkinson-plus syndrome should be referred immediately to a SLP experienced in swallowing disorders for evaluation and treatment recommendations for maintaining safe oral intake.

Summary

Swallowing disorders are a significant problem for most people with PD, at any stage of the disease, and pose potential health risks that range from interfering with taking oral medications to aspiration pneumonia that leads to death. Evaluation of dysphagia should occur as early as possible to identify the underlying impairments that contribute to the dysphagia using clinical and instrumental evaluations.

The benefits of pharmacologic and neurosurgical management on dysphagia remain unclear, and there appear to be both positive and negative effects on swallowing function. Consequently, direct therapeutic intervention is needed to improve swallowing impairments in persons with PD. In addition to traditional management of swallowing disorders with diet modification and compensatory strategies, a number of behavioral interventions are available for targeting the underlying neurologic/physiologic deficit associated with PD. Principles of neuroplasticity suggest that task-specific and intensive intervention with a sensory recalibration component can improve swallowing function in disordered individuals. As with any treatment of dysphagia, it is important to consider the complexity of each individual. This includes disease state and progression, environment of care (independent living vs. varying levels of assistance), nutrition/hydration status, personal preferences, and compliance with recommendations. An interdisciplinary team approach is needed and includes the patient, caregivers, physicians, nurses, dieticians, SLPs, and other health care providers.

It also is clear from this brief review that much additional clinically motivated research is needed to elucidate appropriate intervention strategies and test their specific efficacy in patients with PD. The importance of keeping in mind the nature of the underlying impairment in swallowing function that may be associated with PD, for example, problems in sensory calibration of movement amplitude was stressed. Interventions providing sensorimotor calibration, minimal cognitive load, and task-specific, high-intensity exercise are likely to have great promise in improving or slowing the decline of swallowing impairments in persons with PD. Another promising avenue is the potential cross-system interactions between speech and swallowing and the fact that interventions may have distributed and potentially complementary impacts on these two behaviors (El Sharkawi et al., 2002; McFarland & Tremblay, 2006).

One of the major challenges of appropriate treatment is early detection and channeling of patients into appropriate behavioral treatments for swallowing and other impairments. Another major challenge is that there are insufficient resources (e.g., SLPs) to treat the potentially millions of PD patients who are likely to have swallowing (and speech) impairments during the course of their disease. This emphasizes the need to think of alternative methods of contact and intervention with patients, including advanced technologic solutions.

References

Alberts, J. L., Voelcker-Rehage, C., Hallahan, K., Vitek, M., Bamzai, R., & Vitek, J. L. (2008). Bilateral subthalamic stimulation impairs cognitive-motor performance in Parkinson's disease patients. *Brain, 131*(Pt. 12): 3348–3360.

Ali, G. N., Wallace, K. L., Schwartz, R., DeCarle, D. J., Zagami, A. S., & Cook, I. J. (1996). Mechanisms of oral-pharyngeal dysphagia in patients with Parkinson's disease. *Gastroenterology, 110,* 383–392.

Anstrom, K. K., Schallert, T., Woodlee, M. T., Shattuk, A., & Roberts, D. C. (2007) Repetitive vibrissae-elicited forelimb placing before and immediately after unilateral 6-hydroxydopamine improves outcome in a model of Parkinson's disease. *Behavioural Brain Research, 179,* 183–191.

Ashford J., McCabe, D., Wheeler-Hegland, K., Frymark, T., Mullen, R., Musson, N., . . . Hammond, C. S.(2009). Evidence-based systematic review: Oropharyngeal dysphagia behavioral treatments. Part III—impact of dysphagia treatments on populations with neurological disorders. *Journal of Rehabilitation and Research Development, 46,* 195–204.

Baijens, L. W., & Speyer, R. (2009). Effects of therapy for dysphagia in Parkinson's disease: Systematic review. *Dysphagia, 24,* 91–102.

Barichella, M., Cereda, E., & Pezzoli, G. (2009). Major nutritional issues in the management of Parkinson's disease. *Movement Disorders, 24,* 1881–1892.

Bejjani, B. P., Damier, P., Arnulf, I., Papaedopoulos, S., Bonnet, A. M., Vidailhet, M., Agid, Y., Pidoux, B., Cornu, P., Dormont, D., & Marsault, C. (1998). Deep brain stimulation in Parkinson's disease: Opposite effects of stimulation in the pallidum. *Movement Disorders, 13,* 969–970.

Benabid, A.L., Chabardes, S., Mitrofanis, J., & Pollak P. (2009). Deep brain stimulation of the subthalamic nucleus for the treatment of Parkinson's disease. *Lancet Neurology, 8,* 67–81.

Beyer, M. K., Herlofson, K., Arsland, D., & Larsen, J. P. (2001). Causes of death in a community-based study of Parkinson's disease. *Acta Neurologica Sandanavia, 103,* 7–11.

Bird, M., Woodward, M., Gibson, E. M., Phyland, D., & Fonda, D. (1994). Asymptomatic swallowing disorders in elderly patients with Parkinson's disease: A description of findings on clinical examination and videofluoroscopy in 16 patients. *Age and Ageing, 23*, 251–254.

Buchholz, D. W., & Robbins, J. (1997). Neurologic diseases affecting oropharyngeal swallowing. In A. L. Perlman & K. Schulze-Delrieu (Eds.), *Deglutition and its disorders* (pp. 319–342). San Diego, CA: Singular.

Bushman, M., Dobmeyer, S. M., Leeker, L., & Perlmutter, J. S. (1989). Swallowing abnormalities and their response to treatment in Parkinson's disease. *Neurology, 39*, 1309–1314.

Ciucci, M. R., Barkmeier-Kraemer, J. M., & Sherman, S. J., (2008). Subthalamic nucleus deep brain stimulation improves deglutition in Parkinson's disease. *Movement Disorders, 23*, 676–683.

Clarke, C. E., (2000). Mortality from Parkinson's disease. *Journal of Neurology, Neurosurgery, and Psychiatry, 68*, 254–255.

Clarke, C. E., Gullaksen, Macdonald, S., & Lowe, F. (1998). Referral criteria for speech and language therapy assessment of dysphagia caused by idiopathic Parkinson's disease. *Acta Neurologica Scandinavica, 97*, 27–35.

Cohen, A. D., Tillerson, J. L., Smith, A. D., Schallert, T., & Zigmond, M. J. (2003). Neuroprotective effects of prior limb use in 6-hydroxydopamine-treated rats: possible role of GDNF. *Journal of Neurochemistry, 85*, 299–305.

D'Alatri, L., Paludetti, G., Contarino, M., Galla, S., Marchese, M., & Bentivoglio, A. (2008). Effects of bilateral subthalamic nucleus stimulation and medication on parkinsonian speech impairment. *Journal of Voice, 22*, 365–372.

D'Amelio, M., Ragonese, P., Morgante, L., Reggio, A., Callari, G., Salemi, G., & Savettieri, G. (2006). Long-term survival of Parkinson's disease: A population-based study. *Journal of Neurology, 253*, 33–37.

Davenport, P. (2008). Urge-to-cough: What can it teach us about cough? *Lung, 86* (Suppl. 1), S107–S111.

Doan, J. B., Melvin, K. G., Whishaw, I. Q., & Suchowersky, O. (2008). Bilateral impairments of skilled reach-to-eat in early Parkinson's disease patients presenting with unilateral or asymmetrical symptoms. *Behavioural Brain Research, 194*, 207–213.

Dromey, C., Kumar, R., Lang, A. E., & Lozano, A. M. (2000). An investigation of the effects of subthalamic nucleus stimulation on acoustic measures of voice. *Movement Disorders, 15*, 1132–1138.

Eadie, M. J., & Tyrer, J. H. (1965). Alimentary disorder in parkinsonism. *Australasia Annals of Medicine, 14*, 13–22.

El Sharkawi, E., Ramig, L. O., Logemann, J. A., Pauloski, B. R., Rademaker, A. W., Smith, C. H., . . . Werner, C. (2002). Swallowing and voice effects of Lee Silverman Voice Treatment (LSVT): A pilot study. *Journal of Neurology, Neurosurgery, and Psychiatry, 72*, 31–36.

Ertekin, C. (2002). Physiological and pathological aspects of oropharyngeal swallowing. *Movement Disorders, 17*, S86–S89.

Faherty, C. J., Raviie Shepherd, K., Herasimtschuk, A, & Smeyne, R. J (2005). Environmental enrichment in adulthood eliminates neuronal death in experimental Parkinsonism. *Brain Research Molecular Brain Research, 134*, 170–179.

Farley, B. G., & Koshland, G. F. (2005). Training BIG to move faster: the application of the speed-amplitude relation as a rehabilitation strategy for people with Parkinson's disease. *Experimental Brain Research, 167*, 462–467.

Farley, B. G., Fox, C. M., Ramig L. O., & McFarland D. H., (2008). Intensive amplitude-specific therapeutic approaches for Parkinson disease: Toward a neuroplasticity-principled rehabilitation model. *Topics in Geriatric Rehabilitation, 24*, 99–114.

Fontana, G. A., Pantaleo, T., Lavorini, F., Benvenuti, F., & Gangemi, S. (1998). Defective motor control of coughing in Parkinson's disease. *American Journal of Respiratory and Critical Care Medicine, 158*, 458–464.

Fox, C. M., Ramig, L. O., Ciucci, M. R., Sapir, S., McFarland, D. H., & Farley, B. G. (2006). The science and practice of LSVT/LOUD: Neural plasticity-principled approach to treating individuals with Parkinson disease and other neurological disorders. *Seminars in Speech and Language, 2*, 283–299.

Friedlander, A. H., Mahler, M., Norman, K. M., & Ettinger, R. L. (2009). Parkinson disease: Systemic and orofacial manifestations, medical and dental management. *Journal of the American Medical Association, 140*, 658–669.

Fuh, J., Lee, R., Wang, S. J., Lin, C., Wang, P. N., Chiang, J., & Liu, H. (1997). Swallowing difficulty in Parkinson's disease. *Clinical Neurology and Neurosurgery, 99*, 106–112.

Gentil, M, Garcia-Ruiz, P., Pollak, P., & Benabid, A. L. (1999). The effect of stimulation of the subthalamic nucleus on oral control of patients with parkinsonism. *Journal of Neurology, Neurosurgery and Psychiatry, 67*, 329–333.

Harel, B. T., Cannizaro, M. S., Cohen, H., Reilly, N., & Snyder, P. J. (2004). Acoustic characteristics of parkinsonian speech: A potential biomarker of early disease progression and treatment. *Journal of Neurolinguistics, 17*, 439–453.

Hartelius, L., & Svensson, P. (1994). Speech and swallowing symptoms associated with Parkinson's disease and multiple sclerosis. *Folia Phoniatrica et Logopedia, 46*, 9–17.

Higo, R., Tayama, N., Watanabe, T., Nitou, T., & Ugawa, Y. (2003). Videofluoroscopic swallowing function in patients with multiple system atrophy. *Annals of Otology, Rhinology, and Laryngology, 112*, 630–636.

Hirsch, M. A., & Farley, B. G. (2009). Exercise and neuroplasticity in persons living with Parkinson's disease. *European Journal of Physical Rehabilitation Medicine, 45*, 215–229.

Ho, A. K., Bradshaw, J. L., Iansek, R., & Alfredson, R. (1999). Speech volume regulation in Parkinson's disease: Effects of implicit cues and explicit instructions. *Neuropsychologia*, 37, 1453–1460.

Ho, A. K., Iansek, R., & Bradshaw, J. L. (1999). Regulation of parkinsonian speech volume: The effect of interlocutor distance. *Journal of Neurology, Neurosurgery, and Psychiatry, 67*, 199–202.

Hunter, P. C., Crameri, J., Austin, S., Woodward, M. C., & Hughes, A. J. (1997). Response of Parkinsonian swallowing dysfunction to dopaminergic stimulation. *Journal of Neurology, Neurosurgery, and Psychiatry, 63,* 579–583.

Jean, A. (1990). Brainstem control of swallowing: Localization and organization of the central pattern generator for swallowing. In A. Taylor (Ed.), *Neurophysiology of the jaws and teeth.* London, UK: MacMillan Press.

Jobges, E. M., Spittler-Schneiders, H., Renner C. I., & Hummelsheim, H. (2007). Clinical relevance of rehabilitation programs for patients with idiopathic Parkinson syndrome II: Symptom-specific therapeutic approaches. *Parkinsonism and Related Disorders, 13,* 203–213.

Kieser, J., Jones, G., Borlase, G., & MacFadyen, E. (1999). Dental treatment of patients with neurodegenerative disease. *New Zealand Dental Journal, 95,* 130–134.

Kleim, J. A., & Jones, T. A. (2008). Principles of experience-dependent neural plasticity: Implications for rehabilitation after brain damage. *Journal of Speech, Language and Hearing Research, 51,* S225–S239.

Kompoliti, K., Wang, Q. E., Goetz, C. G., Leurgans, S., & Raman, R. (2000). Effects of central dopaminergic stimulation by apomorphine on speech in Parkinson's disease. *Neurology, 54,* 458–462.

Langmore, S., Terpenning, M. S., Schork, A., Chen, Y. Murray, J. T., Lopatin, D., & Loesche, W. J.. (1998). Predictors of aspiration pneumonia: How important is dysphagia? *Dysphagia, 13,* 69–81.

Leonard, R., & Kendall, K. (2008). *Dysphagia assessment and treatment planning: A team approach,* (2nd ed.). San Diego, CA: Plural.

Leopold, N., & Kagel, M. (1997). Pharyngo-esophageal dysphagia in Parkinson's disease. *Dysphagia, 12,* 11–18.

Logemann, J. A. (1998). *Evaluation and treatment of swallowing disorders* (2nd ed.). Austin, TX: Pro-Ed.

Logemann, J. A., Blonsky, E. R., & Boshes, B. (1975). Editorial: Dysphagia in parkinsonism. *Journal of the American Medical Association, 231,* 69–70.

Logemann, J. A., Gensler, G., Robbins, J., Lindblad, A. S., Brandt, D., Hind, J. A., . . . Miller Gardner, P. J. (2008). A randomized study of three interventions for aspiration of thin liquids in patients with dementia or Parkinson's disease. *Journal of Speech, Language, and Hearing Research, 51,* 173–183.

Mahler, L., Ramig, L. O., & Logemann, J., (2008). *Description of subjective and objective swallow characteristics of people with PD.* Poster session presented at the International Movement Disorders Society, Chicago, IL.

Mancini, F., Zangaglia, R., Cristina, S., Sommaruga, M, Martignoni, E., Nappi, G., & Pacchetti, C. (2003). Double-blind placebo-controlled study to evaluate the efficacy and safety of botulinum toxin type A in the treatment of drooling in parkinsonism. *Movement Disorders, 18,* 685–688.

Martin, B. J., & Corlew, M. M. (1990). The incidence of communication disorders in dysphagic patients. *Journal of Speech and Hearing Disorders, 55,* 28–32.

Martin-Harris, B., Brodsky, M. B., Michel, Y., Lee, F. S., & Walters, B. (2007). Delayed initiation of the pharyngeal swallow: Normal variability in adult swallows. *Journal of Speech, Language and Hearing Research, 50,* 585–594.

Martin-Harris, B., Michel, Y., & Castell, D. O. (2005). Physiologic model of oropharyngeal swallowing revisited. *Otolaryngology-Head and Neck Surgery, 133,* 234–240.

McFarland, D., & Tremblay, P. (2006). Clinical implications of cross-system interactions. *Seminars in Speech and Language, 27,* 300–310.

Miller, A. J. (1999). *The neuroscientific principles of swallowing and dysphagia.* San Diego, CA: Singular.

Miller, A. J. (2002). Oral and pharyngeal reflexes in the mammalian nervous system: Their diverse range in complexity and the pivotal role of the tongue. *Critical Reviews in of Oral Biology and Medicine, 13,* 409–425.

Miller, N., Allcock, L., Hildreth, A. J., Jones, D., Noble, E., & Burn, D. J. (2009). Swallowing problems in Parkinson disease: Frequency and clinical correlates. *Journal of Neurology, Neurosurgery and Psychiatry, 80,* 1047–1049.

Miller, N., Noble, E., Jones, D., & Burn, D. (2006) Hard to swallow: Dysphagia in Parkinson's disease. *Age and Ageing, 35,* 614–618.

Monte, F. S., da Silva-Junior, F. P., Braga-Neto, P., Nobred e Souza, M. A., & de Bruin, V. M. (2005). Swallowing abnormalities and dyskinesia in Parkinson's disease. *Movement Disorders, 20,* 457–462.

Nagaya, M., Kachi, T., Yamada, T., & Igata, A. (1998). Videofluorographic study of swallowing in Parkinson's disease. *Dysphagia, 13,* 95–100.

Nixon, G. M., Charbonneau, I., Kermack, A. S., Brouillette, R. T., & McFarland, D. H.. (2008). Respiratory-swallowing interactions during sleep in premature infants at term. *Respiratory Physiology and Neurobiology, 160,* 76–82.

Pereira, E. A., Muthusamy, K. A., De Pennington, N., Joint, C. A., & Aziz, T. Z. (2008). Deep brain stimulation of the pedunculopontine nucleus in Parkinson's disease. Preliminary experience at Oxford. *British Journal of Neurosurgery, 22*(Suppl. 1), S41–S44.

Pinto, S., Thobois, W., Costes, N., Le Bars, D, Benabid, A., Broussolle, E., . . . Gentil, M. (2004). Subthalamic nucleus stimulation and dysarthria in Parkinson's disease: A PET study. *Brain, 127,* 602–615.

Pitts, T., Bolser, D., Rosenbek, J., Troche, M., Okun, M., & Sapienza, C. (2009). Impact of expiratory muscle strength training on voluntary cough and swallow function in Parkinson's disease. *Chest,* Epub ahead of print.

Pitts, T., Bolser, D., Rosenbek, J., Troche, M., & Sapienza, C. (2008). Voluntary cough production and swallow dysfunction in Parkinson's disease. *Dysphagia, 23,* 297–301.

Potulska, A., Friedman, A., Krolicki, L., & Spychala, A. (2003). Swallowing disorders in Parkinson's disease. *Parkinsonism and Related Disorders, 9,* 349–353.

Proulx, M., de Courval, F. P., Wiseman, M. A., & Panisset, M. (2005). Salivary production in Parkinson's disease. *Movement Disorders, 20,* 204–207.

Ramig, L. O., Sapir, S., Countryman, S., Pawlas, A., O'Brien, C., Hoen, M., & Thompson, L. (2001a). Intensive voice treatment (LSVT®) for individuals with Parkinson's disease: A two-year follow-up. *Journal of Neurology, Neurosurgery, and Psychiatry, 71,* 493–498.

Ramig, L. O., Sapir, S., Fox, C. M., & Countryman, S. (2001b). Changes in vocal loudness following intensive voice treatment (LSVT) in individuals with Parkinson's disease: A comparison with untreated patients and normal age-matched controls. *Movement Disorders, 16,* 79–83.

Robbins, J., Gangnon, R. E., Theis, S. T., Kays, S. A., Hewitt, A. L., & Hind, J. A. (2005). The effects of lingual exercise on swallowing in older adults. *Journal of the American Geriatric Society, 53,* 1483–1489.

Robbins, J. A., Logemann, J. A., & Kirshner, H. S. (1986). Swallowing and speech production in Parkinson's disease. *Annals of Neurology, 19,* 283–287.

Rosenbek, J. C., & Jones, H. (2009). *Dysphagia in movement disorders.* San Diego, CA: Plural.

Sapir, S., Ramig, L., & Fox, C. (2008). Speech and swallowing disorders in Parkinson disease. *Current Opinion in Otolaryngology, Head and Neck Surgery, 16,* 205–210.

Schwarz, J., Heimhilger, E., & Storch, A. (2006). Increased periodontal pathology in Parkinson's disease. *Journal of Neurology, 253,* 608–611.

Solomon, N. P., McKee, A. S., Larson, K. J., Nawrocki, M. D., Tuite, P. J., Eriksen, S., . . . Maxwell, R. E. (2000). Effects of pallidal stimulation on speech in three men with severe Parkinson's disease. *American Journal of Speech-Language Pathology, 9,* 241–256.

Stefani, A., Lozano, A. M., Peppe, A., Stanzione, P., Galati, S., Tropep, D., . . . Mazzone, P. (2007). Bilateral deep brain stimulation of the pedunculopontine and subthalamic nuclei in severe Parkinson's disease. *Brain, 130,* 1596–1607.

Sung, H. Y., Kim, J. S., Lee, K. S., Kim, Y. I., Song, I. U., Chung, S. W., . . . Choi, M. G. (2010). The prevalence and patterns of pharngoesophageal dysmotility in patients with early stage Parkinson's disease. *Movement Disorders,* Epub ahead of print.

Swain, R. A., Harris, A. B., Wiener, E. C., Dutka, M. V., Morris, H. D., Theien, B. E., . . . Greenough, W. T. (2003). Prolonged exercise induces angiogenesis and increases cerebral blood volume in primary motor cortex of the rat. *Neuroscience, 117,* 1037–1046.

Tillerson, J. L., Caudle, W. M., Reveron, M. E., & Miller, G. W. (2003). Exercise induces behavioral recovery and attenuates neurochemical deficits in rodent models of Parkinson's disease. *Neuroscience, 119,* 899–911.

Tillerson, J. L., Cohen, A. D., Caudle, W. M., Zigmond, M. J., Schallert, T., & Miller, G. W. (2002) Forced non-use in unilateral parkinsonian rats exacerbates injury. *Journal of Neuroscience, 22,* 6790–6799.

Tillerson, J. L., Cohen, A. D. Philhower, J., Miller, G. W., Zigmond, M. J., & Schallert, T. (2001). Forced limb-use effects on the behavioral and neurochemical effects of 6-hydroxydopamine. *Journal of Neuroscience, 21,* 4427–4435.

Trail, M., Fox, C., Ramig, L. O., Sapir, S., Howard, J., & Lai, E. C. (2005). Speech treatment for Parkinson's disease. *NeuroRehabilitation, 20,* 205–221.

Troche, M. S., Sapienza, C. M., & Rosenbek, J. C. (2008). Effects of bolus consistency on timing and safety of swallow in patients with Parkinson's disease. *Dysphagia, 23,* 26–32.

van Praag, H., Shubert, T., Zhao, C., & Gage, F. H. (2005). Exercise enhances learning and hippocampal neurogenesis in aged mice. *Journal of Neuroscience, 25*(38), 8680–8685.

Wintzen, A. R., Badrising, U. A., Roos, R. A., Vielvoye, J., & Liauw, L. (1994). Influence of bolus volume on hyoid movements in normal individuals and patients with Parkinson's disease. *Canadian Journal of Neurological Sciences, 21*, 57–59.

Index

D

E

P

T

V

W